Hearing Loss: Causes, Prevention and Treatment

Hearing Loss: Causes, Prevention and Treatment

Editor: Branson Scott

MURPHY & MOORE
www.murphy-moorepublishing.com

www.murphy-moorepublishing.com

MURPHY & MOORE

Cataloging-in-Publication Data

Hearing loss : causes, prevention and treatment / edited by Branson Scott.
p. cm.
Includes bibliographical references and index.
ISBN 978-1-63987-298-5
1. Deafness. 2. Deafness--Etiology. 3. Deafness--Prevention. 4. Deafness--Treatment. 5. Ear--Diseases.
6. Hearing disorders. I. Scott, Branson.
RF290 .H43 2022
617.8--dc23

Murphy & Moore Publishing,
1 Rockefeller Plaza,
New York City, NY 10020, USA

ISBN 978-1-63987-298-5 (Hardback)

Contents

Preface

Hearing loss refers to the loss of hearing in one or both ears. It is broadly categorized into three categories, namely, sensorineural, conductive and a mixture of the two. Sensorineural hearing loss is connected to the inner ear while conductive hearing loss involves the outer or middle ear. Major causes of hearing loss are infections in the ear, excessive buildup of earwax, injury to the inner ear, and rupture in the eardrum. Hearing loss can be prevented by following steps such as regularly getting the hearing tested if one works in a high risk environment, protecting the ears from damaging noise, and avoiding risks from recreational activities which can affect the hearing. This book includes some of the vital pieces of work being conducted across the world, on various topics related to the loss of hearing and its causes. It also elucidates new techniques on its prevention and management. The extensive content of this book provides the readers with a thorough understanding of the subject.

This book has been the outcome of endless efforts put in by authors and researchers on various issues and topics within the field. The book is a comprehensive collection of significant researches that are addressed in a variety of chapters. It will surely enhance the knowledge of the field among readers across the globe.

It gives us an immense pleasure to thank our researchers and authors for their efforts to submit their piece of writing before the deadlines. Finally in the end, I would like to thank my family and colleagues who have been a great source of inspiration and support.

Editor

1

Hearing Screening around the World

Piotr Henryk Skarżyński and Maciej Ludwikowski

Abstract

Newborn hearing screening programs for congenital disorders and chronic diseases are expanding worldwide, and children are identified at the earliest possible stage. However, the practice is limited or absent in much of the developing world, such as Africa. Recent epidemiological studies show significant increase of hearing impairments in school-age children (around 20 in 100). Hearing disorders disturb the child's perception of sound, as well as the development of speech which in consequence negatively affects the child relations in society. The early detection of hearing impairments in children enables the effective implementation of medical and rehabilitation procedures or preventive treatment. According to the guidelines of the European Scientific Consensus on Hearing, the detection and treatment of hearing disorders in early school-age children are of the highest importance. That idea was one of the priorities during Polish Presidency of the Council of the European Union (the second half of 2011). The Institute team, in collaboration with numerous national centers, has laid the groundwork for screening programs and developed methods, procedures, and devices for carrying them out. In addition, the Institute was the coordinator and producer of many programs. Based on this, two screening models have been created—newborn and school-age children.

Keywords: hearing screening, hearing impairment, school-age children

1. Introduction

Nowadays, audiology and otolaryngology, which are included in preventive medicine, have many possibilities to assist patients with hearing impairment. However, in order to make full use of these opportunities, hearing disorders or damage should be detected in the early stages. Hence, screening programs for early detection of hearing defects are of great importance. In an optimal healthcare system, hearing screening should be conducted not only during the neonatal or infancy but also in the subsequent years of the child's life. In this way, both congenital and acquired hearing defects can be detected.

Timely intervention is an important component of Early Hearing Detection and Intervention (EHDI) screening program. In Poland, neonatal screening program (NHS) is carried out. The first projects were performed over 25 years ago [1]. The result of the Polish EHDI/NHS program shows that the prevalence of congenital hearing impairment ranges from 2 to 7 per 1000 births [2]. The National Institute on Deafness and Other Communication Disorders (NIDCD) adduces that 6–7/1000 children have permanent hearing loss in addition to the 3/1000 likely to be diagnosed in short period after birth [3]. From the official database of the National Health & Nutrition Evaluation Studies (NHANES) for screened children who are 6–19 years, it is indicated that approximated 3/1000 prevalence of permanent hearing loss in infants can be expected to increase to 9–10/1000 children in the school-age population.

In years 2007–2016, the Institute of Physiology and Pathology of Hearing screened over million pupils from class I to VI primary school in Poland and approximately~ million children around the world [4]. This experience provided an opportunity to screen a significant number of school-age children and also created the international infrastructure for screening which makes it a suitable solution for place even in remote rural areas.

2. Etiology of hearing loss in school-aged children

Moderate-to-profound degrees of hearing loss are targeted in our newborn screening programs; however, lesser degrees of loss are often not identified until school age. The late age of identification of mild hearing loss may contribute to our lack of knowledge about causative factors. That is, in some cases, a delay in identification of hearing loss may limit our ability to interpret etiologic evaluations reliably or may affect parental memory of possible illnesses or injuries that could account for the loss [5].

As discussed by Ross et al. [6], newborn screening programs are designed to identify hearing losses that are of moderate degree or greater. As such, the equipment and protocols used for newborn screening (e.g., otoacoustic emission (OAE)) are dedicated to identify impairment greater than approximately 40 dB HL. Moreover, a lot of factors appear after newborn screening:

1. Genetic—connexin [7], mitochondrial [8]
2. Enlarged vestibular aqueduct (EVA) syndrome [9]
3. Sudden idiopathic [10]
4. Auditory neuropathy/dyssynchrony [11]
5. Noise inducted [12]
6. Viral/bacterial—mumps [13], otitis media with effusion [13]; meningitis, measles, chicken pox, influenza, encephalitis, rubella
7. Head trauma

8. Ototoxic (damaging to the auditory system) drugs

Acquired hearing loss is a hearing loss which appears after birth, at any time in one's life, as a result of a disease, a condition, or an injury. In fact, the most common cause of hearing loss in young children is otitis media. Fluctuating conductive hearing loss nearly always occurs with all types of otitis media [14]. Symptoms, severity, frequency, and length of the condition vary. At one extreme is a single short period of thin, clear, no infected fluid without any pain or fever but with a slight decrease in hearing ability. At the other extreme are repeated bouts with infection, thick "glue-like" fluid, and possible complications such as permanent hearing loss. Therefore, a hearing screening in school-age children is very important [15].

3. The impact of hearing loss on child's development

It is recommended that hearing loss in infants be identified, and when possible treated, prior to 6 months of age. This recommendation is based on studies that have shown that children identified with hearing loss prior to 6 months of age have a better chance of developing skills equivalent to their peers by the time they enter kindergarten.

Following the guidelines for hearing screening, hearing deficits in children can interfere with normal speech and language development, communication, and the ability to learn.

Failure to identify children with congenital or acquired hearing impairment can lead to lifelong consequences including deficits in speech and language abilities, cognition delays [16], poor academic performance [17], insufficient psychosocial skills, underemployment, and psychological distress [18].

Classroom is an auditory verbal environment where precise transmission and reception of speech is critical for effective learning to occur [19]. For instance, being able to hear all sounds is fundamental when learning to read. The behavioral effects of hearing impairment are frequently subtle and look similar to those of children who experience attention-deficit disorders, learning disabilities, language, and cognitive delays. Commonly cited behaviors include the following [20]: difficulty attending to spoken or other auditory information; often requests repetition; tired easily when listening; gives not suitable answer; avoids contacts with peers; difficulty with reading skills and written language; and easily frustrated. Children with mild unilateral hearing impairment can cause difficulties in sound-source location and problem with speech perception in background noise. In addition, problem associated with the loss of binaural summation and sound localization is delays in speech-language development and school achievements. Lack of binaural hearing may decrease accidental learning due to background noise interferes with overheard speech. Therefore, only such early identification results in early intervention via hearing aids, cochlear implants, and various assistive listening devices. The intervention allows for speech and language development and academic achievements to remain on target.

What is important, there are many factors that affect the speech and language acquisition, academic achievements of each child. Level of hearing loss (mild, moderate, severe, or profound) based on the pure-tone threshold does not predict handicap or success in school. Some children have severe hearing loss; however, their speech is comprehensible and they get good grades. But on the other hand, other children with mild hearing loss and lack of family support exhibit considerable academic failure. Therefore, any hearing impairment, no matter how mild, needs to be assessed in order to assert confidently attention to any barrier of learning.

Children with unilateral hearing loss (UHL) appear to have an increased rate of grade failures, need for additional educational assistance, and perceived behavioral issues in the classroom. Possible risk factors include lower cognitive ability, right-ear hearing loss, and severe-to-profound hearing loss. Speech and language development may be delayed in some children with UHL, but it is unclear if children "catch up" as they grow older.

4. Screening methods around the world

As part of a hearing evaluation, child's healthcare provider will do a complete medical history and physical exam. In addition, there are many different types of hearing tests. Some of them may be used on all ages, while others are used based on child's age and level of understanding. Moreover, a variety of objective tools have been developed for screening tools. Hearing screening test should be conducted in a quiet area where visual and auditory distractions are minimal.

4.1. Questionnaires

Newton et al. [21] developed an eight-item questionnaire for hearing screening of children in Kenya. This tool is based on typical behavioral reaction to sound and communication ability. The main aim of this questionnaires was to identify children who may have bilateral hearing loss of a moderate degree or greater. It was designed for children of 3–8 years old and completed by teachers, parents, or community nurses, but authors recommended this tool for use only when administered by community health nurses. This questionnaire showed a high sensitivity of 100% but lower specificity of 75%. In addition, all young patients were invited to have an evaluation by ear-nose-throat physician and to have pure-tone audiometry completed.

Olusanya [22] created a questionnaire to screen children at school entry in Nigeria, Lagos. In this study was compared audiometry to results of questionnaires, otoscopy, and also tympanometry for each child. First step was a full physical exam on the children and then the parents were interviewed using a structured questionnaire that explored past medical/developmental history and family history of hearing loss. The parent questionnaire showed high specificity of 94% but low sensitivity of only 10%. The author noted that given limited resources in developing countries there is a need for a low-cost method that requires minimal training and that a questionnaire is a feasible approach. Moreover, the authors recommended the use of the questionnaire for mass screening when administered by trained teachers.

Samelli et al. [23] developed a 14-item questionnaire to identify children at risk for screening in Sao Paulo in Brazil. This tool is dedicated to children of 2–10 years old. In this study, a parent-completed questionnaire was compared with the results of an audiological assessment.

Conduction analyses show that this questionnaire from all of the children identified only with permanent severe-to-profound hearing loss. This tool showed low sensitivity of 44% and specificity of 87%. Researchers recommended the questionnaire for use in healthcare settings.

To conclude, all questionnaires were designed as a tool to identify children with hearing problems so that appropriate treatment and/or intervention could be provided; there were differences in the extent of hearing loss being targeted by the questionnaire. The purpose of population-based hearing screening is to identify those who need further testing from those who do not, with a minimum of false positives (failing the questionnaire when hearing is normal) and false negatives (passing the questionnaire when hearing loss exists).

4.2. Evoked otoacoustic emission

Physiologic test specifically measures outer hair cell response to presentation of a click stimulus (transient evoked OAEs). The test is that acoustic signals generated from within the cochlea travel in a reverse direction through the middle-ear space and tympanic membrane out of the ear. OAEs use a tiny, flexible plug that is inserted into the baby's ear. Sounds are sent through the plug. A microphone in the plug records the otoacoustic emissions (responses) of the normal ear in reaction to the sounds. There are no emissions in a baby with hearing loss. This test is painless and usually takes just a few minutes, while the baby sleeps.

1. **Advantages:** quick time test; ear-specific results; not dependent on whether patient is asleep or awake

2. **Limitations:** infant or child must be relatively inactive during the test; not a comprehensive test of hearing, because it does not assess cortical processing of sound; OAEs are very sensitive to middle-ear effusions and cerumen or vernix in the ear canal

3. **Average time:** 10-min test

4.3. Automated auditory brainstem response

Auditory brainstem responses (ABR) are measures of electrical events generated within the auditory brainstem pathway. These ABRs are used to assess brainstem function at different levels of the auditory pathway and are typically evoked by rapid multi-frequency clicks or chirps. Small metal discs with thin electrodes (wires) are placed on the baby's scalp, and then send signals to a computer to record the results. One objective physiologic means of screening hearing is the automated ABR. This instrument measures cochlear response in the 1- to 4-kHz range with a broadband click stimulus in the ear. While the baby sleeps, clicking sounds are made through tiny earphones in the baby's ears. As in OAEs, this test is painless.

1. **Advantages:** ear-specific results; responses not dependent on patient cooperation

2. **Limitations:** infant or child must remain quiet during the test (sedation is often required); not a comprehensive test of hearing, because it does not assess cortical processing of sound

3. **Average time:** 15-min test

4.4. Play audiometry

Behavioral test of auditory thresholds in response to speech and frequency-specific stimuli is presented through earphones and/or bone vibrator. This test is dedicated to children of 2–4 years old. A test that uses a special audiometer which is able to transmit sounds at different volumes and pitches into child's ears. This test is modified slightly in the toddler age group and made into a game. The toddler is asked to do something with a toy (such as touch or move a toy) every time when a sound is heard through earphones. Air-conduction hearing threshold levels of greater than 20 dB at any of these frequencies indicate possible hearing impairment. This test relies on the cooperation of the child, which may not always be given.

1. **Advantages:** ear-specific results; assesses auditory perception of child
2. **Limitations**: attention span of child may limit the amount of information obtained
3. **Average time:** 15–30 min test

4.5. Pure-tone audiometry

Behavioral test measuring auditory thresholds in response to frequency-specific stimuli is presented through earphones for children of 4 years and older. A test that uses a audiometer which is able to produces sounds at different frequently and intensity into child's ears. The child usually wears some type of earphones. Each ear should be tested at 500, 1000, 2000, and 4000 Hz. Results greater than 20 dB at any frequencies indicate possible hearing loss. In this age group, the child is simply asked to respond in some way when the tone is heard in the earphone. In that test, the most important is the cooperation of the child.

1. **Advantages:** ear-specific results; assesses auditory perception of child
2. **Limitations**: depends on the level of understanding and cooperation of the child
3. **Average time:** 15- to 30-min test

5. Hearing screening programs around the world

The major aim of hearing screening program is to detect a disease at a stage when treatment can be effective in reducing long-term complications [24]. According to the estimates provided by the World Health Organization (WHO), nearly 7.5 million children suffer from hearing loss [25]. Around 80% of them live in low- to middle-income countries [26].

In the absence of a systematic effort to screen infants with hearing loss, the average age of detection is well over 2 years, and detection may be as late as 6 years in sub-Saharan Africa [27]. In Kenya, many children with hearing impairment are not identified until 5–7 years old due to stigma, while some are hidden and are never diagnosed [28].

India launched the National Programme for Prevention and Control of Deafness. Under this program, the following two-part protocol for infant hearing screening is being complemented: institution- and community-based screening. First, screen every baby born in a hospital or admitted there soon after birth using OAE and second, screen babies who are not born in a hospital; screening is carried out using a brief questionnaire and behavioral testing.

In 2011, 97.9% of babies born in the United States had their hearing screened in the first few weeks of life according to Centers for Disease Control and Prevention (CDC) [29].

In Europe and England, two models are used: first, in hospital before discharge, if discharge takes place before the test is completed, a letter is sent asking the mother to attend an appointment for the screening test and second, in some areas, the test is done at home by a health visitor nurse.

Although newborn hearing screening programs have greatly improved outcomes for those diagnosed with hearing loss in the immediate newborn period, there is no objective universal screening protocol in place during the critical early development years [28]. Unfortunately, school-age children are rarely screened for hearing loss during routine clinical examination, and health authorities pay little attention to audiometric evaluation particularly in primary schools.

5.1. Comprehensive approach to hearing screening in Poland

One of the priority activities of the Institute of Physiology and Pathology of Hearing in Kajetany is a screening program for children of all ages. The Institute team, in collaboration with numerous national centers, has laid the groundwork for screening programs and developed methods, procedures, and devices for carrying out them. He was the coordinator and producer of many programs. Based on this, two screening models have been created—newborn and school-age children.

5.1.1. Newborn hearing screening

The foundation on which the modern screening system was based was a research program for 150,000 newborns with funds in 15 neonatal and infants' centers in Warsaw. It was realized in 1992–1994 under the direction of Professor Maria Góralowna, and we cooperate with the team Diagnostic-Therapeutic and Rehabilitation Center "Cochlear Center" headed by Professor H. Skarżyński.

In the years 1995–1998, under the direction of Professor H. Skarżyński, a grant awarded to the Minister of Health, "Development of a unified screening program for neonates with hearing defects" was implemented. As part of the program, methods and procedures for screening hearing in newborns were developed, as well as their models - universal and intended for newborns at risk. At the end of the project, a draft of the Minister of Health was prepared for hearing screening in neonates.

In 1998, the grants were awarded the team award of the Minister of Health first degree. Another important initiative was implemented in 1996-1998, when the Institute of Physiology and Pathology of Hearing participated in the European program "European Concerted Action AHEAD (*Advancement of Hearing Assessment Methods and Devices*). This program aimed to develop a common European position on hearing screening for newborns.

In 1998, in Milan, a consensus on universal screening of hearing in newborns in Europe was signed. The signature on the Polish side was by Professor H. Skarżyński.

In the years 1998–2001, in the framework of the Government Action Plan for Disability Achievement, in which several dozen centers participated, hearing screening were disseminated and enriched. Alternative diagnostic, therapeutic, and rehabilitation facilities have been created for future screening programs. In 70 centers, more than 60,000 newborns and infants were examined.

5.1.2. School-aged children hearing screening

In 1999, the team of the Institute of Physiology and Pathology of Hearing collaborated with Brigham Young University of the United States and University of Michigan. M. Curie-Skłodowska from Lublin conducted pioneering screening of hearing in various regions of the country in a group of about 6000 children and adolescents in school age. Studies have shown that every 5 children aged 6–18 have hearing problems.

As part of the implementation of various programs (e.g., the Ministry of Health—the "Program for the Care of Persons with Hearing Loss in Poland"—the Mazovian Regional Health Service, the Ministry of National Education and Sport) conducted by the Institute of Physiology and Hearing Pathology in the years 2000–2006 in cooperation with the dozens of centers around the country, modern multimedia tools are developed for hearing screening. To use the program "I hear …" has trained over 3500 people and screened many centers. In cooperation with the Gdansk University of Technology, highly specialized systems such as "I can hear…," "I can see…," and "I can speak…" have been developed. About 16 million people from 62 countries have used the Internet.

Since 2007, a hearing screening program has been launched in Warsaw for children in class VI. Since 2011, the program also includes children in first grades. In total, these programs have covered up to now more than 56,000 children in Warsaw.

In the years 2008–2011, the programs were conducted by the Institute of Physiology and Pathology of Hearing in cooperation with the Contribution Fund of Social Insurance of Farmers and the Agricultural Insurance Fund Social screening in rural centers and small towns. Within these programs, nearly 300,000 children were studied.

In 2008, new multimedia tool—Platform for Sense Examination—used in screening was developed by the Institute of Physiology and Hearing Pathology in cooperation with the Institute of Sensory Organs. In addition, local screening programs were implemented, within the Ministry of National Education, which involved around 500 psychological and pedagogical clinics throughout the country.

In June 2007, the Institute team organized an exhibition at the European Parliament in Brussels. "HEAR-VISION-SPEAK" is the basis of communication and integration of the young generation of Europe. The exhibit was accompanied by a series of lectures, and numerous audiophiles and audiologists were examined by MEPs. The abovementioned actions aimed to draw Europeans' attention to the major social problem of communication disorders.

The exhibition was an introduction to further European activity. More than 3 years of negotiations and preparations resulted in the signing of the European Consensus on Audiology, Vision and Speech Screening in preschool and school children on June 22, 2011. There was great support during the Polish Presidency and an important argument for the adoption of the

"EU Council Conclusions on Early Detection and Treatment of Communication Disorders in Children, including the use of eHealth tools and innovative solutions".

Thanks to all these activities, Poland is currently at the forefront of countries that perform hearing screening in children of all ages.

5.1.3. System of integrated communication operations "SZOK"®

Every large-scale project involving children or adults is a great opportunity for early detection of congenital or acquired defects. In response to social needs related to the early detection of birth defects and acquired by detection and prevention, the Institute of Physiology and Hearing Pathology was involved in the implementation of the project, which was named System of Integrated Communication Operations "SZOK"®.

The project's innovation is the use of a system to assist patients with remote diagnosis and to transfer the results of their research to the health services sector. Integrating patient data into the "SZOK"® system will allow for quick service and thus shorten patient waiting times for visits to IFPS or other specialized facilities and as a comprehensive patient medical base. The system can also be successfully used in other healthcare and other medical fields. It is a unique solution in the field of telemedicine and e-health and is an excellent starting point for the Center for Screening.

Moreover, a standard for the transmission of audiological screening results has been implemented in the "SZOK"® system, which is developed within the Institute's project, so that it is adapted to obtain research results from other institutions and collect them in one place (**Figure 1**).

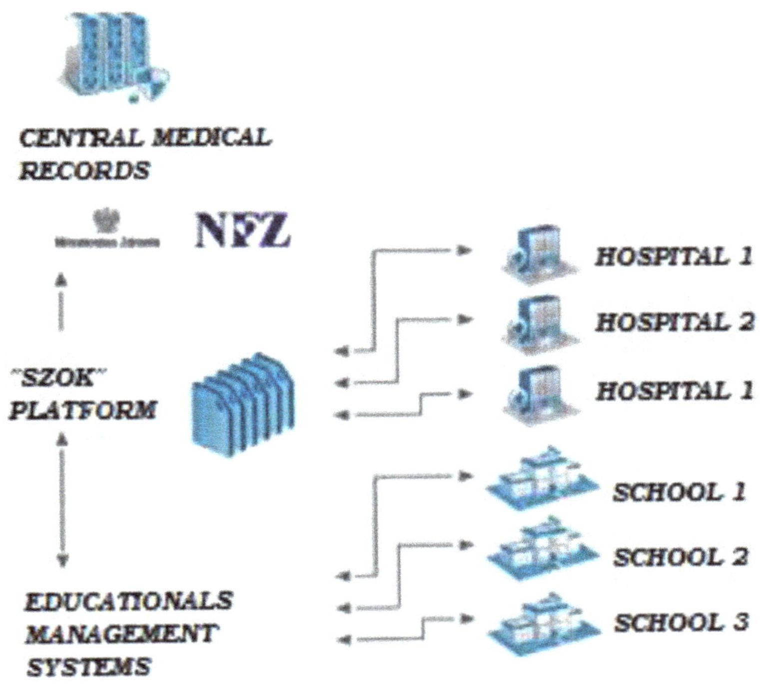

Figure 1. System of integrated communication operations "SZOK"®.

5.1.4. Platform for sense organ examination

In 2008, new multimedia tool used in screening—Platform for Sense Organs Screening—was developed by the Institute of Physiology and Hearing Pathology in cooperation with the Institute of Sensory Organs(**Figure 2**).

The platform is built around an Internet network solution, interfacing a central computer system and a series of portable computers (remote client devices) equipped with audiometric headphones and a response-button interface. The platform allows the user to conduct the following tests:

1. **Audiometric testing**: This feature allows the user to perform air conduction audiometric testing for each ear separately, in a tone frequency range from 250 to 8000 Hz, and for hearing threshold levels not exceeding 80 dB HL.
2. **Speech screening:** The speech test is carried out to obtain reliable information on: (1) the quality of verbal behavior of the child and (2) the degree of speech development (or of any potential delays) and any pathological linguistic phenomena occurring in the speech of the child.
3. **Audiological survey:** This module allows the user to conduct a general survey regarding the hearing, sight, and speech of a patient. The surveys were developed by specialists based on years of experience in specific areas, and they provide reliable information on the tested person.
4. **Test module DDT**: This is a dichotic listening test. During the test, pairs of sounds are presented to each ear and the task of the tested subjects is to repeat what they heard in one or both ears.
5. **Test module FPT**: This is a frequency pattern test. The test items are sequences of three tone bursts that are presented to one or both ears. In each of the sequences, two tone bursts

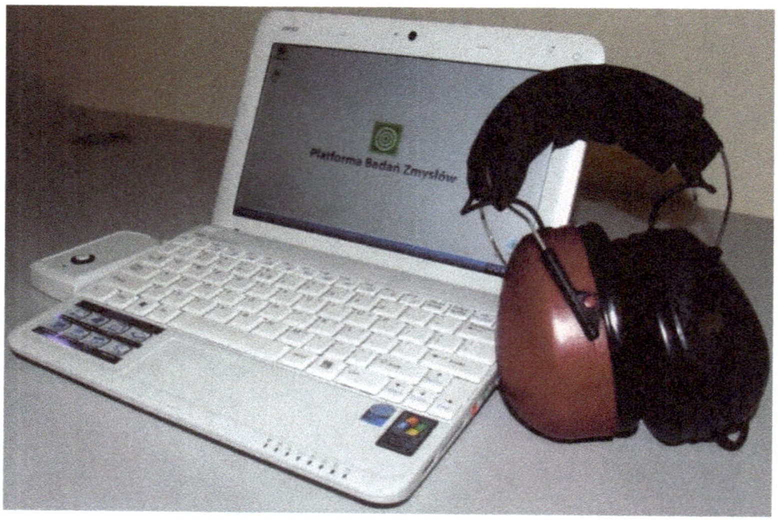

Figure 2. Platform for sense organs examinations.

are of the same frequency, while the third tone is of a different frequency. There are just two different frequencies used in this test: one is a high-frequency sound and the other a low-frequency sound pattern test.

6. **Test module DPT:** This is a duration pattern test. Test consists of sequences of three tones, one of which differs from the other two in the sequences by being either longer or shorter.
7. **Test module GIN**: This test allows assessment of the potential of perception of gaps in noise. During the test, the noise is presented with constantly emerging gaps of varying lengths.

5.2. Protocol used in the hearing screening in school-age children around the world conducted by world hearing Centre in Kajetany, Poland

Large-scale hearing screening experience called for a European Scientific Consensus agreement, which was defined and signed during the European Federation of Audiology Societies (EFAS) meeting in 2011 under auspices of the Institute of Physiology and Pathology of Hearing. As a result of this, a number of pilot hearing screening programs were started in various countries. Countries in which the team from the Institute of Physiology and Pathology of Hearing in Kajetany conducted hearing screening were presented in the **Table 1**.

Country in which IFPS conducted hearing screening	Children's age	Number of tested children	Universal Newborn Hearing Screening in this country
Armenia	6–9	200	No information
Azerbaijan	6–8	200	No screening program
Cameroon	5–15	220	No screening program
Columbia	6–8	150	In some district
Congo	6–8	200	No screening program
Ivory Coast	6–8	130	No screening program
Kazakhstan	7–8	212	No screening program
Kyrgyzstan	6–7	300	No screening program
Moldova	6–7	179	No information
Nigeria	4–7	200	Pilot project
Romania	6–7	130	No screening program
Russia	6–12	166	No screening program
Rwanda	6–15	195	No screening program
Senegal	6–10	200	No screening program
Tajikistan	7–8	143	No screening program
Tanzania	6–11	200	No screening program
Ukraine	6–11	184	No screening program

Table 1. Overview of hearing screening around the world conducted by the Institute Physiology and Pathology of Hearing.

School-entry hearing screening is especially important. That screening may actually be the first point of access to detect childhood hearing impairment.

Prior to testing, the children's parents were informed of the testing procedures and provided their written consent. The results of the audiometric tests were supplemented by the results of the questionnaire completed by the parents. This questionnaire included questions concerning data on the potential causes of the child's hearing problems, medical history, possible presence of tinnitus, and any presence of learning difficulties.

A hearing screening protocol used by a team from the Institute of Physiology and Pathology of Hearing in Kajetany, while screening in different countries includes three steps (**Figure 3**).

The first step is video-otoscopy. In this test, the specialist otolaryngologist views the middle ear on the monitor. This is the most accurate visual cure repair method and structure of the outer ear. This examination allows the diagnose change in the outer and middle ear such as excessive earwax, acute or chronic otitis media, fungal infection and changes in the tympanic membrane.

Second step is otoacoustic emission (OAE). It is an objective method of assessment—technically not a test of hearing but rather a reflection of inner ear mechanism. OAEs are sounds detected in the external ear canal that are generated by the outer hair cells within the cochlea. If the otoacoustic emission is absent, then we perform the third step—pure-tone audiometry.

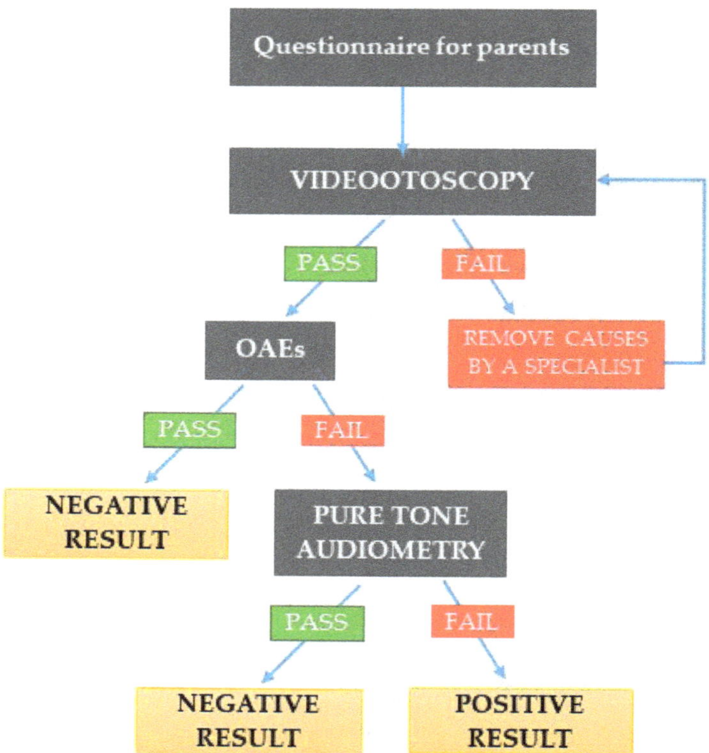

Figure 3. Schema of hearing screening protocol in school-age children used in the institute physiology and pathology of hearing.

Pure-tone audiometry (PTA) was performed using the modern platform elaborated by the Institute of Sense Organs and is fundamental for the inexpensive and universal screening in large populations of children—a platform for sense organs' screening. In addition, PTA was performed using SZOK described previously. The threshold for air conduction in the frequency range of 500–8000 Hz was determined. For abnormal test results, a hearing threshold value of 25 dB and above was used for at least one frequency in at least one ear.

The proposed screening procedure allows the detection not only of children with hearing loss but also of those with other hearing disorders, such as tinnitus. According to data study conducted by the team, led by Professor H. Skarżyńskiego, the incidence of tinnitus in school-age children is approximately 13–37.7% [30].

Moreover, the Institute of Physiology and Pathology of Hearing has their own truck that they are currently using for running a rural hearing health study—called Mobile Hearing Center. Inside, the truck functions as a regular audiology clinic, only on a much smaller scale. The larger of the two booths has a typical audiology setup with video-otoscopy. They were able to conduct assessment of the external and middle ears. The smaller booth is strictly used for testing adults. It may appear to be a small space; however, it is relatively spacious inside for the patient. Currently, we conduct only hearing screening, but in future, they hope to have Internet on the truck, so when they encounter a situation (e.g., with video otoscopy), they can evaluate the patient remotely. In that case, it would be a combination of two delivery types. Right now, it is a completely contained mobile audiology clinic, delivering the same level of service as you would expect in a brick-and-mortar clinic, except that they are able to bring hearing care services to the local community.

6. Summary

The positive impact of early identification and intervention for children with hearing loss is well established, and the primary care provider plays a vital role in screening children who require such services. Without prompt intervention, hearing loss in early childhood can cause significant delays in speech development, socioemotional growth, and school achievement.

Index of technical terms

Acute Otitis Media—painful type of ear infection. It occurs when the area behind the eardrum called the middle ear is inflamed and infected.

Auditory Brainstem Response (ABR)—neurologic test which gives information about the inner ear and brain pathways for hearing. The ABR is performed by pasting electrodes on the head—similar to electrodes placed around the heart when an electrocardiogram is run—and recording brain wave activity in response to sound.

Auditory Neuropathy/Dyssynchrony—hearing disorder in which sound enters the inner ear normally but the transmission of signals from the inner ear to the brain is impaired. People with auditory neuropathy may have normal hearing, or hearing loss ranges from mild to severe but they always have poor speech-perception abilities.

Behavioral Test–test investigates propensities toward certain kinds of behavior and styles of interaction with others.

Cerumen (Earwax)—brown, gray, or yellowish waxy substance secreted in the ear canal. It protects the skin of the human ear canal, assists in cleaning and lubrication, and also provides some protection against bacteria, fungi, insects, and water.

Chickenpox (Varicella)—a virus infection, commonly of children, caused by the varicella zoster virus and characterized by mild headache and fever, malaise, and eruption of blisters on the skin and mucous membranes.

Chronic Otitis Media—a long-standing, persistently draining perforation of the eardrum.

Cochlea—the auditory portion of the inner ear situated in the temporal bone. The cochlea interacts with the middle ear via two holes that are closed by membranes: the oval window, which is located at the base of the scala vestibuli and which undergoes pressure from the stapes, and the round window, which seals the base of the tympanic membrane and is used to relieve pressure. The cochlea is filled with a watery liquid, the perilymph, which moves in response to the vibrations coming from the middle ear via the oval window.

Cochlear Implant—a device that provides direct electrical stimulation to the auditory (hearing) nerve in the inner ear. Children and adults with a severe-to-profound sensorineural hearing loss who cannot be helped with hearing aids may be helped with cochlear implants. Cochlear implants have external (outside) parts and internal (surgically implanted) parts that work together to allow the user to perceive sound.

Congenital Hearing Impairment—it means that the hearing impairment is present at birth. Congenital hearing loss can be caused by genetic or nongenetic factors.

Connexin—structurally related transmembrane proteins that assemble to form vertebrate gap junctions.

Dichotic Listening Test—a psychological test commonly used to investigate selective attention within the auditory. Specifically, it is used as a behavioral test for hemispheric lateralization of speech sound perception. During a standard dichotic listening test, a participant is presented with two different auditory stimuli simultaneously (usually speech). The different stimuli are directed into different ears over headphones.

Duration Pattern Test—standard version is an auditory processing disorder test for ages 11 and over using nonverbal stimuli. The duration patterns are composed of three 1000-Hz tones and two 300-ms intertone intervals.

Ear Canal—it is a tube running from the outer ear to the middle ear. The adult human ear canal extends from the pinna to the eardrum and is about 2.5 cm (1 in) in length and 0.7 cm (0.3 in) in diameter.

Encephalitis—inflammation of the brain tissue. The most common cause is viral infections. In rare cases, it can be caused by bacteria or even fungi. Symptoms may include headache, fever, confusion, a stiff neck, and vomiting.

Enlarged Vestibular Aqueduct (EVA) Syndrome—a syndromic form of hearing loss, caused by the enlargement of the vestibular aqueduct in the inner ear. It is one of the most common inner ear deformities, which results in hearing loss during childhood.

Evoked Otoacoustic Emission (OAE)—sounds of cochlear origin, which can be recorded by a microphone fitted into the ear canal. They are caused by the motion of the cochlea's sensory hair cells as they energetically respond to auditory stimulation.

Frequency Pattern Test—an auditory processing disorder test for ages 8 and over using nonverbal stimuli. The frequency pattern test consists of 880 Hz (low) and 1122 Hz (high) tones that are 200 ms in duration and have an interstimulus interval of 150 ms and a 10-ms rise fall time.

Fungal infection—fungal infections occur when an invading fungus takes over an area of the body and is too much for the immune system to handle.

Gaps in noise—test auditory processing disorder test for ages 7 and older using nonverbal stimuli. It is designed to measure temporal resolution which resolution refers to the ability to detect changes in either the duration of an auditory stimulus and/or the time intervals or gaps of silence embedded within an auditory stimulus. The ability to detect small silent intervals is an important factor in speech perception.

Head trauma—any injury that results in trauma to the skull or brain.

Hearing aid—a device designed to improve hearing. Hearing aids are incapable of truly correcting a hearing loss; they are an aid to make sounds more accessible.

Hearing deficits—it is a partial or total inability to hear.

Influenza—an infectious disease caused by an influenza virus. It is characterized by a sudden onset of fever, cough (usually dry), headache, muscle and joint pain, severe malaise (feeling unwell), sore throat, and a runny nose. The cough can be severe and can last 2 or more weeks.

Measles—a highly contagious infection caused by the measles virus. Initial signs and symptoms typically include fever, often greater than 40°C (104.0°F), cough, runny nose, and inflamed eyes. Two or three days after the start of symptoms, small white spots may form inside the mouth. A red, flat rash which usually starts on the face and then spreads to the rest of the body typically begins 3–5 days after the start of symptoms.

Medical History—information gained by a physician by asking specific questions, either of the patient or of other people who know the person and can give suitable information with the aim of obtaining information useful in formulating a diagnosis and providing medical care to the patient. The medically relevant complaints reported by the patient or others familiar with the patient are referred to as symptoms, in contrast with clinical signs, which are ascertained by direct examination on the part of medical personnel.

Meningitis—an acute inflammation of the protective membranes covering the brain and spinal cord, collectively known as the meninges. The most common symptoms are fever, headache, and neck stiffness. The inflammation may be caused by infection with viruses, bacteria, or other microorganisms, and less commonly by certain drugs.

Middle Ear—the portion of the ear internal to the eardrum, and external to the oval window of the inner ear. The mammalian middle ear contains three ossicles, which transfer the vibrations of the eardrum into waves in the fluid and membranes of the inner ear. It joins the tympanic cavity with the nasal cavity, allowing pressure to equalize between the middle ear and throat. The hollow space of the middle ear is also known as the tympanic cavity. The primary function of the middle ear is to efficiently transfer acoustic energy from compression waves in air to fluid-membrane waves within the cochlea.

Mitochondrial Hearing Loss—nonsyndromic deafness caused by mutations in both nuclear and mitochondrial genes. Nonsyndromic mitochondrial hearing loss is characterized by moderate to profound hearing loss, and a maternally inherited mutation in either the MTRNR1 or MTTS1 gene.

Mumps—a viral disease caused by the mumps virus. Initial signs and symptoms often include fever, muscle pain, headache, and feeling tired. This is then usually followed by painful swelling of one or both parotid salivary glands. Symptoms typically occur 16—18 days after exposure and resolve after 7–10 days. Symptoms in adults are often more severe than those in children. Complications may include meningitis, pancreatitis, permanent deafness, and testicular inflammation, which uncommonly results in infertility.

Noise-induced Hearing Loss—hearing impairment resulting from exposure to loud sound. People may have a loss of perception of a narrow range of frequencies, impaired cognitive perception of sound, or other impairment, including sensitivity to sound or ringing in the ears. Hearing may deteriorate gradually from chronic and repeated noise exposure or suddenly from a short high intensity noise. In both types, loud sound overstimulates delicate hearing cells, leading to the permanent injury or death of the cells.

Otitis Media with Effusion—when there is thick or sticky fluid behind the eardrum in the middle ear, but there is no ear infection. Normally, the Eustachian tube drains fluid from your ears to the back of your throat. If it clogs, otitis media with effusion (OME) can occur. This condition most often affects children. Muffled hearing is a common symptom.

Ototoxic Drugs—medications which can damage the ear, resulting in hearing loss, ringing in the ear, or balance disorders. The effects of ototoxicity can be reversible and temporary, or irreversible and permanent. Ototoxic drugs include, for example, antibiotics (gentamicin), loop diuretics (furosemide), and platinum-based hemotherapy (cisplatin). Outer hair cells.

Outer Hair Cells—called acoustical preamplifiers. In mammalian outer hair cells, the receptor potential triggers active vibrations of the cell body. This mechanical response to electrical signals is termed somatic electromotility and drives oscillations in the cell's length, which occur at the frequency of the incoming sound and provide mechanical feedback amplification. They also improve frequency selectivity.

Platform for Sense Examination—a portable device for screening hearing, sight and speech and hearing and speech rehabilitation in children (also with special educational needs), adolescents and adults. The device is built on the basis of an advanced central computer system and a portable computer equipped with additional accessories enabling the test.

Play Audiometry—it allows an audiologist to test the hearing of very young toddlers and preschoolers. CPA uses behavioral conditioning to get kids to respond to sounds. It is designed for children usually between 2 and 5 years of age. It measures hearing sensitivity to determine both a child's type and degree of hearing loss, if any. The audiologist can then refer parents to another specialist, if necessary.

Pure Tone Audiometry (PTA)—the key hearing test used to identify hearing threshold levels of an individual, enabling determination of the degree, type and configuration of a hearing loss, thus providing the basis for diagnosis and management. PTA is a subjective, behavioral measurement of hearing threshold, as it relies on patient response to pure tone stimuli. Therefore, PTA is used on adults and children old enough to cooperate with the test procedure.

Questionnaire—a research instrument consisting of a series of questions (or other types of prompts) for the purpose of gathering information from respondents. Although questionnaires are often designed for statistical analysis of the responses, this is not always the case.

Rubella—is an infection caused by the rubella virus. This disease is often mild with half of people not realizing that they are sick. A rash may start around 2 weeks after exposure and last for 3 days. Complications may include bleeding problems, testicular swelling, and inflammation of nerves. Infection during early pregnancy may result in a child born with congenital rubella syndrome (CRS) or miscarriage.

Sensitivity—the ability of an organism or organ to respond to external stimuli. For example, auditory hypersensitivity occurs when a person has a collapsed tolerance to normal environmental sound. The term commonly used to describe this condition is "hyperacusis."

Sound-source location—a listener's ability to identify the location or origin of a detected sound in direction and distance. The auditory system uses several cues for sound source localization, including time and level differences (or intensity-difference) between both ears, spectral information, timing analysis, correlation analysis, and pattern matching.

Specificity—In medicine, it means the extent to which a diagnostic test is specific for a particular condition, trait, and so on.

Sudden Idiopathic Hearing Loss—defined as greater than 30 dB hearing reduction, over at least three contiguous frequencies, occurring over a period of 72 h or less. Some patients describe that the hearing loss was noticed instantaneously in the morning, and others report that it rapidly developed over a period of hours or days. Only one ear is usually affected. About half of people recover some or all of their hearing spontaneously, and some people need a treatment from an otolaryngologist.

System of Integrated Communication Operations "SZOK"®—a world-class solution—is a revolution in the creation of IT infrastructure and data management. The project's innovativeness is based on the use of a system supporting patient diagnosis at a distance and the transfer of research results to the health services sector. Integrating patient data into the system platform will allow for better and faster service and will reduce patient waiting times for visits to an institute.

Teleaudiology—it is the utilization of telehealth to provide audiological services and may include the full scope of audiological practice. The innovation that is currently being developed broadens teleaudiology and hearing care practice to virtual care modalities such as clinical video telehealth, store-and-forward telehealth, home telehealth, mobile health applications, secure messaging, and electronic consults.

Telemedicine—the use of telecommunication and information technology to provide clinical healthcare from a distance. It has been used to overcome distance barriers and to improve access to medical services that would often not be consistently available in distant rural communities. It is also used to save lives in critical care and emergency situations.

Tinnitus—the hearing of sound when no external sound is present. While often described as a ringing, it may also sound like a clicking, hiss, or roaring. Rarely, unclear voices or music are heard. The sound may be soft or loud, low pitched or high pitched and appear to be coming from one ear or both. Most of the time, it comes on gradually. In some people, the sound causes depression or anxiety and can interfere with concentration.

Tympanic Membrane—a thin, cone-shaped membrane that separates the external ear from the middle ear. Its function is to transmit sound from the air to the ossicles inside the middle ear and then to the oval window in the fluid-filled cochlea. Hence, it ultimately converts and amplifies vibration in air to vibration in fluid. Rupture or perforation of the eardrum can lead to conductive hearing loss.

Unilateral Hearing Loss (UHL)—a type of hearing impairment where there is normal hearing in one ear and impaired hearing in the other ear. Patients with unilateral hearing loss have difficulty in hearing conversation on their impaired side, localizing sound, understanding speech in the presence of background noise, interpersonal and social relations. Using for example CROS hearing aids or BAHA implant can help to resist better hearing functioning.

Universal Screening Protocol—it is the largest preventive health program in Poland. Its primary goal is to examine each newborn baby to except possible hearing impairment and to analyze risk factors that predispose to hearing loss.

Vernix—the waxy or cheese-like white substance found coating the skin of newborn human babies. It is produced by dedicated cells and is thought to have some protective roles during fetal development and for a few hours after birth. Vernix is theorized to serve several purposes, including moisturizing the infant's skin, and facilitating passage through the bacteria. It serves to conserve heat and protect the delicate newborn skin from environmental stress.

Video-otoscopy—video-otoscopy is the use of an otoscope (this is an instrument used to look in the ears) that has a very tiny video camera that transmits images to a television screen. These scopes use fiber optics to transmit a very bright light that illuminates the ear canal. The video otoscope allows the doctor to see in the ear much better than a traditional handheld otoscope. With the irrigating function, debris can be cleaned deep within the ear that would be impossible to remove any other way.

Author details

Piotr Henryk Skarżyński[1,2,3,4*] and Maciej Ludwikowski[1]

*Address all correspondence to: p.skarzynski@medincus.pl

1 World Hearing Center, Institute of Physiology and Pathology of Hearing, Department of Teleaudiology, Kajetany/Warsaw, Poland

2 Institute of Sensory Organs, Kajetany, Poland

3 Heart Failure and Cardiac Rehabilitation, Department of the Medical University of Warsaw, Poland

4 Center of Hearing and Speech, MEDINCUS, Kajetany, Poland

References

[1] Skarżyński PH, Kochanek K, Skarżyński H, Senderski A, Wysocki J, Szkiełkowska A. Hearing screening program in school-age children in western Poland. The Journal of International Advanced Otology. 2011;**7**(2):194-200

[2] Skarżyński PH, Świerniak W, Piłka A, Skarżyńska MB, Włodarczyk AW, Kholmatov, et al. A hearing screening program for children in primary schools in Tajikistan: A telemedicine model. Medical Science Monitor. 2016;**22**:2424-2430. DOI: 10.12659/MSM.895967

[3] Anderson KL. http://successforkidswithhearingloss.com. 2012. Retrieved from Supporting Success for Children with Hearing Loss: https://successforkidswithhearingloss.com/wp-content/uploads/2011/12/Handout-Hearing-Screening-in-Early-Childhood.pdf

[4] Skarżyński PH, Piłka A, Ludwikowski M, Skarżyńska MB. Comparison of the frequency of positive hearing screening outcomes in schoolchildren from Poland and other countries of Europe, Central Asia, and Africa. Journal of Hearing Science. 2015, February;**51-58**

[5] Tharpe AM, Sladen DP. Causation of permanent unilateral and mild bilateral hearing loss in children. Trends in Amplification. 2008, March;**12**(1):17-25

[6] Ross DS, Holstrum WJ, Gaffney M, Green D, Oyler RF, Gravel JS. Hearing screening and diagnostic evaluation of children with unilateral and mild bilateral hearing loss. Trends in Amplification. 2008, March;**12**(1):27-34

[7] Liu XZ, Pandya A, Angeli S, Telischi FF, Arnos KS, Nance, et al. Audiological features of GJB2 (connexin 26) deafness. Ear and Hearing. 2005, June;**26**(3):361-369

[8] Marazita G, Ploughman LM, Rawlings B, Remington E, Arnos KS, Nance WE. Genetic epidemiological studies of early-onset deafness in the U.S. school-age population. American Journal of Medicine Genetics. 1993, June 15;**46**(5):486-491

[9] Arjamand EM, Webber A. Audiometric findings in children with a large vestibular aqueduct. Archives of Otolaryngology - Head & Neck Surgery. 2004, October;**130**(10):1169-1174

[10] Wynne MK, Diefendorf AO, Fritsch MH. Sudden hearing loss. The ASHA Leader. 2001;**6**:6-8

[11] Foerst A, Beutner D, Lang-Roth R, Huttenbrink KB, van Wedel H, Walger M. Prevalence of auditory neuropathy/synaptopathy in a population of children with profound hearing loss. International Journal of Pediatric Otorhinolaryngology, 2006;**70**(8):415–1422

[12] Niskar AS, Kieszak SM, Holmes AE, Esteban E, Rubin C, Brody DJ. Estimated prevalence of noise-induced hearing threshold shifts among children 6 to 19 years of age: The third National Health and nutrition examination survey. Pediatrics. 2001, July;**108**(1):40-43

[13] Unal M, Katircioglu S, Karatay MC, Suoglu Y, Erdamar B, Aslan I. Sudden total bilateral deafness due to asymptomatic mumps infection. International Journal of Pediatric Otorhinolaryngology. 1998, October 2;**45**(2):167-169

[14] Paparella MM, Morizono T, Le CT, Choo YB, Mancini F, Lidén G, et al. Sensorineural hearing loss in otitis media. Annals of Otology, Rhinology % Laryngology. 1984:623-629

[15] Wake M, Tobin S, Cone-Wesson B, Dahl HH, Gillam L, McCormick L, et al. Slight/mild sensorineural hearing loss in children. Pediatrics. 2006:1842-1851

[16] Yoshinaga-Italona C. Levels of evidence: Universal newborn hearing screening (UNHS) and early hearing detection and intervention systems (EHDI). Jounal of Communication Disorders. 2004:451-465

[17] Patel H, Feldman M. Universal newborn hearing screening. Paediatrics Child Health. 2011, 5;**16**(5):301-305

[18] Mason A, Mason M. Psychologic impact of deafness on the child and adolescent. Primary Care. 2007, June;**34**(2):407-426

[19] Davis JM, Elfenbein J, Schum R, Bentler RA. Effects of mild and moderate hearing impairments on language, educational, and psychosocial behavior of children. The Journal of Speech and Hearing Disorders. 1986;**51**(1):53-62

[20] Johnson CD, Seaton JB. Educational Audiology Handbook with CD. 2nd ed. Clifton Park, New York: Cengage Learning; 2011

[21] Newton VE, Macharia I, Mugwe P, Ototo B, Kan SW. Evaluation of the use of a questionnaire to detect hearing loss in Kenyan pre-school children. International Journal of Pediatric Otorhinolaryngology. 2001, March 1;**53**:229-234

[22] Olusanya B. Early detection of hearing impairment in a developing country: What options? Audiology: Official Organ of the International Society of Audiology. 2001, May-June;**40**(3): 141-147

[23] Samelli AG, Rabelo CM, Vespasiano AP. Development and analysis of a low-cost screening tool to identify and classify hearing loss in children: A proposal for developing countries. Clinics (Sao Paula, Brazil). 2011;**66**(11):1943-1948

[24] Herman CR, Gill HK, Eng J, Fajardo LL. Screening for preclinical disease: Test and disease characteristics. American Journal of Roentgenology. 2002, October;**179**(4):825-831

[25] Olusanya BO, Neumann K, Saunders JE. The global burden of disabling hearing impairment: A call to action. Bulletin of the World Health Organization. 2014;**92**:367-373

[26] Ravi R, Gunjawate DR, Yerraguntla K, Lewis LE, Driscoll C, Rajashekhar B. Follow-up in newborn hearing screening - a systematic review. International Journal of Pediatric Otorhinolaryngology. 2016, November;**90**:29-36

[27] Olusanya BO, Wirz SL, Luxon LM. Hospital-based universal newborn hearing screening for early detection of permanent congenital hearing loss in Lagos, Nigeria. International Journal of Pediatric Otorhinolaryngology. 2008, July;**72**(7):991-1001

[28] Bhatia P, Mintz S, Hecht BF, Deavenport A, Kuo A. Early identification of young children with hearing loss in federally qualified health centers. Journal of Developmental & Behavioral Pediatrics. 2013, January;**34**(1):15-21

[29] Prevention, Centers for Disease Control. Guide to Infection Prevention in Outpatient Settings: Minimum Expectations for Safe Care. 2016, September. Retrieved from cdc.gov/hai/pdfs/guidelines/ambulatory-care-04-2011.pdf.

[30] Raj-Koziak D, Piłka A, Bartnik G, Fabijańska A, Kochanek K, Skarżyński H. The prevalance of tinnitus in 7-year-old children in estern of Poland. The Polish Otolaryngology. 2011: 106-109

2

Intratympanic Steroid Treatment in Méniére Disease

Fatih Oghan, Ibrahim Erdim, Metin Çeliker,
Muhammet Fatih Topuz, Ahmet Uluat,
Onur Erdogan and Sinan Aksoy

Abstract

Méniére disease (MD) is characterized by vertigo attacks, hearing loss, tinnitus, and aural fullness. Although the exact treatment of MD is lacking, several treatment options including conservative, medical, and surgical aim to control symptoms. Recently, an increasingly used treatment method called intratympanic steroid (ITS) treatment is applied to patients suffering from MD. In which step the ITS takes part for MD treatment protocol is not certain. But common wisdom is that ITS can be used in patients with intractable MD to conservative and medical treatment before applying intratympanic gentamicin and surgical treatments.

Keywords: Méniére Disease, Steroid Treatment, Vertigo

1. Introduction

Méniére disease (MD) is characterized by vertigo attacks, hearing loss, tinnitus, and aural fullness. Several treatment options include conservative, medical, and surgical aims to control symptoms. Recently, an increasingly used treatment method called intratympanic steroid (ITS) treatment is applied to patients suffering from MD. In this chapter, we mention this alternative treatment option.

2. Pathophysiology

After Mc Cabe's report on auto-immune depended on sensorineural hearing loss in 1979, immunological mechanisms about inner ear pathologies started to be investigated [1]. Many studies showed that MD is an immune system-related disease. Autoantibody for the Raf-1 protein in the membranous labyrinth is found in patients with MD [2]. Elevated IgG immune complexes, auto-immune response to type II collagen, and focal inflammation with intraepithelial invasion caused by mononuclear cells are shown in endolymphatic sac. This phenomenon is also called "endolymphatic sacitis" [3, 4].

Rarey and Curtis found glycocorticoid receptors on the cochlea and vestibule (especially on the spiral ligament) [5]. Lohuis also showed cell atrophy on stria vascularis after adrenal steroid defects [6]. Glycocorticoid receptors are also found in the lateral wall of cochlea, organ of Corti, modiolus, vestibule, and stria vascularis [7].

It is already shown that steroids regulate inner ear fluid balance with potassium transport channels by mineralocorticoid receptor genes and aquaporin regulation [8, 9]. Cochlear blood flow is also positively affected by topical steroid application [10, 11].

According to these information and steroids' anti-inflammatory/immunosuppressive effects, we can say that ITS treatment is helpful for MD control.

3. Intratympanic steroid injection protocol

Procedure is done under operation microscope. Head is turned 45° to the opposite side. EMLA® 5% cream (lidocaine Hcl + prilocaine) or 88% phenol can be used for local anesthesia. Twenty-two or 25 gauge spinal needle can be used for injection. Myringotomy is made anterosuperior part of tympanic membrane to fill middle ear as long as possible. After intervention, the patient has to wait for 30–40 min as the head is turned 45° to the opposite side. During this time, the patient is requested not to speak and not to swallow as much as possible [12, 13].

4. Application features (steroid types, daily usage time, dosage, and time duration)

Despite many studies, there is no consensus for ITS application [14]. Three different types of steroids are used for ITS: hydrocortisone (short-acting), methylprednisolone (intermediate-acting), and dexamethasone (long-acting). Methylprednisolone and dexamethasone are generally preferred types in studies (**Table 1**). In some studies, it is claimed that methylprednisolone reaches inner ear tissues and fluids in shorter time (2 h), and maximum concentration continues by 6 h [4, 15]. However, other studies have claimed that dexamethasone reaches inner ear tissues and fluids in shorter time than methylprednisolone [15, 16].

Three different application ways are used for ITS: injection, ventilation tube, and perfusion with catheter. Daily intervention is recommended regardless of application ways. Methylprednisolone stays for 6 h at maximal concentration in blood and descends as basal level at 24 h. Dexamethasone also descends as basal level at 6 h. We recommend using a ventilation

Types of ITS in MD	Hydrocortisone	Methylprednisolone*	Dexamethasone*
Efficiency period	**Short-acting**	**Intermediate-acting**	**Long-acting**
Dosage		62.5 mg/ml, 3 weeks [3]	4 mg/ml, three times with 3 days interval [14, 18]
			17.5 mg, 0.3–0.8 ml applied each day for 5 days [12]
			4 mg/cc, 4 weeks [13]
			24 mg/cc [20]
			0.20 mg/cc, five drops in each day for 3 months [19]

*Preferred steroid types in studies, ITS: intratympanic steroid, MD: Méniére disease.

Table 1. Types, efficiency period, and dosage of ITS using in MD.

tube or catheter application for daily intervention that provides less patient pain and prevents time lost for both doctor and patient [15, 17].

Both the dosing of the steroid types and the daily usage protocols are also different in the studies. Dexamethasone (4 mg/ml) is used for three times at 3 days interval in two studies [14, 18]. In another study, 17.5 mg dexamethasone in 0.3–0.8 ml was applied each day for 5 days [12]. Ventilation tube application was made toward posteroinferior cadrane to 20 patients with MD in another study. In that study, 1 mg/cc dexamethasone was distilled to 0.20 mg/cc with water. Five drops were applied to 20 patients in each day for 3 months (**Table 1**) [19]. Barr et al. administered 4 mg/cc dexamethasone for 4 weeks [13]. Hamid et al. applied 24 mg/cc dexamethasone (**Table 1**) [20]. Nathalie Gabra et al. used methylprednisolone (62.5 mg/ml) each week for 3 weeks (**Table 1**) [3]. The reason for not performing daily intervention in these studies is the difficulty of injection application way [14]. All studies mentioned earlier show that vertigo control rates get higher when drug concentration increases.

5. Advantages

Steroids are permeable to round window and across blood-labyrinthine barrier [13] so drug concentration in inner ear fluids (both perilymph and endolymph) is higher with ITS application than systemic administration [3, 13]. ITS application also prevents steroid side effects.

6. Disadvantages and side effects

Tympanic membrane perforation may occur after ITS. Its incidence seems low and changes between 0 and 5.1%. If the tympanic membrane perforation develops after ITS, it may recover or be permanent [12, 14, 18, 21]. To reduce the likelihood of development perforation, it needs attention to not penetrate tympanic membrane from thinned areas.

Pain and burn sensation in the ear and pharynx are other problems. These resolve approximately 0.5–1 h later. Mild dizziness and transient vertigo may be seen due to inner ear content concentration change [4, 13, 18].

7. Treatment effects

Patients with MD suffer from vertigo attacks, hearing loss, tinnitus, and aural fullness. Life is also unbearable during MD attacks. We mention each symptom recovering rate by ITS treatment in subsequent text (**Table 2**).

	Vertigo	Hearing loss	Tinnitus	Aural fullness	Quality of life
Albu et al. [14]	46% class A 21.2% class B 24.2% class C/D 3% class E	PTA: Pretreatment 57.4 ± 14.7 After 1 year 55.8 ± 15.5	THI: Pretreatment 28.6 ± 14.3 Posttreatment 23.5 ± 12.4	–	DHI: Pretreatment 53.2 ± 13.4 Posttreatment 40.7 ± 16.5
Casani et al. [18]	42.9% class A 17.9% class B 32.2% class C/D 7% class E/F	PTA: Pretreatment 66.6 ± 16.4 After 1 month 67.5 ± 17.7 After 1 year 67.1 ± 17.6 After 2 years 65.0 ± 18.7	–	–	–
Gabra and Saliba [3]	**Number of attack** Before therapy: 5.3 ± 6.41 After 0–6 months: therapy 1.4 ± 1.87 After 6–12 months: therapy 1.4 ± 1.87	PTA: Pretreatment 41.89 ± 14.92 After 1 yeary 49.51 ± 17.9	Decreased to: 78% at 0–6 months therapy 68% at 6–12 months therapy	Pretreatment: 95.2% Posttreatment: 65%	–
Paragache et al. [19]	85% class A 10% class C/D 5% class E/F	PTA:15% improved 10% dropped SDS:15% improved 85% same	10% recovery 60% improved	15% Disappeared 65% Improved	–
Ren et al. [12]	48.8% class A 20.9% class B 9.3% class C/D 20.9% class E	–	Disappeared 11.6% Decreased 48.8% Same 23.3% Improved 16.3%	16.7%: Disappeared 45.8%: Alleviated 35.7%: Intensive	–
Barr et al. [13]	At 3rd month of therapy: 52% class A At 6th month of therapy: 43% class A	At 6th month of therapy: An average loss of 2.7 dB	–	–	–

	Vertigo	Hearing loss	Tinnitus	Aural fullness	Quality of life
Garduño-Anaya et al. [22]	82% class A 18% class B	PTA: Pretreatment 55.7 After 2 years 53.4 SDS: Pretreatment 68.5% After 2 years 66.7%	THI: 61 pretreatment 22.3 at 2 years therapy GTS: 3.2 pretreatment 1.6 at 2 years therapy	48% subjective improvement	DHI: Pretreatment 68.7 Posttreatment 8.3

ITS: Intratympanic steroid, MD: Ménière disease, PTA: Pure tone average, SDS: Speech discrimination score, THI: Tinnitus Handicap Inventory, GTS: Grading of Tinnitus Severity, DHI: Dizziness Handicap Inventory.

Table 2. Symptom relief success of ITS on MD.

7.1. Vertigo

Vertigo control is generally reported according to the 1995 AAO-HNS guidelines or Sakata's criteria in the studies about ITS treatment.

Albu et al. investigated 66 patients with definite unilateral MD. Thirty-three of them received IT dexamethasone. Fourteen patients (46.6%) were free from vertigo attack (class A), seven patients (21.2%) had substantial control (class B), and eight patients (24.2%) had limited control (classes C and D) at 1-year follow-up. Vertigo control couldn't be obtained in one patient (class E). Failures were planned for intratympanic gentamicin (ITG), which did not benefit enough from the ITC [14].

In Casani et al.'s study, 12 patients (42.9%) had full vertigo control (class A), 5 patients (17.9%) had substantial control (class B), 9 patients (32.2%) had limited control (class C or D) despite 1 or 2 additional intratympanic dexamethasone (ITD). Two patients (7%) couldn't get vertigo control (class E or F) and were scheduled for ITG therapy [18].

In a study, Gabra and Saliba had evaluated the effect of intratympanic methylprednisolone and gentamicin injection on MD. In this study, the number of patient's vertigo attacks per month before ITS (for methylprednisolone) was 5.3 ± 6.41 ($n = 42$). In 0–6 months after the ITS, the number of attacks decreased to 2.3 ± 3.20 ($n = 41$). Finally, 6–12 months after ITS, attack frequency was 1.4 ± 1.87 ($n = 27$). In the first period after treatment, 41.5% of the patients achieved complete control of vertigo. In the second period after treatment, 48.1% of the patients achieved complete control of vertigo ($P = 0.004$). There was a statistically significant decrease in the number of vertigo attacks in the first period ($P = 0.025$) and no difference between the 0- to 6-month and 6- to 12-month periods after ITS ($P = 0.95$) [3].

Paragache et al. reported 85% (17 of 20 patients) control of vertigo with intratympanic dexamethasone therapy. Two patients (10%) had only limited control. One patient (5%) had worsening of vertigo during treatment [19].

Boleas-Aguirre et al. reported 91% "acceptable" vertigo control using 12 mg/ml dexamethasone. Most of the patients (63%) needed more than one series of treatment for achieving remission of MD [21].

Ren et al. reported complete control of vertigo in 21 of 43 patients (48.8%), substantial control in 9 patents (20.9%), limited control in 4 patients (9.3%), and no exact response in 9 patients (20.9%) with intratympanic dexamethasone injections for refractory MD after 18 months follow-up [12].

In a retrospective analysis of 17 intractable MD patients treated with ITD, short-term (after 6 months) and long-term (after 24 months) vertigo control rates were 94 and 81% [4].

Barrs's et al. reported that 21 patients with intractable MD underwent intratympanic injections of 4 mg/ml dexamethasone over a period of 4 weeks as an office procedure. Eleven (52%) of 21 patients were free for vertigo attack at the 3rd month of treatment. However, vertigo attacks relapsed in two patients and success rate decreased to 43% at the 6th month. At 1-year follow-up, six of remaining nine patients had no vertigo attack. Recurrent injections applied to five patients who responded at the beginning but repeated vertigo attacks later. Vertigo was controlled in three of those five patients. One patient got only one additional injection but two patients got multiple injections for each month up to 6 months [13].

In another prospective, randomized, double-blind study with a 2-year follow-up, the effect of five consecutive daily intratympanic injections of dexamethasone on 22 patients having definite MD was investigated. Complete control of vertigo (class A) was achieved in 9 of 11 patients (82%) and substantial control of vertigo (class B) in the remaining 2 patients (18%) [22].

In a retrospective study including 129 patients diagnosed with unilateral MD still having vertigo despite medical therapy, patient's satisfaction with vertigo attack control using ITD (12 mg/ml) was assessed. Vertigo control was obtained in 117 (91%) of 129 patients. One injection was enough for 48 patients (37%), two injections were needed for 26 patients (20%), three injections for 18 patients (14%), and four injections for 10 patients (8%). More than four injections were needed for 15 patients (21%). Ninety-six patients were followed for 2 years. Vertigo control was obtained in 87 (91%) patients with ITD. After 2 years, additional injection wasn't needed in 61 patients but repeated injections were required in 23 patients. Three patients requested ITG treatment because of repeated ITD injections [21].

Different vertigo control rates were given in studies mentioned earlier. This may be related to steroid type, concentration, time duration, and frequency of therapy. Also keep in mind that each drug has different personal effect.

7.2. Hearing loss

Sensorineural hearing loss is another symptom of MD. It may be transient or permanent. The success of any treatment about MD on hearing improvement is a change of 10 dB or more in pure tone average (PTA) or a change of 15% in speech discrimination score (SDS) according to 1995 AAO-HNS guidelines [3, 14, 18].

Paragache et al. observed hearing improvement in only three patients (15%) with two patients (10%) having a 20-dB improvement in threshold and one patient (5%) having a 10-dB improvement in threshold. In 10% of patients, the hearing level was observed to decrease. The speech discrimination score improved in three patients (15%). For the rest, the SDS remained the same with the intratympanic dexamethasone applications [19].

Albu et al. found the mean pretreatment PTA as 57.4 (standard deviation (SD), 14.7) with the intratympanic dexamethasone injection. After 12 months of therapy, the PTA values were 55.8 (SD, 15.5). Hearing was unchanged in 14 patients, improved in 4 patients and worsened in 12 patients. With reference to hearing outcomes, they had demonstrated that hearing conservation was only able to be maintained in patients reporting vertigo, which was well controlled. As previously stated [18], hearing loss is associated with the evolution of MD [14, 23].

Casani et al. found the mean pretreatment PTA as 66.6 (SD, 16.4). After 1 month with ITD injection, the PTA values changed on average to 67.5 (SD, 17.7). The mean PTA was 67.1 (SD, 17.6) at 1 year and 65.0 (SD, 18.7) at 2-year follow-up with the intratympanic ITD injection. No significant variations of SDS were observed during each follow-up period ($P > 0.05$) [18]. Hearing improved in 3 patients (10.7%) and did not worsen in 13 patients (46.4%). Vertigo was detected as class A and class B in those 16 patients. Hearing deterioration on PTA was more than 10 dB in remaining 10 patients who couldn't obtain vertigo control [18]. It pays attention that a correlation was found between hearing deterioration and vertigo attack persistence.

Gabra et al. found the mean PTA as 41.89 ± 14.92 dB before intratympanic methylprednisolone injection (ITM). There was a slight increase in PTA at 6 months. This was followed by an increase in PTA at 12 months after ITM, the mean PTA was 49.51 ± 17.9 dB. There was no statistically significant difference in the evolution from before to after treatment ($P = 0.456$ for the 0- to 6-month period and $P = 0.06$ for the 6- to 12-month period) [3]. In the first 0–6 months, the SDS decreased and remained stable in the second period. There was no statistically significant difference in the evolution of SDS after ITM [3].

Another retrospective analysis was conducted on 17 MD patients treated with ITM. Sixteen patients were followed up for more than 2 years. The PTA was 53 ± 14 dB before treatment, and 50 ± 16 dB at 6 months and 52 ± 20 dB at 24 months after ITM. Thus, a significant improvement in PTA after 6 months had returned to the pretreatment baseline after 2 years and there were no significant differences in clinical stage, based on hearing changes at the 6- and 24-month follow-up [4].

Garduño-Anaya et al. found the mean initial PTA as 55.7 dB and after receiving the ITD the mean PTA was 53.4 dB at 2-year follow-up. Only one patient's hearing (9%) improvement, 10 dB or more according to the 1995 AAO-HNS criteria, was considered to be clinically significant. One of 11 patients was demonstrated to have hearing deterioration of 10 dB at 2-year follow-up [22]. The mean SDS was 68.5% at the beginning of treatment and 66.7% after 2 years of ITD. According to 1995 AAO-HNS criteria, 15% or higher improvement on SDS was provided in two patients (18%). Only one (9%) of 11 patients got 15% or higher deterioration at 2 years follow-up. They reported a subjective improvement of 35% in hearing loss [22].

Kaplan et al. investigated 30 patients (20 women and 10 men, aged 28–85 years) with MD who underwent intratympanic dexamethasone perfusion. Six patients obtained 10 dB or higher improvement at PTA and six patients obtained 15% or higher improvement at SDS at short-term period (4 weeks after perfusion). Those patient numbers decreased to 5 and 2 at 12 months later, respectively [23].

Arriaga and Goldman demonstrated that only 33% of patients had hearing improvement, and 20% of patients had hearing deterioration after ITD with hyaluronan. However, Hillman et al. [24] reported 40% of patients who had hearing improvement after ITD [21].

7.3. Tinnitus

In Paragache et al.'s study, 2 patients (of 20, 10%) showed complete relief from tinnitus and tinnitus improved in 12 patients (60%) [19]. In Gabra et al.'s study, all patients suffered from tinnitus before ITM injections. Tinnitus rate decreased to 78% for 0–6 month period and 68% for 6–12 months period [3]. Tinnitus symptom disappeared in 5 (11.6%) of 43 patients, decreased in 21 (48.8%) patients, didn't change in 10 (23.3%) patients, and increased in 7 (16.3%) patients after ITD in Ren et al.'s study [12].

In a retrospective analysis of 17 intractable MD patients treated with ITM perfusion, 16 patients were followed up for more than 2 years. Tinnitus was controlled in three patients and improved in two patients at the 24-month follow-up, and patient without tinnitus worsened over this interval [4].

Another study measured tinnitus severity with "Tinnitus Handicap Inventory" score and the "Grading of Tinnitus Severity." Eleven patients with unilateral MD were treated with ITD. The initial mean handicap score was 61 and after receiving ITD was 22.3 at 2 years of follow-up. At 2 years of follow-up, a handicap score of 0 was found in 4 of 11 patients (36%) [22]. The initial "Grading of Tinnitus Severity" score was 3.2 and after receiving ITD injection was 1.6 at 2 years of follow-up. Grade 1 of the Grading of Tinnitus Severity (THI 0–16) at 2-year follow-up was achieved by 8 of 11 patients (72%). At 2-year follow-up, 1 of 11 patients (9%) in the dexamethasone group reported improvement of 100% and 1 other patient (9%) reported 90% improvement. Five of 11 patients (45%) reported 0% improvement. The mean subjective improvement at 2-year follow up was 48.1% [22].

7.4. Aural fullness

Garduno-Anaya et al. pointed out a 48% subjective improvement in aural fullness with ITD [21]. In Ren et al.'s study, aural fullness was complained in 24 of 43 patients. It was disappeared in 4 of 24 patients (16.7%), alleviated in 11 patients (45.8%), and even intensive in 9 patients (37.5%) after ITD injection [12].

Another study included 20 patients with MD; aural fullness was completely resolved in 3 patients (15%) and showed some improvement in 13 patients (65%) after ITD application from ventilation tube by the end of 6 months [19]. In other study including 42 patients treated with ITM, 95.2% had aural fullness before ITM and 65% after ITM by the end of 1-year period [3].

7.5. Live functional activity/quality of life

She et al. found improvement in 94% at 6 months and 87% at 24 months on functional activity after ITM perfusion [4].

In Garduño-Anaya et al.'s study, the initial mean "Dizziness Handicap Inventory" score was 68.7. After receiving ITD, the score was 8.3 at 2 years of follow-up [22].

In Kyrodimos et al.'s study, 30 patients (20 women and 10 men, aged 28–85 years) with MD underwent intratympanic 24 mg/ml of dexamethasone perfusion, and were assessed with the assistance of the Glasgow Benefit Inventory (GBI) questionnaire. Follow-up ranged from 12 to 48 months (mean 30 months) with regard to the GBI responses, nine patients (50%) expressed an overall benefit, while six (33%) expressed no benefit and three patients (17%) complained of negative effect after the intervention [25].

Albu et al. investigated 30 patients with intractable unilateral MD. Before therapy, Dizziness Handicap Inventory (DHI) was 53.2 ± 13.4 and after 12 months follow-up, it was 40.7 ± 16.5. Tinnitus Handicap Inventory (THI) was 28.6 ± 14.3 before therapy and 23.5 ± 12.4 after therapy. Both DHI and THI scores were statistically significant with pre- and posttreatment comparison ($P < 0.001$). At 12 months follow-up, level 1 of Functional Level Score (FLS) was attained in 14 (46.7%) patients and level 2 in 9 (30%) patients [14].

8. Comparison with other treatment methods

Although the exact treatment for MD is still not discovered, several treatment options are available. Caffeine, alcohol, theine and salt (CATS) restriction, diuretics, vasodilators, betahistine, intratympanic injection of gentamicin or corticosteroids, and surgery are most accepted treatment strategies [26].

The initial treatment for MD is diet restriction and oral/parenteral medications. Resistance to this therapy, minimal invasive procedures like intratympanic injections are attempted. The last chance to control symptoms is surgery despite complications (**Figure 1**) [13]. In this section, we compare ITS with other treatment options.

First of all, it must be searched whether ITS has a placebo effect or not. Hu et al. disputed the importance of placebo treatment in MD patients [27]. A double-blind randomized crossover trial using ITD (8 mg/ml) showed no benefit over placebo [28].

Hirvonen et al. also used intratympanic and systemic dexamethasone in 17 patients with MD. They claimed that symptoms of aural fullness, hearing loss, tinnitus, and vertigo did not improve significantly and the clinical use of dexamethasone in MD needs further investigation [16].

On the contrary, another randomized placebo controlled trial showed complete control of vertigo attacks in 82% of patients treated with ITD compared with 57% of those receiving placebo [22].

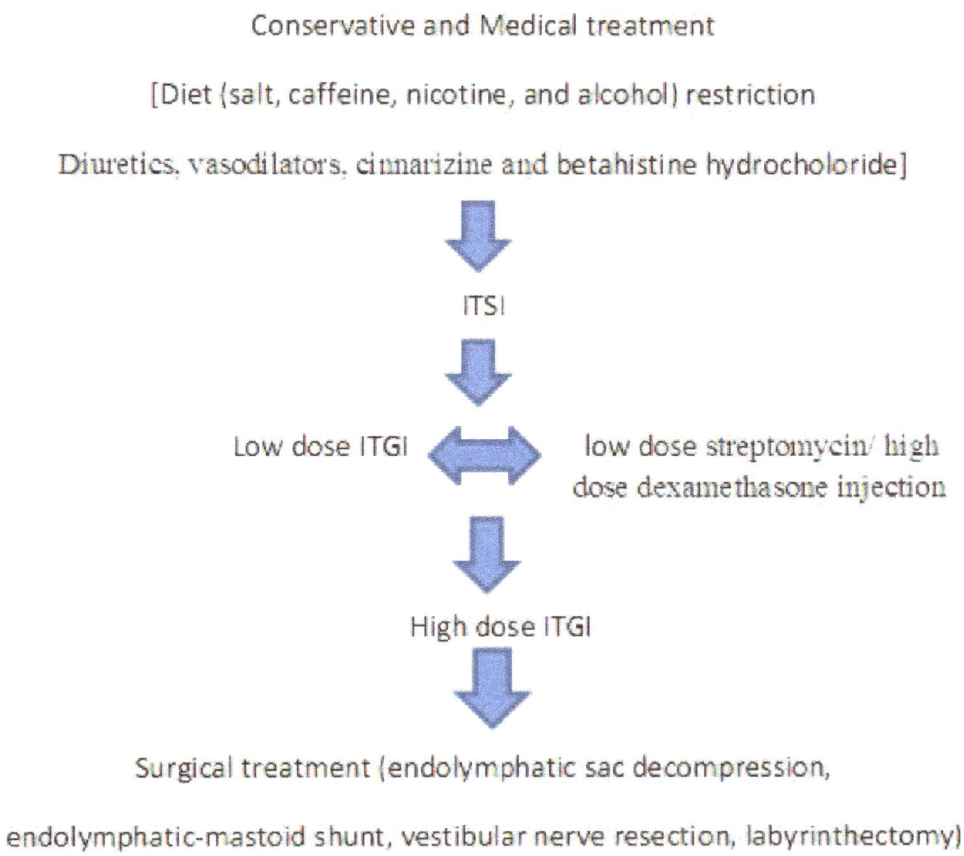

Figure 1. The initial treatment for MD.

Several studies also compare the efficacy of conventional medical treatment and ITS. In Paragache et al.'s study, study group was constituted from 20 patients who was applied ITS and control group was also constituted from 20 patients. Control group patients' diet was free from salt, caffeine, nicotine, and alcohol. Medical management was formed from cinnarizine 25 mg tablets TDS for acute episodes and betahistine hydrochloride 16 mg tablets TDS for continuous treatment. All patients were followed up for 6 months, and results were assessed at 1st, 2nd, 3rd, and 6th months. Vertigo control was 85% at study group and 80% at control group. Hearing loss recovered in three (15%) patients in study group and two (10%) patients in control group. An improvement on SDS was obtained in three (15%) patients in study group and two (10%) patients in control group. Other patients' SDS values were the same. Tinnitus disappeared in two patients in study group and three patients in control group. Tinnitus severity decreased in 12 patients in study group and 10 patients in control group. Aural fullness disappeared in three patients in study group and five patients in control group. Aural fullness severity decreased in 13 patients in study group and 11 patients in control group. They found that both modalities of therapy have almost equal efficacy on MD symptoms, and ITS therapy has an edge over conventional therapy in cases with severe attacks and shorter duration of symptoms [19].

Albu et al. compared the efficacy of ITD and high-dosage betahistine 144 mg/day (48 mg tid). Sixty-six patients with definite unilateral MD were randomly divided in two groups, each comprising 33 patients: Group A received a combination of ITD and identical appearing placebo pills, while Group B received a combination of high-dosage betahistine and IT saline. Fifty-nine patients completed the study and were available at 12 months for analysis, while seven patients (three in Group A and four in Group B) were excluded because of insufficient compliance. The mean number of vertigo attacks per month was recorded at baseline, at 1, 3, and then every 3 months for up to 1 year. Vertigo control was complete (class A) in 14 (46.6%) patients, partial (class B) in 7 (21.2%) patients, and limited (class C or D) in 8 (24.2%) patients in Group A. Vertigo couldn't be controlled in one (3%) patient (class E) in Group A. Vertigo control was complete (class A) in 12 (36.4%) patients, partial (class B) in 5 (15.2%) patients, and limited (class C or D) in 10 (30.4%) patients in Group B. Vertigo couldn't be controlled in two (6.1%) patients (class E) in Group B. Patients whose vertigo attacks couldn't be controlled in both groups were scheduled for ITG therapy. Vertigo control rate wasn't statistically different between two groups. But vertigo attack frequency was 8.6 in Group A and 7.9 in Group B before treatment. It was 1.8 in Group A and 4.3 in Group B after 1 month of treatment. It became 1.5 for Group A and 2.4 for Group B after 3 months of therapy.

According to those results while ITD has a rapid effect to prevent vertigo attack, betahistine and ITD have similar effect on vertigo attack at the end of 3rd month. [14]. Regarding quality of life, while FLS was found level 1 in 14 patients and level 2 in 9 patients in group A, it was found level 1 in 10 patients and level 2 in 9 patients in group B. There was no statistical significance about FLS for both groups [14]. The mean PTA was 57.4 ± 14.7 dB in Group A and 58.2 ± 13.9 dB in Group B before treatment. It became 55.8 ± 15.5 dB for Group A and 56.1 ± 12.5 dB for Group B after 1-year treatment. There was no statistical significance on hearing level and SDS for both groups. A significant reduction in tinnitus assessed by THI at the end of the follow-up was reported in both treatment groups. The difference among the two groups was not significant [14]. They demonstrated that ITD has an immediate effect while higher dosage of betahistine (144 mg/day) is able to get the same outcome only after 3 months of treatment [14].

Intratympanic gentamicin is a traditional treatment for resistant MD. Despite effective vertigo attack control, ototoxicity is a feared complication. Low-dose ITG protocol was used to overcome this complication in some studies [29–31].

Casani et al. compared the effectiveness of ITG and ITD in a study. In this study, patients were randomized and divided into two groups: 32 patients were treated with ITG and 28 patients were treated with ITD. All measurements were obtained immediately before the treatment and were repeated after 1 month, 1 year, and 2 years following the procedure. Vertigo control was complete (class A) in 26 (81.3%) patients, partial (class B) in four (12.5%) patients, and limited (class D) in one (3.2%) patient in ITG group. Vertigo control couldn't be obtained in one patient and vestibular neurectomy was recommended. Vertigo control was complete (class A) in 12 (42.9%) patients, partial (class B) in 5 (17.9%) patients, limited (class C or D) in 9 (32.1%) patients in ITD group. Vertigo control couldn't be obtained in two patients and they were scheduled for gentamicin treatment. There was no statistical significance for vertigo control in both groups ($P < 0.001$) [18]. Level 1 FLS was obtained in 13 (40.6%) patients in ITG group and 11 (39.3%) patients in ITD group at 1-year follow-up. But level 1 FLS was obtained in 22 (71%) patients in ITG group and in 12 (46.1%) patients in ITD group at 2-year follow-up. Although there was no statistical significance at 1-year follow-up, significance was found at 2-year follow-up ($P < 0.05$) [18]. The mean PTA was 58.7 ± 13.3 dB in ITG group and 56.5 ± 13.4 dB in ITD group before treatment. It was 61.3 ± 14.6 and 53.7 ± 15.6 dB in ITG and ITD groups, respectively, after 1 month treatment. At first year, it became 62.3 ± 15.3 and 54.6 ± 16 dB, at second year 64.5 ± 15.5 and 56 ± 17.3 dB for both groups, respectively. There was statistical significance on PTA for both groups ($P > 0.05$) [18]. SDS was found to be 67 ± 19 before treatment, 63.1 ± 20 after 1 month treatment, 61.1 ± 21.1 after 1 year treatment, and 60.3 ± 22.6 after 2 year treatment for ITG group. It was found to be 66.6 ± 16.4 before treatment, 67.5 ± 17.7 after 1 month treatment, 67.1 ± 17.6 after 1 year treatment, and 65.0 ± 18.7 after 2 year treatment for ITD group. The only one value for SDS that reached statistical significance was the difference between pretreatment and after 1 month treatment in ITG group ($P < 0.05$). In the ITD group, no significant variations of SDS were observed during each follow-up ($P > 0.05$) [18]. According to 1995 AAO-HNS criteria, hearing got worse in four (12.9%) patients, not changed in 27 (84.4%) patients, and improved in one (3.1%) patient in ITG group after 2-year treatment. Hearing became worse in 12 (42.9%) patients, not changed in 13 (46.4%) patients, and improved in 3 (10.7%) patients in ITD group after 2-year treatment. Vertigo control was classes A and B in 16 patients in ITD group whose hearing didn't get worse [18]. Total or partial vertigo attack control (class A or B) was over 90% for ITG group and 61% for ITD group after 2-year treatment. According to this study, low-dose ITG therapy was more successful than ITD for vertigo attack control [18]. Regarding the hearing outcome, no statistically significant differences were verified between the two groups in terms of mean PTA and SDS values. On the whole, the mean PTA and SDS values were slightly better for the patients treated with ITD [18]. The authors claimed that low-dose ITG was safe for hearing and efficient for vertigo attack on resistant MD cases [18].

Gabra et al. compared ITM and ITG treatments. There were 89 patients with MD, 47 of them treated with ITG and 42 of them treated with ITM. Two groups were compared for vertigo attack, tinnitus, aural fullness, PTA, and SDS at 0–6 months and 6–12 months. Both groups had similar vertigo attack number before treatment (P: 0.883). Complete vertigo control was obtained in 82.9% in ITG group and 48.1% in ITM group after 6–12 months of treatment (P: 0.004). Tinnitus and aural fullness control were higher in ITG group than in ITM group (P: 0.002). PTA and SDS values were better in ITM group at pretreatment period ($P < 0.001$). But those values became worse in ITM group at 6–12-month control, and difference disappeared between groups ($P > 0.05$) [3]. According to that study, ITG was more effective than ITM to control MD symptoms [3].

Shea et al. suggested a combination of streptomycin and dexamethasone perfusion for MD. The hearing changes and quality-of-life outcomes of 393 cases of streptomycin/dexamethasone inner ear perfusion were searched retrospectively. All patients underwent one or more 3-day treatments consisting of daily intratympanic injections of a low-dose streptomycin (10 mg/ml)/high-dose dexamethasone (24 mg/ml) mixture plus 16 mg of intravenous dexamethasone. The end point for treatment was adequate control of vertigo. The mean PTA change was 0.89 ± 11 dB and the mean SDS change was 0.49 ± 17 after 3-day treatment. Significant hearing loss was detected in 62 (15.7%) patients and hearing loss was severe in 20 (5%) of those patients. Ninety percent of the patients had improved quality of life after treatment and 88% of the patients showed improvement in their "vertigo subscore," a domain within the survey that focuses on vertigo control. According to their results, streptomycin/dexamethasone inner ear perfusion is as safe as other aminoglycoside regimens in the hearing of patients with MD and provides good control of vertigo and a significant improvement in quality of life [32].

Sennaroglu et al. compared three methods to control MD symptoms: ITD, ITG, and decompression of the endolymphatic sac (ESD). Dexamethasone was applied to 24 patients and gentamicin was applied to 16 patients by the ventilation tube way. Surgery of ESD was performed in 25 patients. Vertigo control rates of ITD, ITG, and ESD were 72, 75, and 52%, respectively. Total hearing lost was detected in two patients in ITG group. Hearing level decreased in 9 (38%) patients, improved in 4 (16%) patients, and didn't change in 11 (46%) patients in ITD group. They suggested ITD for patients with the vertiginous symptoms still persisting after 6 months of medical treatment. If patients are resistant to this intervention, ITG could be planned for patients with profound sensorineural hearing loss and ESD could be recommended for patients with normal hearing. Vestibular nerve section could be planned as a last chance to control vertigo attacks for patients with good hearing and labyrinthectomy for patients with profound sensorineural hearing loss [33].

Vestibular nervectomy could be planned as a last chance to control vertigo attacks for good hearing.

Quaranta et al. investigated 38 patients with intractable MD with a minimum of 7 years of follow-up. Twenty patients were treated with endolymphatic-mastoid shunt (EMS) surgery and the remaining eighteen patients refused surgery (natural history, NH group). At the last control, 85% of the patients in EMS group and 74% of the NH patients had complete or substantial control of vertigo. The difference between the two groups was not significant. However, it was significant at 2 and 4 years of follow-up. At 2 years, 65% of the EMS patients had complete or substantial control of vertigo and at 4–6 years in 85% of the cases. Only 32% of the NH patients had complete or substantial control of vertigo at 2 years. This percentage had increased to 50% in the fourth year and to 74% in the sixth year. Hearing results in the two groups were not significantly different. Tinnitus disappeared or decreased in 56% of the EMS patients and in 18% of the NH patients. Sixty-seven percent of the EMS patients and twenty-nine percent of the NH patients reported that their aural fullness disappeared. Consequently, vertigo attack reduction was observed earlier in EMS patients than in those who refused surgery [34].

9. Conclusions

Although the fact that definitive treatment of MD has not been found yet, several treatment options are used to control the MD symptoms. Different success rates of symptom relief are given in literature for each option. However, common agreed decision is that ITS can be used in patients with intractable MD to conservative and medical treatment before intratympanic gentamicin and surgical treatments.

Author details

Fatih Oghan[1]*, Ibrahim Erdim[2], Metin Çeliker[3], Muhammet Fatih Topuz[4], Ahmet Uluat[4], Onur Erdogan[4] and Sinan Aksoy[4]

*Address all correspondence to: fatihoghan@hotmail.com

1 Faculty of Medicine, Department of ORL&HNS, Dumlupinar University, Kutahya, Turkey

2 Tokat Erbaa Hospital, Tokat, Turkey

3 Recep Tayyip Erdogan University Research Hospital, Rize, Turkey

4 SB DPU Evliya Celebi Research Hospital, Kutahya, Turkey

References

[1] McCabe BF. Autoimmune sensorineural hearing loss. Annals of Otology & Rhinology. 1979;**88**:585-590

[2] Cheng KC, Mastsvoka H, Lee KM, Kim NS, Krug MS, Kwon SS, et al. Proto-oncogene Raf-1 as an autoantigen in Méniére's disease. Annals of Otology, Rhinology & Layngology. 2000;**109**:1093-1098

[3] Gabra N, Saliba I. The effect of intratympanic methylprednisolone and gentamicin injection on Méniére's Disease. Otolaryngology—Head and Neck Surgery. 2013;**148** (4):642-647

[4] She W, Lv L, Du X, Li H, Dai Y, Lu L, Ma X, Chen F. Long-term effects of intratympanic methylprednisolone perfusion treatment on intractable Ménière's disease. The Journal of Laryngology & Otology. 2015;**129**:232-237

[5] Rarey KE, Curtis LM. Receptors for glucocorticoids in the human inner ear. Otolaryngology—Head and Neck Surgery. 1996;**115**:38-41

[6] Lohuis PJ, Ten Cate WJ, Patterson KE. Modulation of rat stria vascularis in the absence of circulating adrenocorticosteroids. Acta Otolaryngologica (Stockh). 1990;**110**:348-356

[7] Tomiyama S, Nonaka M, Gotoh Y, Ikezono I, Yagi I. Immunological approach to Méniére's disease: Vestibular immune injury following immune reaction of the endolymphatic sac. The Journal of Otorhinology & Laryngology. 1994;**56**:11-18

[8] Merchant SN, Adams JC, Nadol JB Jr. Pathophysiology of Méniére's syndrome: Are symptoms caused by endolymphatic hydrops? Otology & Neurotology. 2005;**26**:74-81

[9] Fukushima M, Kitahara T, Fuse Y, et al. Changes in aquaporin expression in the inner ear of the rat after i.p. injection of steroids. Acta Oto-Laryngologica Supplementum. 2004;**553**:13-18

[10] Shirwany NA, Seidman MD, Tang W. Effects of transtympanic injection of steroids on cochlear blood flow, auditory sensitivity and histology in guinea pigs. American Journal of Otolaryngology. 1998;**19**:230-235

[11] Otake H, Yamamoto H, Teranishi M, Sone M, Nakashima T. Cochlear blood flow during occlusion and reperfusion of the anterior inferior cerebellar artery: Effect of topical application of dexamethasone to the round window. Acta Otolaryngology. 2009;**129**:127-131

[12] Ren H, Yin T, Lu Y, Kong W, Ren J. Intratympanic dexamethasone injections for refractory Méniére's disease. International Journal of Clinical and Experimental Medicine. 2015;**8**(4):6016-6023

[13] Barrs DM, Keyser JS, Stallworth C, McElveen JT. Intratympanic steroid injections for intractable Méniére's disease. Laryngoscope. 2001;**111**:2100-2104

[14] Albu S, Chirtes F, Trombitas V, Nagy A, Marceanu L, Babighian G, Trabalzini F. Intratympanic dexamethasone versus high dosage of betahistine in the treatment of intractable unilateral Méniére disease. American Journal of Otolaryngology. 2015 Mar–Apr;**36**(2):205-209

[15] Parnes LS, Sun AH, Freeman DJ. Corticosteroid pharmacokinetics in the inner ear fluids: An animal study followed by clinical application. Laryngoscope. 1999;**109**:1-17

[16] Hirvonen TP, Peltomaa M, Ylikoski J. Intratympanic and systemic dexamethasone for Méniére's disease. ORL Journal of Otorhinolaryngology and its Related Specialties. 2000;**62**:117-120

[17] She W, Dai Y, Du X, Yu C, Chen F, Wang J et al. Hearing evaluation of intratympanic methylprednisolone perfusion for refractory sudden sensorineural hearing loss. Otolaryngology—Head and Neck Surgery. 2010;**142**:266-271

[18] Casani AP, Piaggi P, Cerchiai N, Seccia V, Franceschini SS, Dallan I. Intratympanic treatment of intractable unilateral Méniére disease: Gentamicin or dexamethasone? A randomized controlled trial. Otolaryngology—Head and Neck Surgery. 2012 Mar;**146**(3):430-437

[19] Paragache G, Panda NK, Ragunathan M, Sridhara. Intratympanic dexamethasone application in Méniére's disease—Is it superior to conventional therapy? Indian Journal of Otolaryngology—Head and Neck Surgery. 2005 Jan;**57**(1):21-23

[20] Hamid MA. Intratympanic dexamethasone perfusion in Méniére's. In: Presented at the Spring Meeting of the American Neurotology Society; Palm Desert, CA; May 2001. p. 12

[21] Boleas-Aguirre MS, Lin FR, Della Santina CC, Minor LB, Carey JP. Longitudinal results with intratympanic dexamethasone in the treatment of Ménière's disease. Otology & Neurotology. 2008;**29**(1):33-38

[22] Garduño-Anaya MA, Couthino De Toledo H, Hinojosa-González R, Pane-Pianese C, Ríos-Castañeda LC. Dexamethasone inner ear perfusion by intratympanic injection in unilateral Ménière's disease: A two-year prospective, placebo-controlled, double-blind, randomized trial. Otolaryngology—Head and Neck Surgery. 2005 Aug;**133**(2):285-294

[23] Kaplan DM, Hehar SS, Bance ML, Rutka JA. Intentional ablation of vestibular function using commercially available topical gentamicin-betamethasone eardrops in patients with Méniére's disease: Further evidence for topical eardrop ototoxicity. Laryngoscope. 2002 Apr;**112**(4):689-695

[24] Hillman TM, Arriaga MA, Chen DA. Intratympanic steroids: Do they acutely improve hearing in cases of cochlear hydrops? Laryngoscope. 2003;**113**:1903-1907

[25] Kyrodimos E, Aidonis I, Skalimis A, Sismanis A. Use of Glasgow benefit inventory (GBI) in Méniére's disease managed with intratympanic dexamethasone perfusion: Quality of life assessment. Auris Nasus Larynx. 2011 Apr;**38**(2):172-177

[26] Coelho DH, Lalwani AK. Medical management of Méniére's disease. Laryngoscope. 2008;**118**:1099-1108

[27] Hu A, Parnes LS. Intratympanic steroids for inner ear disorders: A review. Audiology and Neurotology. 2009;**14**:373-382

[28] Silverstein H, Isaacson JE, Olds MJ, Rowan PT, Rosenberg S. Dexamethasone inner ear perfusion for the treatment of Méniére's disease: A prospective, randomized, double-blind, crossover trial. American Journal of Otolaryngology. 1998;**19**:196-201

[29] Longridge NS, Mallinson AI. Low-dose intratympanic gentamicin treatment for dizziness in Méniére's disease. Journal of Otolaryngology. 2000;**29**:35-39

[30] Harner SG, Drisco CL, Facer GW, et al. Long-term follow-up of transtympanic gentamicin for Méniére's syndrome. Otology & Neurotology. 2001;**22**:210-214

[31] Quaranta A, Scaringi A, Aloidi A, Quaranta N, Salonna I. Intratympanic therapy for Méniére's disease: Effect of administration of low concentration of gentamicin. Acta Otolaryngology. 2001;**121**:387-392

[32] Shea PF, Richey PA, Wan JY, Stevens SR. Hearing results and quality of life after streptomycin/dexamethasone perfusion for Méniére's disease. Laryngoscope. 2012 Jan;**122**(1):204-211

[33] Sennaroglu L, Sennaroglu G, Gursel B, Dini FM. Intratympanic dexamethasone, intratympanic gentamicin, and endolymphatic sac surgery for intractable vertigo in Méniére's disease. Otolaryngology—Head and Neck Surgery. 2001 Nov;**125**(5):537-543

[34] Quaranta A, Marini F, Sallustio V. Long-term outcome of Méniére's disease: Endolymphatic mastoid shunt versus natural history. Audiology and Neuro-otology. 1998;**3**:54-60

3

Genetic Basis of Hearing Loss

Agnieszka Pollak and Monika Ołdak

Abstract

Etiology of hearing impairment (HI) is complex and comprises genetic and environmental factors. Currently, the background of genetic hearing impairment is an area of intensive research and we are witnessing fast progress in this field. The story has begun in 1997 when the DFNB1 locus was discovered with *GJB2* and *GJB6* genes causative for almost 50% of cases of recessive, profound, prelingual hearing loss. Nowadays, we have much more possibilities for dissecting the reason of HI, but proper assessment of clinical symptoms is essential for selecting the most optimal diagnostic pathway. In the first stage, the detailed characteristic of hearing loss including its level established by pure tone audiometry (PTA) or auditory brainstem responses (ABR), age of onset, and other helpful features as progressive or no progressive type should be provided. Subsequently, the presence or absence of accompanying symptoms should be established and followed by a detailed analysis of pedigree. In addition, modern assistive algorithms such as AudioGene, Face2Gene, and POSSUM are also discussed. Taking into account the variety of causative genes and pathogenic variants underling hearing loss, searching for causative genes, after exclusion of the DFNB1 variants, should be performed with multigenic panels based on next-generation sequencing technology.

Keywords: gene, pathogenic variant, phenotype, diagnostic, pedigree, next-generation sequencing

1. Introduction

The dynamic development of new DNA sequencing technologies in recent years has given us unprecedented insight into the information encoded in the human genome. Introduction of these techniques into a clinical practice has put the diagnosis of genetic disorders to a much more advanced level with a very high detection rate of pathogenic variants. Hearing loss (HL) has also greatly benefited from the technological revolution as it is a genetically heterogeneous condition with more than 100 different genes being involved in its pathogenesis, and novel genes are still being discovered (www.herediataryhearingloss.org; accessed 10/2017). As compared to the strategy of sequential analysis of single genes, the application of high-throughput DNA sequencing has increased the diagnostic yield of genetic causes of HL by approximately four times [1].

At the same time, the technological advancements have brought us to a higher level of complexity. Searching for HL-causing variants, often hundreds of genes have to be analyzed and we are flooded by huge amounts of information that are difficult to interpret [2]. It is partially overcome by still-improving computational tools and growing data from population studies, but an indispensable part of better planning of genetic testing and understanding its results is the information gathered from a thorough clinical examination and family history. Sometimes, the primary clinical data collected prior to genetic testing do not completely match the phenotypic features that could be expected from molecular findings. In such cases, clinical reevaluation is needed to better delineate the phenotype and verify whether the identified genetic variants are indeed responsible for the observed clinical features [3, 4].

2. Pedigree construction and analysis

The fundamental and basic element of genetic evaluation in the consultation room is the creation of a precise and accurate family pedigree based on the detailed medical interview. A genetic pedigree is a diagram of genetic relationship enriched with an information about health history, which allows to easily trace the transmission of symptoms, estimate whether symptoms may be caused by genetic reason, and evaluate the risk for other family members (including unborn) of an inherited disorder. Although in the archival literature, readers may encounter many different systems of constructing pedigrees [5], the current, uniform, and precise guidelines in this area should be followed and applied in both clinical practice and publications. Taking into account the dynamic rise of genetic knowledge within the last years, triggered by new technologies such as next-generation sequencing (NGS), clinicians and scientists should be familiar with preparation and interpretation of a pedigree. This allows a proper interpretation of medical and genetic information of the studied family. At the time of writing, an authority dealing with the standardization of the terminology used to describe a pedigree is the National Society of Genetic Counselors (NSGC, http://www.nsgc.org) established in 1979 in the United States of America (USA), with its two official journals: "Journal of Genetic Counseling" and "Perspectives in Genetic Counseling." The Pedigree Standardization Work Group (PSWG) operating within the NSGC established unified recommendations for standardized human pedigree in 1995 [6, 7], and updated it in 2008 [8]. Regarding the fact that no alternative comprehensive, analogous recommendations have been proposed, along with lack of critical comments on the proposed system, the PSWG established rules have become an accepted and international symbolic language of human genetic clinicians and researchers.

The most commonly used pedigree symbols, definitions, and abbreviations in compliance with the PSWG revised recommendations are presented in **Figure 1**.

With the symbols listed in **Figure 1**, a family tree should be created according to the following rules:

- At the beginning, a shaded symbol (square for male, circle for female) denoting the proband (an affected person from a family who came for a medical consultation as first) should be placed. In the bottom left corner, an arrow and letter "P" should be placed to uniquely mark that this individual is the proband.
- Above the symbols for proband's, ancestors starting with parents should be placed. The symbol denoting male partner should be placed to the left of the female's one if possible. Furthermore, symbols denoting both parents should be connected by a horizontal line (relationship line) and doubled if the parents are consanguineous. The line of descent should be placed in the middle of the horizontal line, which connects parents with the offspring (sibship line).
- All symbols representing siblings should be placed in the birth order starting from the left side, at the same height as the proband's symbol. Vertical lines (individual's line), linking symbols to the horizontal line (sibship line) above the symbols, must be placed for all siblings' symbols.
- According to the above-described rules, symbols representing all remaining family members should be placed and joined with the appropriate lines.
- Some additional, useful information such as disease, age, age at death, initials, or the first name may be placed below appropriate symbols.

The pedigree line definitions and rules of placing them within the pedigree are presented in **Figure 2**.

Additional most common symbols, rules, and family situations are gathered in **Figure 3**.

Since drawing pedigrees, especially for large families, is complicated and time consuming, it is worth to use computer programs that facilitate and accelerate this task. There are many professional and public tools, which are useful in the process of creating accurate family diagrams for both, clinical and educational purposes, e.g., Genial Pedigree Draw (http://www.pedigreedraw.com/), Progeny Online Pedigree Tool (http://www.progenygenetics.com/online-pedigree/), and CeGaT Pedigree Chart Designer (http://www.cegat.de/en/for-physicians/pedigree-chart-designer/).

Understanding the elementary rules of inheritance is the key to appreciate how traits or diseases are passed on within a family. It should be reminded here that every individual has two copies of almost every gene localized on chromosome (autosome), one of them derives from biological mother and the second one from biological father. The situation is different in case of sex chromosomes—every male has only one X (inherited from mother) and Y chromosome (inherited from father). The Y chromosome is transmitted in its entirety exclusively from

	Female	Male	Gender unknown	Remarks
Healthy person				The age of the individuals should be placed below the symbol.
Affected person				The symbols may be partioned and filled with different pattern if ≥ two symptoms occurred. The used patterns must be defined in the legend.
Deceased person				The age at death should be placed below the symbol. If the cause of death is known it also should be indicated.
Proband	P	P		A first affected individual coming to the consultation.
Consultand				The person(s) referred for genetic counseling.
Multiple persons, number known	3	3	3	If the number is unknown or unstated the letter „n" should be used instead of a number.
Pregnancy	P	P	P	For affected individuals light shading should be used. Gestational age and karyotype should be denoted below the symbols.
Spontaneous abortion				Gestational age, gender should be denoted below the symbols
Termination of pregnancy				Gestational age, gender should be denoted below the symbols
Ectopic pregnancy			ECT	ECT should be given below the symbols

Figure 1. Most common pedigree symbols according to Bennett et al. [8].

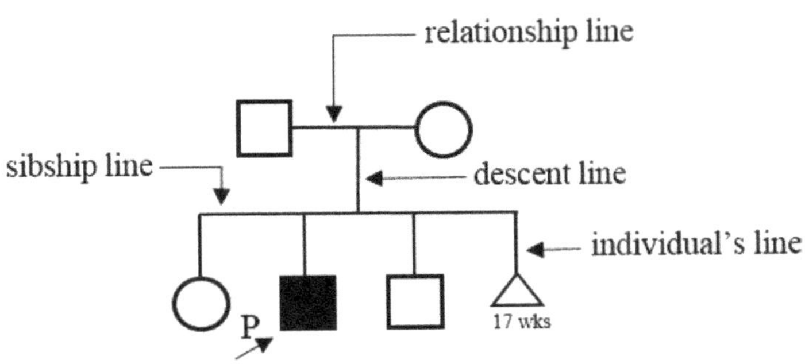

Figure 2. Definition of pedigree lines.

Definition	Symbols	Remarks
Consanguinity	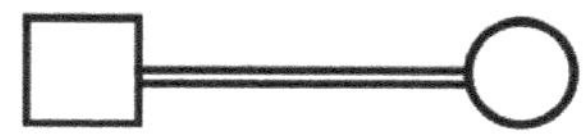	Relationship which is not evident regarding pedigree should be described above relationship line
Relationship	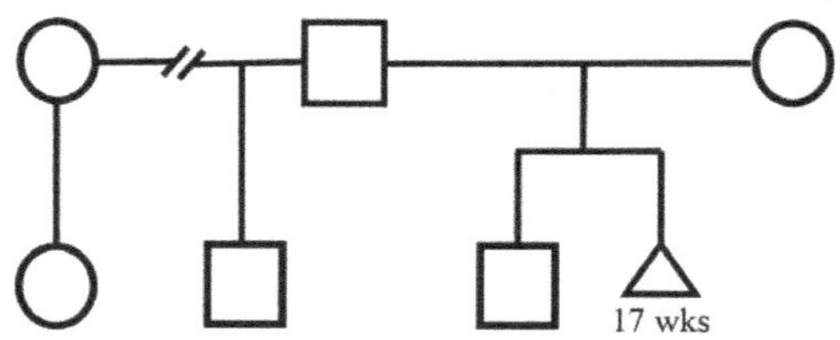	A gap within relationship line denotes that relationship currently is not continued
Multiple gestation	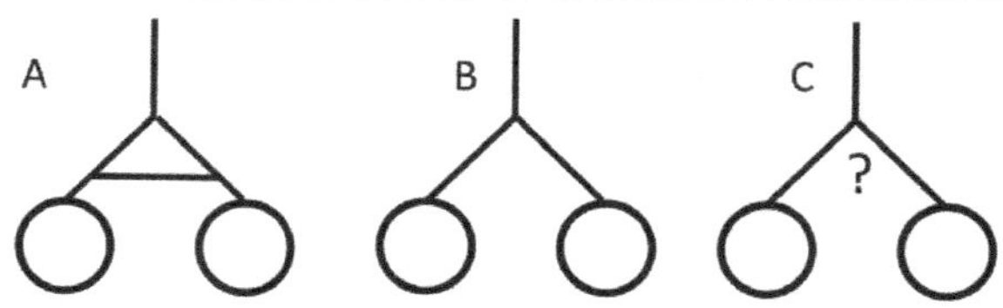	A. Monozygotic B. Dizygotic C. Unknown
Infertility	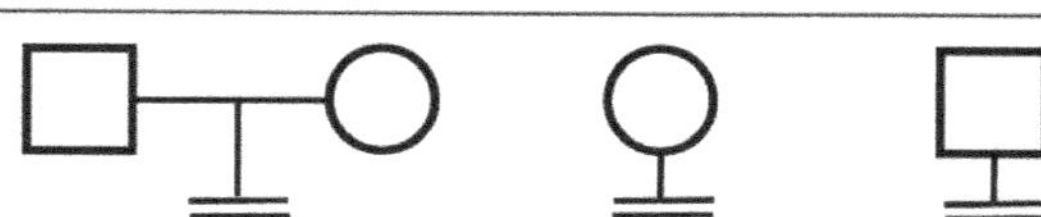	If the reason is known, should be indicated below the symbol
Adoption	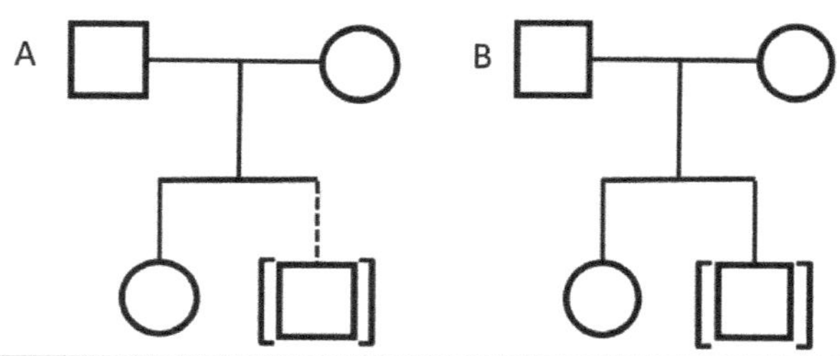	Biological parents are denoted by solid line, adoptive parents are denoted by dashed line. A. In B. Out
Carrier		The disease is not manifested
Asymptomatic or presymptomatic carrier		Individual without clinical symptoms at the time of completing the medical history
Sperm/ovum donor	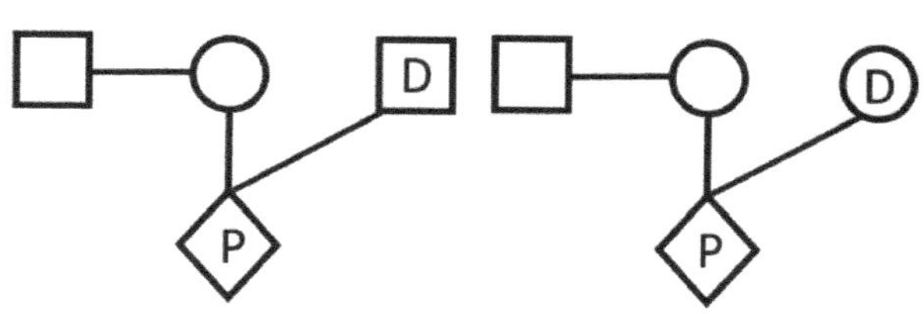	The line of descent is solid denoting biologic relationship which may have influence to the fetus

Figure 3. Symbols useful in uncommon clinical situations.

father to son. In contrast, every female has two X chromosomes (inherited from both parents) [9]. Another derogation from basic inheritance rules is mitochondrial inheritance, in which the entire independent small genome is passed only from mother to offspring [10]. Typically, there are four most common inheritance patterns, depending on the genomic localization and influence on the protein function of pathogenic variants or genes i.e., autosomal dominant (AD), autosomal recessive (AR), sex-linked, and mitochondrial [11]. Diseases caused by pathogenic variants localized in a single gene are mostly inherited in an AD or AR pattern and are referred to as Mendelian inheritance (tribute to Gregor Mendel, who first noted this pattern in pea plants).

The AD mode of inheritance occurs when a single copy of the disrupted (mutated) gene is causative of the disease. It should be emphasized that for AD disorders, a variety of inter and intrafamilial variability of symptoms may occur. Nevertheless, there are few substantial features, which make this mode of inheritance rather simple to distinguish. Dominantly inherited genetic diseases tend to occur in every generation of a family, they affect males and females equally; furthermore, the disorder may be transmitted from males and females. The risk for offspring to inherit the pathogenic variant is 50%. Due to the variability of symptoms severity, characteristic for this type of inheritance, the risk of becoming symptomatic may be less than 50%. A typical family tree representing the AD mode of inheritance is shown in **Figure 4**.

The AR type of inheritance requires two disrupted copies of a gene for a disease to occur. Thus, both parents of an affected individual are obligatory asymptomatic carriers (due to an assumption that heterozygotes do not manifest a disease). Furthermore, the symptoms are not typically seen in every generation. AR diseases are much more common in offspring of consanguineous pairs (which is evident within small, isolated populations e.g., Icelanders, Bedouins, or Amish [12]. In contrast to the AD inheritance mode, affected individuals present more consistent clinical picture. The risk for offspring to inherit both pathogenic variants is 25%, whereas the risk to inherit one heterozygous variant is 50%. It should be also noted that all children of an affected parent and a noncarrier partner, regardless of their gender, will be obligate carriers. A typical family pedigree illustrating the AR mode of inheritance is shown in **Figure 5**.

A sex-linked mode of inheritance consists of three subtypes: X-linked dominant (XLD), X-linked recessive (XLR), and Y-linked. Whereas the Y chromosome contains very limited

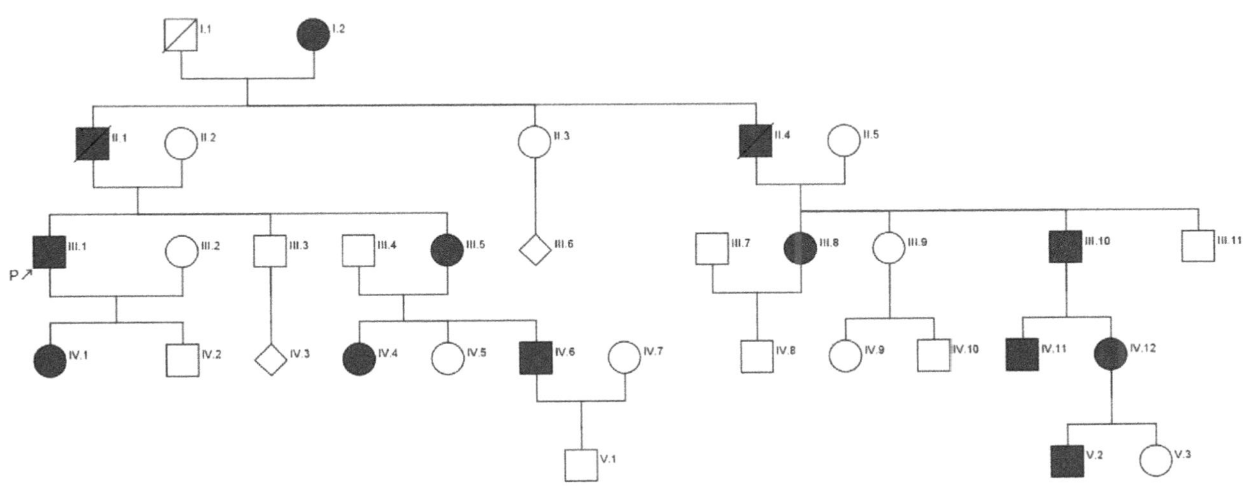

Figure 4. Pedigree of a family with the AD pattern of inheritance.

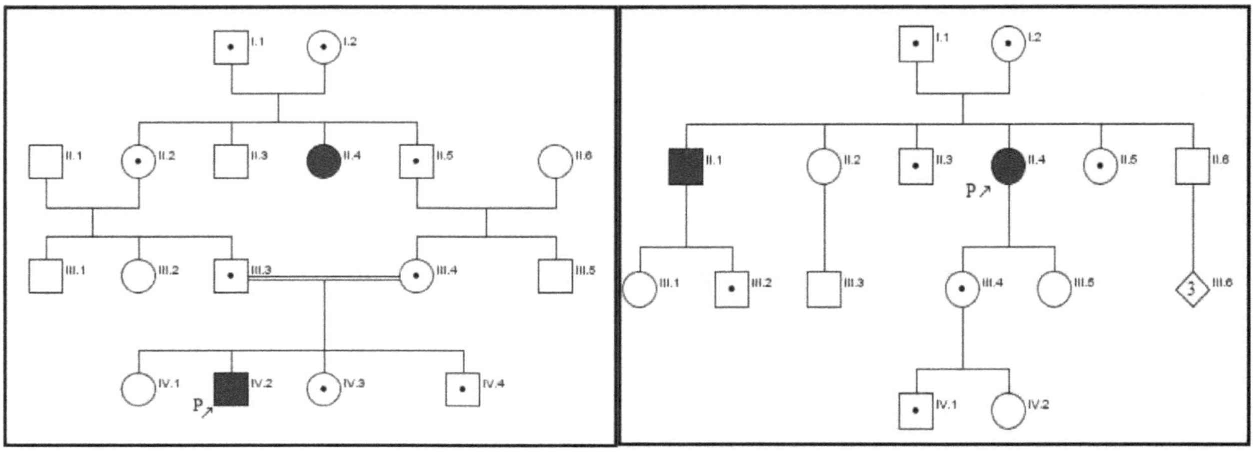

Figure 5. Two typical family trees representing the AR type of inheritance.

number of genes and there are only few Y-linked disorders, none of them related to hearing and speech disorders, this type of inheritance will not be described here. The XLD and XLR type of inheritance relate to genes located on the X chromosome, and for the occurrence of XLD symptoms, only one copy of a disrupted X-linked gene is required. XLD diseases usually manifest very severely in males, which may lead to spontaneous abortion or neonatal death. The characteristic feature for this type of inheritance is that there is no transmission of the disease from male to male, and all of the female offspring of affected male will inherit the pathogenic variant and the disease. A characteristic family tree for the XLD mode of inheritance is shown in **Figure 6**.

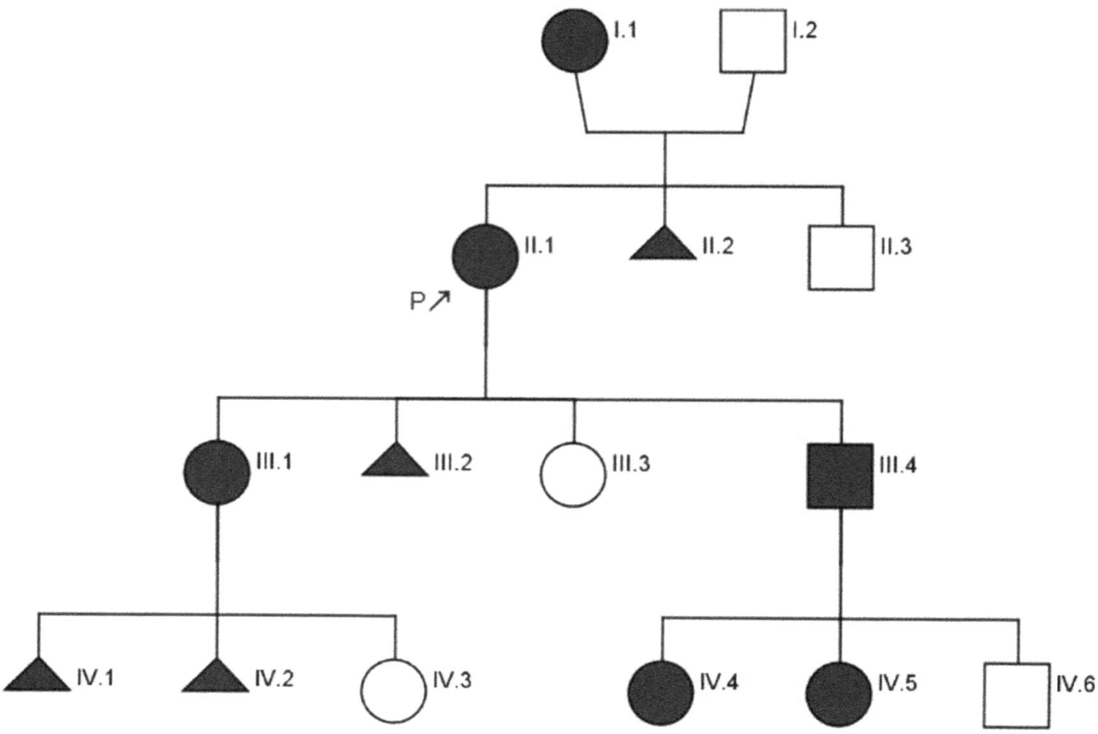

Figure 6. Exemplary pedigree of a family with the XLD type of inheritance.

For an XLR disease to occur in females, both copies of a gene must be impaired. Characteristic features for an XLR inheritance mode are affected males, but an extremely low number or no affected females, in every generation. A distinct feature of the XLR inheritance pattern is that the pedigree tree shows no male to male transmission of the disease. All males harboring a pathogenic variant in an X-linked gene present severe symptoms of the disease, whereas carrier females are in general unaffected or present significantly less severe symptoms. A typical family tree representing the XLR mode of inheritance is shown in **Figure 7**.

Although within small families, which currently are very common, especially in European countries, the recognition of an X-linked inheritance pattern is rather challenging and remains unknown until the results of genetic testing [4].

The mitochondrial mode of inheritance has distinctive features differentiating it from others. Briefly, this unique features come directly from mitochondrial DNA (mtDNA) specificity: mtDNA is a small, independent, circular genome; furthermore, an average human cell contains up to 1000 mitochondria and in every mitochondrion several copies of the mtDNA genome may be present. If all mitochondria in a given individual contain an mtDNA variant it is defined as homoplasmy. In contrast, heteroplasmy indicates the coexistence of more than one mtDNA type within an individual. As all mitochondria of offspring are of maternal origin, the pathogenic variants localized within mtDNA are exclusively passed from mother to children and they may affect males and females equally. Consistently, males do not transmit the mtDNA disorders to their offspring. A representative family tree demonstrating mitochondrial mode of inheritance is shown in **Figure 8**.

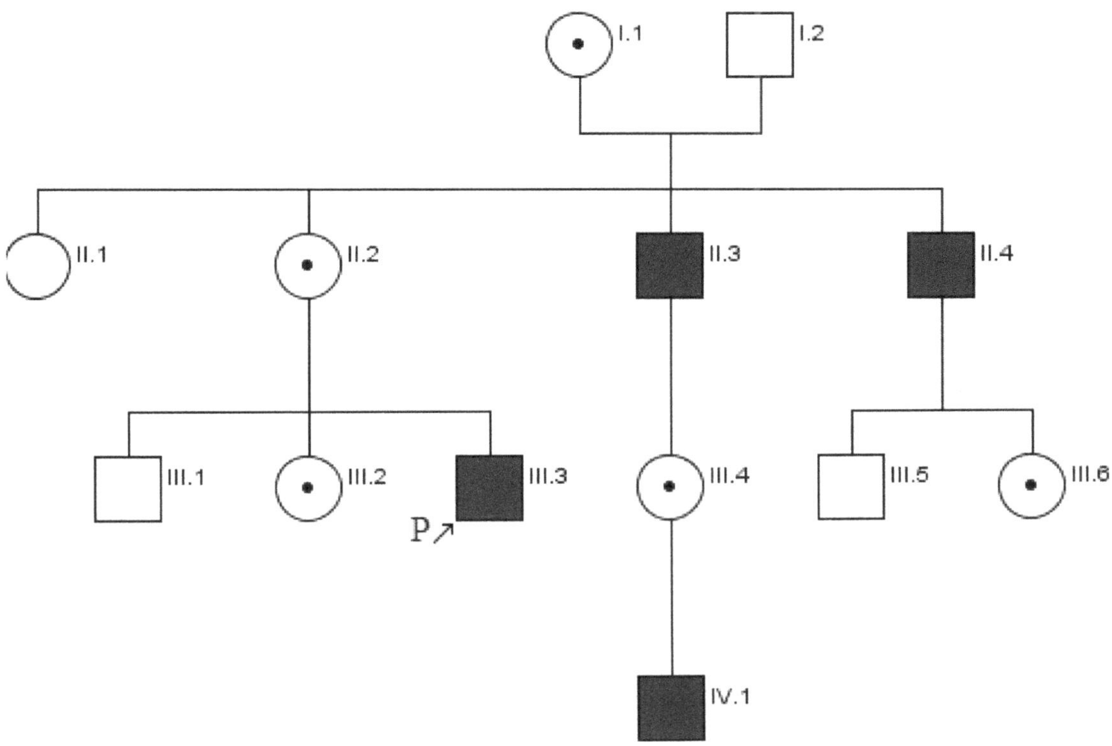

Figure 7. Pedigree of a family with the XLR pattern of inheritance.

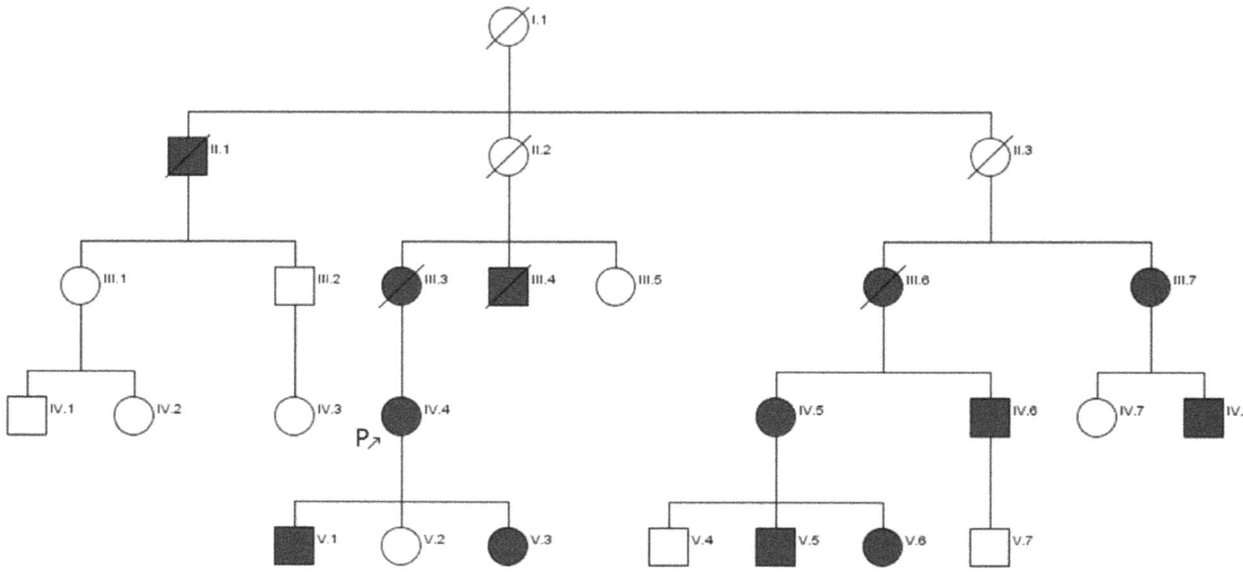

Figure 8. Pedigree of a family with mitochondrial mode of inheritance.

It should be emphasized that in many cases distinction between the mitochondrial and AD inheritance is a difficult task based only on the family tree analysis.

3. Nonsyndromic hearing loss

It has to be stressed that all patients with a positive family history of HL should be referred for genetic counseling. Over generations, an inherited disorder automatically raises a suspicion of a genetic underlying cause. A careful analysis of a family pedigree enables to identify or to presume the mode in which hearing impairment is inherited. This in turn is an important step in directing genetic testing at specific genes that are causally involved in the pathogenesis of autosomal dominant, recessive, X-linked, or mitochondrial HL. In case of marriages between individuals with hearing impairment or between individuals coming from families with hearing impairment, the family pedigrees should be analyzed especially carefully. In the offspring of such couples, different HL causative variants of different genes may be found. Interestingly, in a study of 80 deafness genes, the DNA samples of HL patients were significantly enriched in potentially pathogenic variants [13]. One possible explanation of the phenomenon may the above-mentioned marriages between hearing impaired individuals. Attention should also be paid to the consanguinity between parents, which is common in certain populations. Looking for a genetic cause of HL in offspring of a consanguineous couple, the autosomal recessive mode of inheritance with pathogenic variants in a homozygous state is primarily expected.

A diagnostic challenge represents an HL patient without other affected family members, also referred to as a sporadic case. Here, a family history of HL is negative and a genetic cause is strongly suspected after exclusion of environmental factors, such as prenatal infection (with toxoplasmosis, rubella, cytomegalovirus, and herpesvirus—"TORCH" organisms), postnatal infections (mainly bacterial meningitis, mumps), prematurity, traumatic injury, blood vessels or autoimmune disease, Meniere's disease, acoustic neuroma, exposure to chemical agents, or noise that may be responsible for HL development. While describing HL, four major terms related to its presentation such as (I) the age of onset, (II) the type, (III) the degree of HL, and (IV) stability are usually used. The onset of HL can be congenital, prelingual (before a child develops speech), postlingual (after the acquisition of speech and language, usually after the age of six), adult-onset or age-related late-onset (presbyacusis). The different types of HL (conductive, sensorineural, or mixed) indicate which part of the ear is affected. Genetically determined HL is usually bilateral although families with asymmetric and unilateral HL are also reported [14, 15].

It has been estimated that about 80% of prelingual HL results from genetic factors. It is most often inherited as an autosomal recessive feature without other accompanying medical problems The second most common inheritance pattern of prelingual HL is autosomal dominant (20%), while X-linked and mitochondrial constitute together approximately 1–1.5% [16]. Most of the reported families with nonsyndromic postlingual HL present an autosomal dominant pattern of inheritance. Currently, 36 different genes causally involved in autosomal dominant HL have been identified (www.herediataryhearingloss.org; accessed 10/2017) and only a few of them are associated with prelingual HL [17].

If hearing impairment represents an isolated finding that can be associated with abnormalities of the middle and/or inner ear but is not accompanied by visible abnormalities of the outer ear or any other medical problems, it is referred to as nonsyndromic or isolated. The major cause of prelingual severe-to-profound autosomal recessive nonsyndromic HL in many populations are pathogenic variants of the *GJB*2 gene. The *GJB*2 and *GJB*6 genes, contained within the *DFNB*1 locus, should be tested in the first line in patients with nonsyndromic bilateral sensorineural HL of the prelingual onset [18].

Pathogenic *GJB*2 variants are also identified as the second most frequent cause of mild-to-moderate autosomal recessive HL. The most common causes of HL in this group of patients are pathogenic variants of the *STRC* gene and the third causative gene in this category is *TECTA*, but the prevalences vary among different ethnic groups [13, 19].

Discussing the genetic causes underlying partial deafness, defined as normal or slightly deteriorated thresholds involving low frequencies combined with profound HL in high frequencies [20], pathogenic variants localized within mtDNA and *TMPRSS*3 should be considered for diagnostic purposes [21, 22]. Nevertheless, the contribution of other genes should be also taken into account.

Inheritance pattern	Genes and loci involved
AD	*COCH* (DFNA9), *WFS*1 (DFNA6/14/38), *MYO*6 (DFNA22), *GJB*2 (DFN3A), *MYO7A* (DFNA11)
AR	*GJB*2 (DFNB1A), *SLC26A*4 (DFNB4), *MYO15A* (DFNB3), *TMC*1 (DFNB7/11), *TMPRSS*3 (DFNB8/10), *STRC* (DFNB16)
X-linked	*POU3F*4 (DFNX2), *PRPS*1 (DFNX1), *SMPX* (DFNX4), *COL4A*6 (DFNX6), *AIFM*1 (DFNX5)
Mitochondrial	*MT-TL*1, *MT-TK*, *MT-TS*1, *MT-TE*, *MT-RNR*1

Table 1. Genes involved in the pathogenesis of hearing disorders grouped according to the type of inheritance—examples.

Locus DFNB1, gene *GJB2*, inheritance type: AR		**Remarks**
Truncating pathogenic variants (e.g., c.35delG)	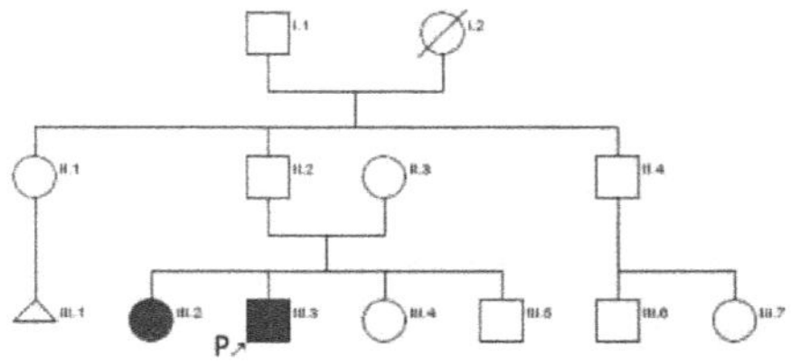	Congenital, bilateral, profound HL [23]
Nontruncating pathogenic variants (e.g., p.Met34Thr)	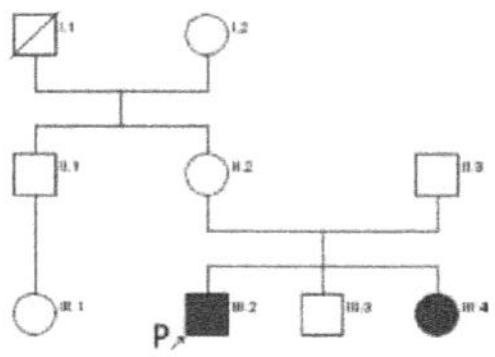	Postlingual, bilateral, mild-to-moderate HL [24]
Locus DFNB4, gene *SLC26A4*, inheritance type: AR		**Remarks**
Nontruncating, pathogenic variants (e.g., p.Glu29Gln)	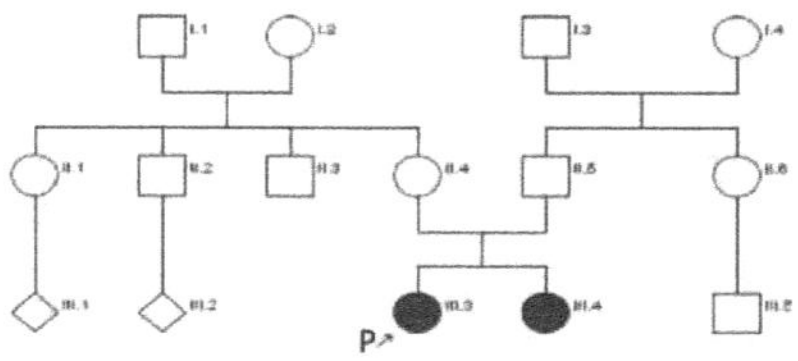	Enlarged vestibular aqueduct, vestibular dysfunction, Mondini malformation, early-onset, fluctuating HL [25]
Locus DFNA6/14/38, gene *WFS1*, inheritance type: AD		**Remarks**
Nontruncating, pathogenic variants (e.g., p.Asp771His)	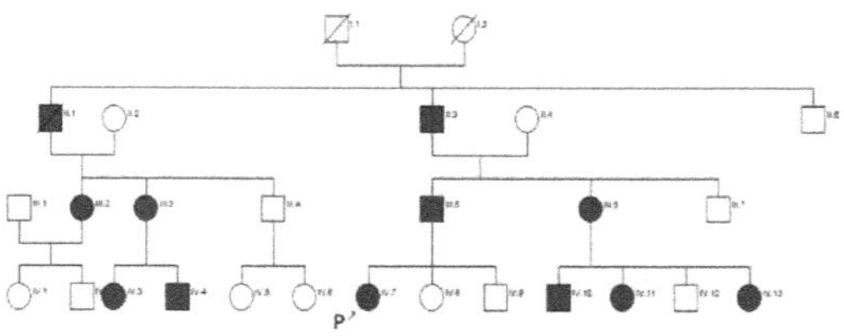	Postlingual, low-frequency HL, deteriorating with time [26]
Locus DFNX2, gene *POU3F4*, inheritance type: X-linked		**Remarks**
Truncating pathogenic variants (e.g., p.Glu187*)	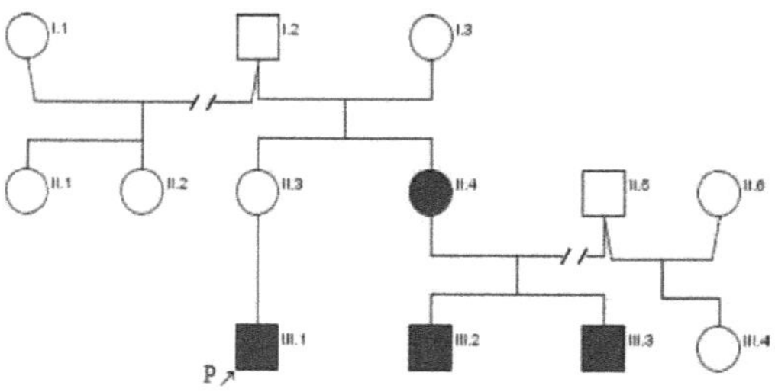	Congenital, profound, sensorineural HL (may be accompanied by a conductive component). Inner ear IP3 type malformation—comprises of enlarged internal auditory canal and vestibular aqueduct, underdeveloped cochlear modiolus and malformations of the vestibule. Due to the inner ear malformation perilymphatic gusher may occur during inner ear surgery [4]
Gene *MT-TS1*, inheritance type: X-linked		**Remarks**
Pathogenic variants (e.g., m.7511T>C)	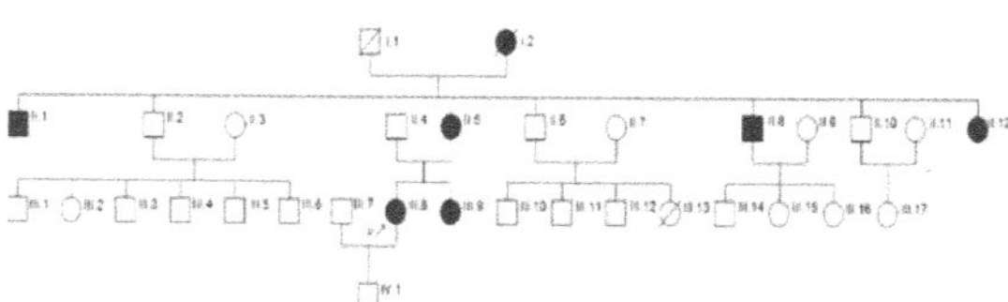	Postlingual, high-frequency HL [27]

Table 2. Pedigrees and audiometric features characteristic for different genes and pathogenic variants causative of HL.

Considering the significant contribution of genetic factors to HL and the recent guideline for clinical evaluation and etiologic diagnosis of HL, one may conclude that single-gene testing is justified if a specific genetic etiology of HL is suspected. If there are no specific clinical indications, testing for the DFNB1-related HL should be performed. If the investigations do not provide conclusive results, HL genes may be analyzed by the NGS approaches such as multigene panels, whole exome or whole genome sequencing [16]. All known nonsyndromic deafness loci (locus denotes the position in the genome linked with the disease) are labeled as DFN (DeaFNess) and classified according to the type of inheritance (DFNA: autosomal dominant; DFNB: autosomal recessive; DFNX: X-linked) followed by a number indicating the order of locus discovery. In **Table 1**, some of the most common HL causative loci are gathered.

As it was previously stated, HL is a genetically heterogenous disease; nevertheless, there are some common, characteristic features, which may be a valuable asset in the process of dissecting the genetic reason of HL. Examples of pedigrees, characteristic audiometric features, and additional remarks for some common HL genes are shown in **Table 2**.

Despite quite a large number of genes causative for HL, the first step in the diagnostic approach should be the analysis of the DFNB1 locus, as the testing is inexpensive and fast [28]. Apart from obvious clinical indications, such as IP3 malformation for the *POU3F4* gene analysis, the remaining cases should be rather streamed to wide, multigenic analysis.

4. Syndromic hearing loss

In contrast to the nonsyndromic hearing impairment, the syndromic hearing impairment is defined as a part of a syndrome, and it is associated with malformations of the external ear, malformations of other organs or other medical problems. HL is identified in more than 400 different syndromes [29]. The most common type of autosomal dominant syndrome with sensorineural HL is **Waardenburg syndrome** (WS types 1-4; OMIM#193500, #193510, #148820, and #277580), an auditory-pigmentary syndrome caused by pathogenic variants in *PAX3*, *MITF*, *EDNRB*, *EDN3*, or *SOX10* genes and characterized by the presence of pigmentary anomalies of skin, hair, and eyes. The second most common are **branchiootorenal spectrum disorders** (OMIM#113650, #610896 #602588, #166780), where conductive/sensorineural HL is accompanied by branchial cleft cysts or fistulas, malformations of outer ear, preauricular pits, and renal anomalies resulting from pathogenic variants in *EYA1*, *SIX1*, or *SIX5*. The third most common cause of autosomal dominant syndromic hearing impairment is **neurofibromatosis type 2** (NF2, OMIM#101000), a multiple neoplasia syndrome with HL secondary to the usually bilateral vestibular schwannomas (acoustic neuroma) and other tumors of the central nervous system (meningioma, schwannoma, glioma, or neurofibroma). NF2 is caused by heterozygous pathogenic variants in a gene-encoding neurofibromin-2 (NF2 gene) [30].

The **Stickler syndrome** (STL) is a connective tissue disorder with eye findings (high myopia, vitreoretinal degeneration, retinal detachment, and cataract) being the most constant traits. Other features are sensorineural or conductive HL, midline clefting (cleft palate, bifid uvula), Pierre Robin sequence, flat midface, mild spondyloephiphyseal dysplasia, and early-onset osteoarthritis [31]. Currently, four types of STL syndrome are distinguished—autosomal dominant STL1 (OMIM#108300) and STL2 (OMIM# 604841) caused by pathogenic variants in *COL2A1* and *COL11A1*, and autosomal recessive STL4 (OMIM#614134) and STL5 (OMIM#614284) due to pathogenic variants in *COL9A1* and *COL9A2* genes, respectively. The **Usher syndrome** (USH) is a combination of HL and visual impairment as a consequence of retinitis pigmentosa. The autosomal recessive condition is classified into three types: USH1 (OMIM#276900) with severe-to-profound deafness and defective vestibular function, USH2 (OMIM#276901) with mild-to-severe hearing impairment and normal vestibular function and USH3 (OMIM#276902) with progressive postlingual HL and vestibular dysfunction. Pathogenic variants in one of six genes (*MYO7A, USH1C, CDH23, PCDH15, USH1G,* or *CIB2*) may lead to USH1 [32], in one of three genes (*ADGRV1, WHRN,* or *USH2A*) to USH2 and in one of two genes (*CLRN1* or *HARS*) to USH3. The second most common autosomal recessive syndrome with sensorineural HL is the **Pendred syndrome** (PDS, OMIM#274600), characterized by severe-to profound deafness that is congenital or develops in early childhood and euthyroid/hypothyroid goiter that arises in early puberty or adulthood. It is associated with developmental abnormalities of the cochlea (Mondini dysplasia or enlarged vestibular aqueduct) that can be diagnosed by a CT examination of temporal bones. The cause of the PDS is pathogenic variants in the *SLAC26A4* gene encoding an anion transporter named pendrin. The third most common autosomal recessive syndrome with deafness is the **Jervell and Lange-Nielsen syndrome** (JLN), which is marked by congenital profound sensorineural HL and prolongation of the QT interval (corrected QT (QTc) > 440 msec), syncopal episodes due to ventricular arrhythmias and a high risk of sudden death. In patients with JLNS1 (OMIM#220400) pathogenic variants in *KCNQ1* and in patients with JLNS2 (OMIM#612347) pathogenic variants in *KCNE1* are found.

The two following autosomal recessive syndromic forms of HL represent rare metabolic disorders that, however, should not be missed out as their symptoms may resolve by appropriate treatment and dietary modifications. The **Biotinidase deficiency** (BTD, OMIM#253260) is a form of multiple carboxylase deficiency characterized by primarily neurologic (seizures, hypertonia, developmental delay, ataxia) and cutaneous (skin rash, dermatitis, alopecia) features. Patients lose vision and three-fourth of those who become symptomatic have some degree of HL. Laboratory findings show organic aciduria, mild hyperammonemia, and biotinidase deficiency. The BTD begins usually within the two first years of life and results from recessive pathogenic variants in the *BTD* gene. Treatment with biotin resolves neurologic and cutaneous manifestations, while HL and optic atrophy are usually irreversible.

The **Refsum disease** (OMIM#266500) is an inborn error of lipid metabolism with anosmia and early-onset retinitis pigmentosa being two universal findings. Other variable clinical features include neuropathy, ataxia, progressive severe HL, ichthyosis, cardiac, and skeletal (metacarpals/metatarsals shortening) involvement. Increased serum concentration of phytanic acid establishes the diagnosis. The symptoms present an insidious onset usually during the late first through third decades of life. Causative recessive variants are found in the *PHYH* and *PEX7* genes. In the medical care, diet modifications aimed at reduction of chlorophyll from the diet (exclusion of green vegetables (phytanic acid), and animal fat (phytol), and plasmapheresis) are used.

Syndromic X-linked HL is represented by the **Alport** (OMIM#301050) and **Mohr-Tranebjaerg** (MTS, OMIM#304700) **syndromes**. The Alport syndrome is characterized by glomerulonephropathy leading to progressive renal failure, varying severity of progressive sensorineural HL (occurs typically after 10 years of age and affects mainly high frequencies), and variable ocular anomalies. In 85% of patients with Alport syndrome, dominant pathogenic variants in the *COL4A5* gene on the X chromosome are found. Approximately 15% of patients develop Alport syndrome due to recessive variants in the *COL4A4* or *COL4A3* genes, cases with autosomal dominant inheritance, have also been occasionally reported.

In the Mohr-Tranebjaerg syndrome, also known as progressive deafness syndrome with blindness, dystonia, fractures and mental deficiency, progressive pre- or postlingual sensorineural deafness occurs in the early childhood and is a presenting symptom. MTS is caused by recessive variants of the *TIMM8A* gene.

Mutations in the **mitochondrial genome** can lead to HL that is an isolated feature or part of genetic syndrome, i.e., mitochondrial encephalomyopathy, lactic acidosis, and stroke-like episodes (MELAS), myoclonic epilepsy with ragged-red fibers (MERFF) or Kearns-Sayre syndrome (KSS), a mitochondrial myopathy, characterized by ptosis, ophthalmoplegia, muscle weakness, cerebellar ataxia, diabetes mellitus, and/or endocrinopathies [33]. Aminoglycoside ototoxicity has been associated with pathogenic variants in *MT-RNR1* [34]. Pathogenic variant m.3243A > G in the *MT-TL1* gene, which is causative of MELAS, was found in patients with diabetes mellitus and HL or HL exclusively [35]. The data raise questions on mitochondrial variant penetrance, tissue specificity, and heteroplasmy level.

5. Assistive algorithms

Regarding the heterogeneity of genetically related HL, the precise evaluation of its cause is a challenging task. Apart from some, rather rare, unquestionable phenotypic manifestations, many of the cases of possibly genetically related HL (syndromic and nonsyndromic) are hard to distinguish. It should be noted that there is a group of useful, assistive algorithms, which are helpful for both: establishing the diagnosis and targeting a diagnostic approach.

The Face2Gene (http://suite.face2gene.com/) is a collection of phenotyping applications, which enable accurate and comprehensive assessment of a patient based on characteristic dysmorphic facial features. As the variations in the face and skull are very common and are present in about 40% of genetic disorders, they are very useful in identification of the disorder. Briefly, the picture of patient face is uploaded to an application, than the quantification of the similarity is calculated with the usage of the algorithm database. The result is the list of syndromes with analogous morphology. The algorithm Face2Gene is accessible free of charge to all healthcare specialists.

The AudioGene (http://audiogene.eng.uiowa.edu/) predicts the genes underling autosomal dominant nonsyndromic hearing loss (ADNSHL) based on the audiometric data. This algorithm also takes into account the age of the patient, which is essential in the ADNSHL study due to characteristic deterioration of hearing during patient's life. The algorithm is based on the computational analysis of specific audiometric data deposited in the database. Furthermore, the machine-learning method is applied to select and prioritize possibly causative genes for pathogenic variant screening [36, 37].

The Pictures of Standard Syndromes and Undiagnosed Malformations (POSSUM) (https://www.possum.net.au/) is a comprehensive dysmorphology database designed for the diagnosis of multiple malformations, metabolic, teratogenic, chromosomal, and skeletal syndromes as well as their images. This database consists of information on over 4000 different syndromes and searching is based on the selected features and results in a specific list of possible diagnoses [38].

6. Next-generation sequencing technology in dissecting the background of hearing loss

In almost all genetically related diseases (included hearing impairment), there is a need for tailored diagnostic strategies in searching for their molecular background. The milestone in this research area was the development of the method for the DNA sequencing by Frederick Sanger in 1975 [39]. Whereas the direct sequencing (called also Sanger sequencing—tribute to its inventor) allows to debunk the molecular cause of disease in a limited number of genes, e.g., when HL background analyses were limited to the *GJB2* gene, there was a significant gap in our knowledge and diagnostic capabilities. This gap has been filled out by introducing NGS technology, also called massive parallel sequencing (MPS) or high-throughput DNA sequencing. The NGS developed over the last decade has revolutionized the genetic research and diagnostic practice, mainly because of reducing costs and time of DNA sequencing. This technology gives a unique opportunity to analyze in one experiment the sequence of more than 1 million base pairs, thus sequencing of the whole genome or thousands of genes simultaneously in a few days has become possible [40]. The most commonly used forms of NGS in searching for pathogenic variants underling HL are whole exome sequencing (WES) and multigene panels.

An undisputable advantage of the WES is the possibility of simultaneous sequencing of the whole coding DNA sequence (protein coding part within all human genes ~20,000) regardless of the disease studied. This makes WES a universal test for almost all known genetic diseases. The multigene panel sequencing is a more economical solution, especially dedicated for the diagnostic purpose. It should be noted that with the panel sequencing, only already known genes associated with a given disease are analyzed. Although the targeted NGS has many advantages, whole-genome sequencing (WGS) is still the state of art approach with its high cost representing a main drawback. The application of high-throughput DNA sequencing methods generates a vast amount of information, which accelerated the discovery of new, causative genes for many diseases. Also in the field of genetically related HL, with the NGS technology, novel genes have been discovered for all modes of inheritance described above. The important, newly discovered genes causative of recessive HL are: *ADCY1*, *BDP1*, *SYNE4*, *ELMOD3*, *CABP2*, *GRXCR2*, *OTOGL*, *TPRN*, and *TSPEAR*. For dominant HL, the *CEACAM16*, *P2RX2*, and *OSBPL2* genes were revealed, also gene for the DFNX4 locus (i.e., *SMPX*) was identified. Another remarkable achievement obtained by the NGS technology is the identification of genes incorrectly classified as pathogenic, the examples of such events are: *MYO1A* and *RAB40AL* [41–43].

For the clinical diagnostic purpose, there are many commercial tests based on NGS, which differ in technologies and numbers of genes included. Heretofore, at least 20 commercially available tests, based on the NGS technology, focused on genetically related HL may be applied [1]. Due to the constant reduction of costs and availability, diagnostic approach based on the NGS technology in the nearest future will become a standard, which will significantly improve the level of patient care.

Index of technical terms

Autosomal dominant inheritance (AD)—type of Mendelian inheritance of a trait in which a defective copy of a gene (localized on autosome) dominates over the normal one. For the symptoms to occur, presence of only one defective copy is sufficient.

Autosomal recessive inheritance (AR)—type of Mendelian inheritance of a trait in which two copies of defective gene (localized on autosomes) are required in order for the disease to develop.

***DFNB*1 locus**—most common locus causative for nonsyndromic hearing loss, containing *GJB*2 and *GJB*6 genes.

Direct sequencing—a technology allowing to determine the sequence of nucleotides in DNA invented in 1977 by Frederic Sanger and Alan R. Coulson, based on the chain-dideoxy terminator method, also called Sanger sequencing.

Genetic pedigree—illustration of genetic relationship of a family, including information about health history of the family members.

Heteroplasmy—coexistence of more than one mtDNA type within an individual.

Homoplasmy—presence of a uniform type of mtDNA within an individual.

Mendelian inheritance—type of transmission of genes according to Gregor Mendel's set of laws, also called classical inheritance. Mendelian inheritance comprises of autosomal dominant, autosomal recessive, and X-linked type of inheritance.

Mitochondrial DNA (mtDNA)—small circular genome localized in the mitochondria.

Mitochondrial inheritance—non-Mendelian type of inheritance, occurring when a defective gene is located within the mitochondrial genome, inheritance of a trait encoded by this gene takes place exclusively from mother to offspring.

Next generation sequencing (NGS)—also known as high-throughput sequencing, a technology allowing to establish the sequence of DNA larger than 1 million base pairs in a single experiment.

Nonsyndromic deafness—deafness not associated with pathological symptoms/signs from other systems.

Partial deafness—hearing loss assessed by an audiometric test as a normal or little elevated hearing threshold within low frequencies and significantly raised hearing threshold in high frequencies.

Post-lingual hearing loss—hearing loss with late onset (after speech development).

Prelingual hearing loss—hearing loss with early onset (before speech development).

Sex-linked inheritance—type of the Mendelian inheritance of a trait in which the defective gene is located on X or Y chromosome.

Syndromic deafness—deafness as a part of a syndrome i.e., associated with pathological symptoms/signs from other organs.

Whole exome sequencing (WES)—approach based on NGS technology, allowing to sequence all protein-coding regions (exons).

Whole genome sequencing (WGS)—approach based on NGS technology allowing to analyze the whole genome DNA sequence.

Author details

Agnieszka Pollak* and Monika Ołdak

*Address all correspondence to: a.pollak@ifps.org.pl

Department of Genetics, Institute of Physiology and Pathology of Hearing, Warsaw, Poland

References

[1] Ołdak M. Chapter 8—Next generation sequencing in vision and hearing impairment. Clinical Applications for Next-Generation Sequencing. Boston: Academic Press; 2016. p. 153-170

[2] Richards S, Aziz N, Bale S, Bick D, Das S, Gastier-Foster J, et al. Standards and guidelines for the interpretation of sequence variants: A joint consensus recommendation of the American College of Medical Genetics and Genomics and the Association for Molecular Pathology. Genetics in Medicine. 2015;**17**(5):405-424

[3] Oldak M, Ozieblo D, Pollak A, Stepniak I, Lazniewski M, Lechowicz U, et al. Novel neuro-audiological findings and further evidence for TWNK involvement in Perrault syndrome. Journal of Translational Medicine. 2017;**15**(1):25

[4] Pollak A, Lechowicz U, Kedra A, Stawinski P, Rydzanicz M, Furmanek M, et al. Novel and de novo mutations extend association of POU3F4 with distinct clinical and radiological phenotype of hearing loss. PLoS One. 2016;**11**(12):e0166618

[5] Resta RG. The crane's foot: The rise of the pedigree in human genetics. Journal of Genetic Counseling. 1993;**2**(4):235-260

[6] Bennett RL, Steinhaus KA, Uhrich SB, O'Sullivan CK, Resta RG, Lochner-Doyle D, et al. Recommendations for standardized human pedigree nomenclature. Journal of Genetic Counseling. 1995;**4**(4):267-279

[7] Bennett RL, Steinhaus KA, Uhrich SB, O'Sullivan CK, Resta RG, Lochner-Doyle D, et al. Recommendations for standardized human pedigree nomenclature. Pedigree standardization task force of the National Society of genetic Counselors. American Journal of Human Genetics. 1995;**56**(3):745-752

[8] Bennett RL, French KS, Resta RG, Doyle DL. Standardized human pedigree nomenclature: Update and assessment of the recommendations of the National Society of genetic Counselors. Journal of Genetic Counseling. 2008;**17**(5):424-433

[9] Charlesworth B. The evolution of sex chromosomes. Science. 1991;**251**(4997):1030-1033

[10] Taylor RW, Turnbull DM. Mitochondrial DNA mutations in human disease. Nature Reviews. Genetics. 2005;**6**(5):389-402

[11] Oxford Desk DABIRT. Reference: Clinical genetics. The Ulster Medical Journal. 2006;**75**(3):235

[12] Chakraborty R, Deka R. Isolated populations. Encyclopedia of Biostatistics. USA: John Wiley & Sons, Ltd. 2005

[13] Vona B, Muller T, Nanda I, Neuner C, Hofrichter MA, Schroder J, et al. Targeted next-generation sequencing of deafness genes in hearing-impaired individuals uncovers informative mutations. Genetics in Medicine. 2014;**16**(12):945-953

[14] Kim SH, Kim AR, Choi HS, Kim MY, Chun EH, Oh SH, et al. Molecular etiology of hereditary single-side deafness: Its association with pigmentary disorders and Waardenburg syndrome. Medicine (Baltimore). 2015;**94**(43):e1817

[15] Zazo Seco C, Serrao de Castro L, van Nierop JW, Morin M, Jhangiani S, Verver EJ, et al. Allelic mutations of KITLG, encoding KIT ligand, cause asymmetric and unilateral hearing loss and Waardenburg syndrome type 2. American Journal of Human Genetics 2015;**97**(5):647-660

[16] Alford RL, Arnos KS, Fox M, Lin JW, Palmer CG, Pandya A, et al. American College of Medical Genetics and Genomics guideline for the clinical evaluation and etiologic diagnosis of hearing loss. Genetics in Medicine. 2014;**16**(4):347-355

[17] Smith RJH, Jones MKN. Nonsyndromic Hearing Loss and Deafness, DFNB1. In: Adam MP, Ardinger HH, Pagon RA, Wallace SE, Bean LJH, Mefford HC, et al., editors. Seattle (WA): GeneReviews(R); 1993

[18] Hoefsloot LH, Roux AF, Bitner-Glindzicz M, contributors to EDbpm. EMQN best practice guidelines for diagnostic testing of mutations causing non-syndromic hearing impairment at the DFNB1 locus. European Journal of Human Genetics. 2013;**21**(11):1325-1329

[19] Sloan-Heggen CM, Bierer AO, Shearer AE, Kolbe DL, Nishimura CJ, Frees KL, et al. Comprehensive genetic testing in the clinical evaluation of 1119 patients with hearing loss. Human Genetics. 2016;**135**(4):441-450

[20] Skarzynski H, Lorens A, Piotrowska A. A new method of partial deafness treatment. Medical Science Monitor. 2003;**9**(4):CS20-CS24

[21] Lechowicz U, Gambin T, Pollak A, Podgorska A, Stawinski P, Franke A, et al. Iterative sequencing and variant screening (ISVS) as a novel pathogenic mutations search strategy - application for TMPRSS3 mutations screen. Scientific Reports. 2017;**7**(1):2543

[22] Iwanicka-Pronicka K, Pollak A, Skorka A, Lechowicz U, Korniszewski L, Westfal P, et al. Audio profiles in mitochondrial deafness m.1555A>G and m.3243A>G show distinct differences. Medical Science Monitor 2015;**21**:694-700

[23] Snoeckx RL, Huygen PL, Feldmann D, Marlin S, Denoyelle F, Waligora J, et al. GJB2 mutations and degree of hearing loss: A multicenter study. American Journal of Human Genetics. 2005;**77**(6):945-957

[24] Pollak A, Skorka A, Mueller-Malesinska M, Kostrzewa G, Kisiel B, Waligora J, et al. M34T and V37I mutations in GJB2 associated hearing impairment: Evidence for pathogenicity and reduced penetrance. American Journal of Medical Genetics. Part A. 2007;**143A**(21):2534-2543

[25] Alasti F, Van Camp G, Smith RJH. Pendred Syndrome/DFNB4. In: Adam MP, Ardinger HH, Pagon RA, Wallace SE, Bean LJH, Mefford HC, et al., editors. Seattle (WA): GeneReviews(R); 1993

[26] Gurtler N, Kim Y, Mhatre A, Schlegel C, Mathis A, Daniels R, et al. Two families with nonsyndromic low-frequency hearing loss harbor novel mutations in Wolfram syndrome gene 1. Journal of Molecular Medicine (Berl). 2005;**83**(7):553-560

[27] Lechowicz U, Pollak A, Frączak A, Rydzanicz M, Stawiński P, Lorens A, et al. Application of nextgeneration sequencing to identify mitochondrial mutations: Study on m.7511T>C in patients with hearing loss. Molecular Medicine Reports. 2018;**17**(1):1782-1790

[28] Pollak A, Prevalence SH. Of DFNB1 hearing loss among cochlear implant users established with the 3-step DFNB1 approach. Journal of Hearing Science. 2017;**7**(1):33-40

[29] Gorlin RJ, Toriello HV, Cohen MM. Hereditary Hearing Loss and its Syndromes: Oxford University Press, USA; 1995

[30] Baser ME, Friedman JM, Aeschliman D, Joe H, Wallace AJ, Ramsden RT, et al. Predictors of the risk of mortality in neurofibromatosis 2. American Journal of Human Genetics. 2002; **71**(4):715-723

[31] Baker S, Booth C, Fillman C, Shapiro M, Blair MP, Hyland JC, et al. A loss of function mutation in the COL9A2 gene causes autosomal recessive stickler syndrome. American Journal of Medical Genetics. Part A. 2011;**155A**(7):1668-1672

[32] Jacoszek A, Pollak A, Ploski R, Oldak M. Advances in genetic hearing loss: CIB2 gene. European Archives of Oto-Rhino-Laryngology. 2017;**274**(4):1791-1795

[33] Van Camp G, Maternally SRJ. Inherited hearing impairment. Clinical Genetics. 2000; **57**(6):409-414

[34] Pandya A. Nonsyndromic Hearing Loss and Deafness, Mitochondrial. In: Adam MP, Ardinger HH, Pagon RA, Wallace SE, Bean LJH, Mefford HC, et al, editors. Seattle (WA): GeneReviews(R); 1993

[35] Iwanicka-Pronicka K, Pollak A, Skorka A, Lechowicz U, Pajdowska M, Furmanek M, et al. Postlingual hearing loss as a mitochondrial 3243A>G mutation phenotype. PLoS One 2012;**7**(10):e44054

[36] Taylor KR, Booth KT, Azaiez H, Sloan CM, Kolbe DL, Glanz EN, et al. Audioprofile surfaces: The 21st century audiogram. The Annals of Otology, Rhinology, and Laryngology. 2016;**125**(5):361-368

[37] Hildebrand MS, DeLuca AP, Taylor KR, Hoskinson DP, Hur IA, Tack D, et al. A contemporary review of AudioGene audioprofiling: A machine-based candidate gene prediction tool for autosomal dominant nonsyndromic hearing loss. The Laryngoscope. 2009;**119**(11):2211-2215

[38] Stromme P. The diagnosis of syndromes by use of a dysmorphology database. Acta Paediatrica Scandinavica. 1991;**80**(1):106-109

[39] Sanger F, Coulson AR. A rapid method for determining sequences in DNA by primed synthesis with DNA polymerase. Journal of Molecular Biology. 1975;**94**(3):441-448

[40] Demkow U, Ploski R. Clinical Applications for Next-Generation Sequencing. USA: Academic Press; 2015

[41] Oldak M, Ruszkowska E, Pollak A, Sobczyk-Kopciol A, Kowalewski C, Piwonska A, et al. A note of caution on the diagnosis of Martin-Probst syndrome by the detection of the p.D59G mutation in the RAB40AL gene. European Journal of Pediatrics. 2015; **174**(5):693-696

[42] Oldak M, Sciezynska A, Mlynarski W, Borowiec M, Ruszkowska E, Szulborski K, et al. Evidence against RAB40AL being the locus for Martin-Probst X-linked deafness-intellectual disability syndrome. Human Mutation. 2014;**35**(10):1171-1174

[43] Eisenberger T, Di Donato N, Baig SM, Neuhaus C, Beyer A, Decker E, et al. Targeted and genomewide NGS data disqualify mutations in MYO1A, the "DFNA48 gene", as a cause of deafness. Human Mutation. 2014;**35**(5):565-570

4

Aging Auditory System and Amplification

Christiane Marques do Couto and
Izabella dos Santos Brites

Abstract

The aging of auditory system determines the physical, sensory, and neural changes in the peripheral and central parts and may cause changes in the reception and sound processing. Age related hearing loss, also called presbycusis, can occur in the elderly population due to aging. The difficulty for compression of speech in the elderly may be due solely to hearing loss, but may be linked to degenerative issues of the central auditory system. Age is a factor that interferes with the central auditory processing. The results of auditory processing may change and more if there is the presence of peripheral hearing loss. It should be considered that the longer an individual has hearing loss, the greater the negative effects on the perception of sound and performance in listening skills. The use of hearing aids favors amplification and modification of the sound stimulus so that it reaches the eardrum with quantity increase and quality, promoting and stimulating the auditory skills. This chapter intends to make a review of the auditory processing disorder and evidence the benefit of the use of amplification in the elderly.

Keywords: hearing aid, auditory system, presbycusis, auditory processing, elderly

1. Introduction

Advancements in health care and technological developments in the areas of preventive medicine and medical technology during the last decades have considerably extended the life expectancy of the human population. As a result, a greater number of people exceed the age of 65. This category of subjects is commonly referred to as seniors or elderly group. With the increasing age, some systems of the human body start to present functional changes such as degeneration or atrophy of neurons or tissues. People older than 65 years show an increased number of nontransmissible diseases, such as cardiac or metabolic ones [1].

Associated with the transformation of the body and with the higher incidence of health complications, the elderly may present sensory, motor, and cognitive alterations. Cellular and molecular damage may also show up due to aging, possibly resulting in sensory loss (hearing or vision) or motor disability. In addition, cognitive changes such as decreased attention and working memory may also be present [1, 2].

All these factors may compromise the quality of life and the independence of the elderly. In addition, these changes can lead this segment of the population to a social isolation and depression [1].

The aging of the auditory system leads to physical, sensory, and neural changes in the peripheral and central portion of the system, which may also cause changes in the sections which receive and process the sound stimuli.

The objective of this chapter is to make a review of hearing loss and auditory processing, while considering the use of amplification technologies (hearing aids) and their intervention in the elderly.

2. Hearing

The concept of hearing is extremely complex and goes beyond the simple act of listening to a particular sound. This is a process in which motor, electrical, and biochemical changes occur along the auditory path inside the human body, which begins in the outer ear (more specifically in the pinna), and ends in the cortex, where the sound information received is decoded [3].

Sound waves generated in the environment are captured by the pinna and driven by the external acoustic meatus to the tympanic membrane, which starts a vibration process, transforming the sound waves into mechanical waves. This vibration moves the ossicles in the middle ear until it reaches the oval window, where stimulation will reach the inner ear.

The movement that begins in the inner ear promotes movement in the liquid (endolymph) that is housed in the cochlea, as well as, a change in its structures, promoting the excitement of the outer and inner hair cells, which in turn stimulate a network of nerve endings, which leads to the stimulation of the cochlear nerve to reach the central nervous system. It will be in the cerebral cortex that the stimulus will be decoded and then spatially interpreted.

As described above, hearing is an extremely complex process. What happens when the auditory system is affected by changes due to aging and it does not work properly?

2.1. Hearing loss and its consequences

When the auditory system presents structural changes, other disorders might be observed first, depending on the location where the hearing complications were first observed. For example, if a problem is observed in the external, middle, or inner ear, it will result in a reversible (or not) hearing loss. If a problem is present in the area of the auditory cortex, it will generate a processing interference, which will affect the understanding and decoding of the incoming sound stimuli.

Aging processes can alter the structures of the auditory system, resulting in hearing loss and a compromise of hearing. This is the most significant and important sensory change in the lives of the elderly, which can generate a social limitation, minimizing the social function and the participation of the elderly in the society [4].

Hearing loss due to aging is called *"presbycusis"* or *age-related hearing loss* (ARHL) [5]. It is usually identified due to complains from the elderly subjects, referring to difficulties in understanding nearby sounds, especially in environments with poor acoustics. In these cases, an audiological assessment usually results in an identification of a mild-to-moderate symmetric sensorineural hearing loss, which worsens in the course of time [6].

It is well known that 80% of the population >85 years present some form of hearing loss [7]. The incidence of the hearing impairment also has gender effects, i.e., elderly men tend to be more affected than elderly women [8].

The data in the literature show that presbycusis can be classified into three types: the **sensory** presbycusis, the **neuronal** presbycusis, and the **metabolic** presbycusis [9, 10]. In the first case, it is possible to observe a lesion in the organ of Corti, which results in an audiogram with sloping configuration. In the **neuronal** presbycusis, there is a loss of spiral ganglion neurons, which leads to a worsening in speech discrimination, which does not seem compatible with hearing loss observed in the audiogram. The **metabolic** presbycusis is caused by a degeneration of the vascular stria, characterized by a vocal discrimination preserved, even in spite of the presence of flat or high frequency configuration [9, 10]. In all the three cases above, the elderly is considered to have a sensory neural hearing loss.

However, it is necessary to account for other factors that may have affected the hearing of the elderly throughout life and that may have worsened the hearing loss, such as exposure to noise, cardiovascular diseases (hypertension or diabetes), or extensive use of antineoplastic drugs. Very often what we call presbycusis is the cumulative effect of aging with cochlear stress caused by other etiologies [11–13].

A decline of the linguistic functions is commonly observed in the elderly presenting hearing loss. Due to this sensorial disorder, an elderly subject loses the quality of sound information in communicating with others, which may generate at first a difficulty or trouble understanding a vocal message, and eventually drives the elderly into social isolation [14]. This situation has an impact in the lives of the elderly as well as in the people who surround the elderly, their caregivers.

These communication difficulties are global and they are changing the life of the elderly, reducing their communication skills with members of the family or friends. This difficulty can even show up with normal environmental sounds such as a telephone ring or the horn of a car, situations that can even put the elderly into a safety hazard [15].

The International Classification of Disability and Health (ICF) (World Health Organization, 2001) considers that a condition of good health depends (i) on the proper functioning of the body and (ii) on social and environmental factors that allow the individual to perform his/her activities and be active socially. Thus, hearing loss should not be a limitation, since it is possible to perform an intervention (hearing aids, implantable hearing aids, and cochlear implants) and to manage positively the hearing impaired adult [16].

2.2. Hearing aids and hearing performance

When hearing loss is diagnosed, an intervention is necessary. The most immediate solution is the use of a hearing aid (**HA**) technology. The HA is a little apparatus placed in the external meatus and that can amplify the sounds that reach the auditory system. With a hearing aid, the person will regain the audibility even of low-intensity sounds, making it possible to resume the activities of daily life. The usage of a hearing aid is the primary treatment option indicated for individuals with nonreversible hearing loss [17].

Since elderly subjects present a symmetrical loss profile in most cases, it is possible to use two hearing aid devices and perform a binaural fitting. Two hearing aids favor a better understanding of the sound messages and a better localization of the sound source [17].

Currently, in the market, there is a wide variety of technologies for hearing aids and resources that can be used to improve hearing. The best hearing aid is indicated for each case, and for it, a process must be followed by the audiologist, thus favoring a better adaptation of the hearing aid.

This process to determine if a hearing aid should be used or not begins with an assessment and the planning of the intervention to be held. Usually, the individual is subjected to the common audiological tests such as tonal and speech audiometry as well as immittance tympanometry tests. However, these procedures can only assess hearing complications in the auditory periphery. The sufficiency of these tests is uncertain and will be further discussed below.

The HA is selected based on desired physical and electroacoustic characteristics. At this stage, the individual complains should be considered, their fine motor skills and even cognitive factors that may influence the use and adaptation of one or other technology.

Since individuals with sensorineural hearing loss have low speech discrimination in the presence of background noise, most hearing aid devices incorporate noise suppressors that amplify the speech signal over noise and directional microphones that capture best sounds from certain directions. Even in these conditions the hearing aid cannot simulate the cochlea function, for all audible sounds. The hearing aid will amplify certain sound frequencies, but still there will be loss of sound signal quality, and a number of individuals still tend to complain about the level of amplification.

The hearing aid should amplify the incoming sounds without being uncomfortable to the person who uses it. This situation is only possible due to the components and digital or electronic operation of the hearing aid, which will amplify the low-intensity sounds, transforming them into audible sounds, without however, causing discomfort in the listener.

Care must be taken in the entire process of fitting, such as the handling conditions of the hearing aid by the elderly, the size of the device, or the occurrence of feedback. If any of these factors were not observed, the chance of the elderly not making effective use of the hearing aid is very high.

After selecting the best hearing aid for the subject case and its characteristics, the specific device performance and the individual performance with this technology must be verified through objective and subjective tests if there was an improvement in the perception of sound stimuli. The next phase consists of providing the user with proper guidance on the usage and handling of the hearing aid, enabling, after one-time use, the validation of the treatment, in other words, the perception of the impact of the intervention in the life of the new user of hearing aids [18]. Throughout this process, the audiologist should consider two important factors: the limitations in activities and participation restriction.

For this reason, even with the existing technological advancements in the field of hearing aids, some elderly subjects still complain about the amplification, signal quality, often failing to make use of this technology. Other elderly subjects, in turn, report great improvement in their lives with the use of hearing aids, accomplishing different listening tasks. So, why does it occur?

3. Auditory processing

In some cases, even if the hearing aid provides audibility of the signal, it cannot improve the listening of the elderly, especially in acoustically unfavorable environments. This may occur because of the listening difficulty caused, including, but not exclusively, by periphery of the auditory system, but also by central portion, in the cortex, thereby generating a difficulty in auditory processing, with consequent difficulty decoding the acoustic signal. This difficulty is not only a result of the increase in hearing thresholds but also of a dysfunction of the auditory processing. This has to be taken into account when selecting hearing aids.

Hearing is a function of the peripheral portion of the auditory system. However, processing and understanding of this sound is a function of the central portion of the auditory system, and incorporates many features and neurological networks, involving aspects like hearing, language, and cognitive.

For a long time, it was believed that only the basic audiological evaluation has been sufficient for diagnosis and intervention in the elderly. Alternatively, the central auditory processing tests should were performed only in individuals with thresholds within normal standard, so that this test is widely used in children with complaints of learning disability without another diagnosis or change detected [19]. However, it is possible to use the auditory processing test with adults and elderly. Several studies [20] on the auditory processing in the elderly or people with hearing loss began to be realized and it looks for the answer of this population, in a way to create a normal answer for this population and investigate if these results can change answer or feeling of the elderly with HA.

It is necessary to consider that it is not only the peripheral portion of the auditory system that is influenced by age, but all the auditory system undergoes aging interference. There may be a drop in auditory skills not only because of a peripheral alteration, but because of a difficulty in working and operating with sounds and auditory skills [21, 22].

Besides the hearing loss, the elderly have trouble in auditory processing. This fact is proven by research showing that older adults with hearing loss perform worse than adults or young people with similar hearing loss. This occurs because there is a deterioration of the central auditory system in the elderly, which generates auditory processing disorder [20]. Especially in the elderly, the acoustic signal that enters the system is distorted due to peripheral hearing loss because of aging (presbycusis) [23], what compromised more the auditory processing. If the whole system is taken into account, only amplification of sound will not be enough, because there can be a change in the processing of this sound in the central portion of the auditory system (cortex). Therefore, this interferes with the fitting of hearing aids, reducing satisfaction and their effective use.

In 1996, the American Speech-Language-Hearing Association characterized and defined "*central auditory process are the auditory system mechanisms and process responsible for the following behavioral phenomenal: sound localization and lateralization, auditory discrimination, auditory pattern recognition, temporal aspects of audition including temporal resolution, temporal masking, temporal integration and temporal ordering, auditory performance decrements with competing acoustic signals and auditory performance decrements with degraded acoustic signals*" [24].

It is important to evaluate what these abilities mean. When someone can detect from which direction the sound is coming, the person is using the sound localization. When someone can organize or memorize auditory information according to the time, they are developing the temporal ordering ability. When someone understands the auditory information in the competitive noise, they are performing the auditory closure. When someone understands the auditory information from the junction of the information provided in each ear, they are doing binaural synthesis.

In children the auditory processing disorder justifies learning or language disorders. When the sound has not been processed properly, dealing with language issues is difficult, resulting in reading and writing problems. In adults, this change can be detected only when specific or elaborate tasks of listening are requested. In the elderly, the auditory processing difficulty is perceived when the individual does not fit to the hearing aid.

3.1. Auditory processing evaluation

Therefore, to detect the presence of auditory processing disorders, it is necessary to perform an evaluation, which is conducted in a soundproof booth, using headphones. The assessment is carried out with different tests, which evaluate the individual auditory skills, such as sound localization, temporal ordering, auditory closure, binaural synthesis, and figure background.

These skills are evaluated using different procedures (**Table 1**), which can be applied in more than one session. Moreover, these tests can be applied in monaural or binaural form, i.e., in order to evaluate just one ear or the binaural integration (both ears). Each test has a specific orientation (purpose) and a specific stimulus. It is not necessary to apply all of the tests. On

Procedure	Skill
Sound localization	Sound localization
Memory for verbal sounds	Temporal ordination
Memory for nonverbal sounds	Temporal ordination
Speech with noise	Auditory closure
Dichotic digits	Integration binaural
Staggered spondaic word (SSW)	Integration binaural
Frequency and duration standard	Temporal processing
Gaps in noise (GIN)	Temporal processing
Identification of synthetic sentences	Figure background

Table 1. Auditory processing tests and auditory abilities.

the other hand, it is necessary to focus on the hearing loss type and its configuration to decide which test is the most important to be performed or can be possibly applied. This analysis is important because the tests are applied with an audible level over the hearing threshold.

Therefore, according to the hearing loss level, one particular test may not be applied because the sound level necessary on that test cannot be reached due to the limitation of the equipment. This aspect will be discussed later on.

3.2. Auditory processing in the elderly

Research comparing young and old individuals, whose hearing level is within the normal range, observed that even with normal thresholds, there is a reduction in speech understanding with background noise with the increase of the age of the individuals for short messages (consonants) or for long messages (phrases) [25].

The main complaint of the elderly is the difficulty to understand speech. There are three hypotheses that justify the difficulty to understand speech in the elderly: peripheral hearing loss, central hearing loss, and cognitive impairment. According to studies, despite being the most accepted hypothesis, only peripheral hearing loss may not generate the difficulties to understand the speech in the elderly [26]. In contrast, it adds that changes in auditory processing could enhance the difficulty that the elderly have to identify speech [27].

It is clear that the elderly has auditory processing disorder, since it is difficult for them to decode phonemes, the perception of rapidly changing speech decoding of verbal and nonverbal sounds and a slowing in interhemispheric transmission [28]. These changes associated with the peripheral hearing loss create a difficulty to understand speech, especially if it occurs in an acoustically unfavorable environment.

In addition to the hearing impairment, either peripheral or central, a decline in cognitive function can also negatively impact the processing of sound information, impairing speech understanding [29]. With the increase of age there is a decrease in attention span and in working memory, slower brain processing, and reduction in the ability to reduce the environmental interference for speech understanding [6].

Factors such as working memory and speech processing speed influence speech recognition in noise. Studies have shown that the elderly who has a good cognitive performance obtained good results, which were better than those who had poorer performance, indicating that for processing the acoustic signal there is a cognitive interference condition [30].

These cognitive changes associated with the decline in hearing thresholds and a worsening in hearing generates a change in perception and speech understanding in noise. These factors result in a decline in the elderly quality of life and can lead to social isolation [31].

3.3. Auditory processing evaluation in the elderly

Nowadays, we have the idea that there is a correlation between auditory processing tests and hearing loss and that the elderly performs worse than adults. Because of that, recent research includes study of the auditory processing and hearing loss, and look for a way to evaluate and intervene with this population.

In the elderly, it is essential to consider the presence of peripheral hearing loss, but as it is a poor signal that reaches the cerebral cortex due to peripheral hearing loss, cognition of the elderly is fundamental for a better understanding of the message. Additionally, the auditory cortex of individuals in this portion of the population tends to atrophy, which causes a change in auditory processing, i.e., the sound that enters the system is already an altered sound, and it worsens because of the way this is processed [31].

Studies show that seniors who have changes in auditory processing tend to perform a self-assessment of the hearing handicap worse than those who have no auditory processing disorder, showing that it is necessary for a better evaluation of each individual [32].

Some researches specify types of responses that can be obtained for each case. Individuals with low- and high-frequency hearing loss show difficulty in monotonic tasks. In turn, the elderly with hearing loss in high frequency or normal hearing can perform well on these tests. Therefore, audiological characteristics of the hearing loss have to be taken into account to select the processing test and understand the results achieved [33].

Many factors have to be considered to assess auditory processing in the elderly. In addition to care in the test selection, it is important to consider the age of the assessed person. It is known that when comparing the performance of adults with the elderly performance, the elderly will have a lower performance than adults, those observed even in the presence of similar hearing loss. This occurs because there is a deterioration of the central auditory system, which generates an auditory processing disorder in the elderly. This context interferes negatively with the hearing aids' fitting, reducing the satisfaction of the elderly in relation to these devices, resulting in a noneffective use [22].

To evaluate how the elderly process this sound, or their listening skills, it can map out a more detailed and correct rehabilitation plan for each case. If there is the presence of peripheral hearing loss, hearing aids must be fitted. However, with a broader look at the elderly's auditory system and their greatest difficulties, a better hearing aid fitting is possible, as well as the indication of a therapy or auditory training.

However, still in the assessment phase, it is important that the evaluator considers the presence of peripheral hearing loss when selecting and evaluating the results of tests of auditory processing, since not all tests can be applied in cases of peripheral hearing loss. It is necessary to select tests that do not suffer interference from hearing loss. Still, there is the degree of limitation of loss, with the possible application in symmetrical hearing loss, from mild to moderate (hearing loss up to 55 dB HL) [34].

Some authors suggest that the battery used to assess auditory processing should have dichotic tests, temporal processing tests, low redundancy monaural tests, and binaural interaction tests [34, 35].

Specifically to evaluate the binaural interaction, it is suggested to use the dichotic digits test. Studies show that there is a drop in performance of the left ear in the dichotic listening in the elderly. This generates a change in interhemispheric transfer of the acoustic signal, which is due to the deterioration of the callosum corpus [36]. This change in dichotic listening can alter also in working memory and selective attention, suggesting cognitive impairment [37, 38].

It is important to explain that in the dichotic test, four numbers are introduced. First of all, two numbers will be shown, at same time, but each one in each ear. Immediately after, other two numbers are shown in the same way. The listener has to pay attention and tell which numbers he listened and/or what numbers were heard in each ear.

In this age group (elderly), more problems are observed with listening skills figure background and closing, which affect the listening speech in noise in acoustically unfavorable environments. In addition, changes in auditory temporal processing are also observed in the elderly and widely discussed in the literature [39]. It is believed that the elderly people experience changes in auditory temporal processing, which can be detected both in frequency and in test duration [6].

In the temporal tests, three stimuli in sequence are presented, and the assessed individual has to name or reproduce the sound, and thick or thin the frequency test, or long and short in duration test.

The hearing performance worsens with the presentation of a complex or an acoustically unfavorable environment stimulus. Added to this, the elderly has great difficulty with sequencing activities, which involve auditory processing and cognition [40].

4. Auditory neuronal plasticity

The elderly with hearing loss suffer from the beginning of the hearing loss installation, sensory deprivation by having hearing restricted to some sounds. Thus, the introduction of sound stimuli, through the hearing aid, even after the privation period, can cause changes in the sensory system responsible for transmitting acoustic information.

The adaptation of hearing aids promotes neuronal plasticity. Neural networks are generated and areas of the brain that were not stimulated become stimulated, favoring the adaptation of the hearing aid and social reintegration of the elderly. In addition, the adaptation of the hearing aid can contribute to the stabilization of the hearing loss, namely, the reintroduction of certain sounds by the hearing aid can promote a positive plasticity (structural and functional reorganization of the central auditory system).

The longer an individual stays with hearing loss and without the use of hearing aids, the greater the negative effects on the perception of sound and performance in listening skills. The use of hearing aids favors amplification and modification of the sound stimulus so that it reaches the eardrum with quantity increase and quality, and promotes and stimulates the auditory skills.

Due to the improvement of the quality of sound that reaches the central auditory system, it is believed that after auditory stimulation for a certain period of time, the elderly tends to improve his auditory perception because there is a greater stimulation of the auditory cortex. This theory is grounded by the theory of brain plasticity, or because of high stimulation, which happens with the use of hearing aids: the brain region responsible for the understanding of the function and process the auditory information creates new neural network (plasticity), thus, generating a better performance of the individual. When this occurs, the elderly has a better hearing performance, because in fact there were positive brain changes.

In some cases, there is indication of auditory training, so that the auditory cortex can be potentially stimulated and thus there will be an improvement in hearing. Several surveys show that the auditory training is suitable for adults and the elderly with hearing loss, since this therapeutic resource improves perception and hearing in noisy or acoustically unfavorable environments.

Even with those seniors who have mild hearing loss, satisfaction with the use of hearing aids will not be great because of auditory processing disorders. Research claim that therein lies the importance of ear training because it will occur with an improvement in electrophysiological response (latency wave III in ABR) in auditory localization and speech understanding in noise [41].

This training becomes complementary to the use of hearing aids. Thus, it will be through training that the individual with hearing loss will be able to hone your listening skills so there is a better understanding of speech [42].

The auditory training can assist in the recognition of sounds that were not already heard and others that can be modified by technology, such as the lowering frequency that seeks to dislocate a high-frequency sound to a lower one.

The professional who will make the indication of the treatment must have concepts of neuroscience and aging, which should be considered at the time of the hearing aid selection and type of auditory training. Moreover, it is necessary to consider that there is brain reorganization and acclimatization with hearing aids and that these processes are closely related to cognition [43].

All this care and to look further, beyond the peripheral hearing loss, is essential for the individual with hearing aid, and notices an improvement in his understanding of speech.

The presence of hearing loss can lead to changes in the mood of the elderly and social change, taking them into isolation. Because of this, it is important to evaluate the benefits of hearing aids and how the technology can change the life and the neurologic system of the elderly.

5. The benefit of hearing aids

Modification is generated by the use of hearing aid. Benefit is the difference in the auditory performance of the individual with and without the use of this technological resource. It is expected that whenever the benefit obtained is positive, an improvement in auditory responses occurs. This is possible, as already mentioned above, due to neuronal plasticity, with no improvement in hearing thresholds or in the response of the cochlear hair cells, but with a change in the cortex, with better auditory responses.

The modification of auditory responses does not happen only by the input of the sound stimulus of higher quality or more audible. Rather, it is this better quality signal entering the hearing system that makes possible a change in neural networks, generating a better response in auditory sensation.

However, a positive benefit is not always observed. In some cases, the benefit is negative or zero, i.e., the elderly does not perceive changes in hearing with the hearing aid or even refers to a worsening. In these cases, the adaptation of the hearing aid becomes more difficult and the elderly will not make proper use of the device.

The benefit can be measured by objective and subjective tests. Objective tests assess quantitatively the improvement in hearing performance with the use of hearing aid. Usually, speech is used in noise test, functional gain, insertion responses, among other tests [44]. Speech in noise test is conducted in a soundproof booth, with calibration and standardization. It is supposed to get better performance with hearing aid.

Alongside, there are the subjective tests, such as self-assessment questionnaire, which are answered by individuals and seek to assess the feeling the individual has about the improvement in their hearing.

For many services, the subjective test has greater influence and relevance than the objective tests, since these show that the elderly are thinking about the hearing aid, as is its performance in communication activities and may differ from the data obtained in objective tests and influence more on whether or not to use the hearing aid.

The main questionnaires are HHIE (Hearing Handicap Inventory for the Elderly) [45], the APHAB (Abbreviated Profile of Hearing Aid Benefit) [46], and the COSI (Client Oriented Scale of Improvement) [47]. These questionnaires can be used alone or in a combined form and should be applied before and after using the device for the measurement of the benefit.

The HHIE seeks to assess the psychosocial effects of hearing deficiency in the elderly. The questionnaire contains 25 questions that are divided into two scales: social and emotional.

By means of these scales it is possible to assess how much the situations of difficult listening affect the individual's behavior and emotional response front to these situations. There are three possible answers: yes, no, and sometimes.

APHAB seeks to assess the hearing disability associated with hearing loss and how it was reduced after using the hearing aid. Therefore, this questionnaire should be applied before the use of hearing aid and after adaptation.

COSI focuses on individual listening difficulties. Before the adaptation, the individual must choose five categories in which I would like to hear well. For evaluation, two scales are used, a relative scale, which assesses the degree of change, and an absolute scale, which records the individual's final skill listening situations.

It is known that even being subjective, the benefit is influenced by cognitive issues, as with cognitive issue preserved, a more effective use of hearing aid will be made, and also the understanding of the auditory information, as well as the ability to understand speech in noisy environments [48]. In others, research is possible to see that the cognitive can change with the benefit of hearing aids [49].

The modification in many categories is just possible to be measured after 1 year of the use of hearing aid [48]. After 4 months of use of the hearing aid, it is possible to see a change in the quality of life of the elderly. Nevertheless, bigger modification in other categories is just perceived after 12 months of the use of this technology [49]. Some research looks for modification in the benefit after this period, like evaluating the benefit after 24 months of use. However, no significant differences have been observed because an acclimatization had occurred [50].

Many researches look for the benefit of the use of hearing aids. All of them show that the elderly have a significant change in their life to return to social activities and trying again new communication activities. In addition, it is possible to see a reduction in the emotional problems or social isolation [51].

One study evaluated the handicap (Hearing Handicap Inventory for Elderly, HHIE) before and after 6 months of use of hearing aids. One hundred and fifteen (115) elderly were divided into two groups according to the result of the dichotic digits test (normal or abnormal result). After 6 months there was a significant improvement only in the group with normal dichotic test digits. The author also states that the differences observed between the groups are not justified by memory issues, attention, or difficulty in fine motor. However, the central auditory processing, which when altered generates negative influence on the process of adaptation in the elderly [52].

Therefore, measuring the benefit is essential for a correct assessment of the hearing aid gains possible, as well as checking how the use of this technology is favoring a new neural network.

6. Final considerations

In assessing the issue and the hearing status in the elderly, many factors have to be taken into consideration so that appropriate amplification will be proposed and so the elderly make actual use of hearing aids and have the proper advantages.

With the beginning of the use of auditory processing tests to assess the elderly with hearing loss, a new scenario in audiology was established and became an integral care for the elderly hearing.

It is not enough to just consider the degree of peripheral hearing loss but also it is necessary to consider how listening skills are changed, so that a better fitting is indicated, as well as the attempted use of complementary technologies.

That way not only searches the degree of peripheral loss, but searches around which hearing abilities are altered. So, this way it is possible to select a better technology for the elderly. Considering what skills are altered, you can check which technology or which feature of the hearing aid can be used, favoring a better listening and speech understanding by the elderly, which will generate an effective use of the device.

In addition, having a better hearing, the elderly tend to relate better with people, not isolating or minimizing their quality of life and autonomy. Rather, they can develop their daily tasks more independently, which favors their mental, cognitive, and economic conditions.

Glossary

Age-related hearing loss (ARHL)	A synonym of presbycusis
Abbreviated Profile of Hearing Aid Benefit (APHAB)	A shortened version of the Profile of Hearing Aid Benefit, self-assessment, disability-based inventory that can be used to document the outcome of a hearing aid fitting
Client Oriented Scale of Improvement (COSI)	It is a clinical tool developed by NAL (National Acoustic Laboratories) for outcomes measurement. It is an assessment questionnaire for clinicians to use which allows them to document their client's goals/needs and measures improvements in hearing ability
Dichotic digits Test	This is an auditory processing test, which evaluates the ability to reproduce four digits (numbers), which are displayed in pairs, one on each ear, simultaneously
Frequency and Duration Standard	This is an auditory processing test, which assesses the ability to distinguish and name bass and treble, long and short stimuli.
GIN (Gaps-in-Noise) Test	This is an auditory processing test that evaluates which the lowest range in which you can see the occurrence of two auditory stimuli
Hearing Aid (HA)	HA is a little apparatus placed in the external meatus and that can amplify the sounds that reach the auditory system
Hearing Handicap Inventory for the Elderly (HHIE)	Is a 25-item self-assessment scale composed of two subscales (emotional and social/situational)
Identification of Synthetic Sentences	This is a test that evaluates the ability to understand speech in environments with competitive speech noise
Memory for verbal sounds	This is an auditory processing test that evaluates the memorizing ability of verbal sounds when they are presented in a particular sequence and must be played in the same sequence

Memory for nonverbal sounds	This is an auditory processing test that evaluates the memorizing ability of nonverbal sounds when they are presented in a particular sequence and must be played in the same sequence
Speech with noise	This is an auditory processing test, which evaluates the ability to understand speech in environments with background noise
Staggered Spondee Word (SSW) test	This is auditory processing test that evaluates the individual's ability to hear four words in sequence, the first in one ear, the second and third, both simultaneously, one in each ear and the last in the contralateral ear to what the first word was presented
Presbycusis	Loss of the hearing acuity in the elderly (i.e. >65 years) subjects
Sound localization	This is an auditory processing test that evaluates the ability to localize sound stimulus

Author details

Christiane Marques do Couto* and Izabella dos Santos Brites

*Address all correspondence to: christianemcouto@hotmail.com

Department of Human Development and Rehabilitation, Faculty of Medical Sciences, University of Campinas – UNICAMP, Campinas, SP, Brazil

References

[1] WHO. World report on ageing and Health. Geneva, Who Press, 2015. 247 p. ISBN 978 92 4 069481 1.

[2] Li, K.Z.H., Lindersberger, U. Relations between sensory/sensorimotor and cognitive function. Neurosci. Biobehav. Rev. 2002;26(7);777–783. DOI: 10.1016/S0149-7634(02)00073-8

[3] Gelfand, S. A. Essentials of Audiology. 4th ed. New York, Thieme, 2015. 639 p. ISBN:9781604068627

[4] Crews, J.E., Campbell, V.A. Vision impairment and hearing loss among community – dwelling older Americans: Implications for health and functioning. Am. J. Public Health. 2004;94(5);823–829. DOI: 10.2105/AJPH.94.5.823

[5] Schmiedt, R.A. The physiology of cochlear presbycusis. In: Gordon-Salant, S. et al. (eds.), The Aging Auditory System. Springer-Verlag, New York. 2010. Vol. 34; pp. 9–38. ISBN:978-1-44190993-0. DOI 10.1007/978-1-4419-0993-0

[6] Wingfield, A., Tun, P.A., McCoy, S.L. Hearing loss in older adulthood – what is and how it interacts with cognitive performance. Curr. Directions Psychol. Sci. 2005;14(3);144–148. DOI:10.1111/j.0963-7214.2005.00356.x

[7] Parham, K. et al. Comprehensive management of presbycusis: central and peripheral. Otolaryngol. Head Neck Surg. 2013;148(4); 537–539. DOI: 10.1177/0194599813477596

[8] Gopinath, B. et al. Prevalence of age-related hearing loss in older adults: Blue Mountain Study. Arch. Intern. Med. 2009;169(4);415–416.DOI:10.1001/archinternmed.2008.597

[9] Schuknecht, H.F. Further observations on the pathology of presbycusis. Arch. Otolaryngol. 1964;80;369–382. Available from: http://dx.doi.org/10.1001/archotol.1964.00750040381003.

[10] Rizk, H.G., Linthicum Jr., F.H. Histopathologic categorization of presbycusis. Otol. Neurotol. 2012;33;23–24. DOI: 10.1097/MAO.0b013e31821f84ee

[11] Martins, K. et al. Genetic and audiologic study in elderly with sensorineural hearing loss. CoDAS. 2013;25(3);224–228. DOI:10.1590/S2317-17822013000300006

[12] Kid III, A.R., Bao, J. Recent advances in the study of age-related hearing loss – a mini review. Gerontology. 2012;58(6);490–496. DOI: 10.1159/000338588

[13] Yamasoba, T. et al. Current concepts in age-related hearing loss: epidemiology and mechanistic pathways. Hear Res. 2013;303;30–38. DOI: 10.1016/j.heares.2013.01.021.

[14] Gilad, C., Glorig, A. Presbycusis: the aging ear. Part I. J. Am. Aud. Soc. 1979;4(5);195–206.

[15] Dalton, D.S. et al. The impact of hearing loss on quality of life in older adults. The Gerontologist. 2003;43(5);661–668. DOI:10.1093/geront/43.5.661

[16] WHO. The International Classification of Disability and Health (ICF). 2001. Available from: http://psychiatr.ru/download/1313?view=name=CF_18.pdf

[17] Dillon, H. Hearing Aids. Thieme. 2014;57(7);493. Available from: http://dx.doi.org/10.3342/kjorl-hns.2014.57.7.493

[18] American Speech-Hearing-Language Association. Guidelines for hearing aid fitting for adults. ASHA. 1997;2;123–130. DOI:10.1044/policy.GL1998-00012.

[19] Moore, D.R. Auditory processing disorder (APD): definition, diagnosis, neural basis and intervention. Audiol. Med. 2006;1(1);4–11. DOI:10.1080/16513860600568573

[20] Stach, B. A. et al. Special hearing aid considerations in elderly patients with auditory processing disorders. Ear Hearing. 1991;12(6);131–138. Available from: http://dx.doi.org/10.1097/00003446-199112001-00007

[21] Humes, L. et al. Central presbycusis: a review and evaluation of the evidence. J. Am. Acad. Audiol. 2012;23;635–666. DOI: 10.3766/jaaa.23.8.5

[22] Gates, G. Central presbycusis: an emerging view. Otolaryngol. Head Neck Surg. 2012;147(1);1–2. DOI: 10.1177/0194599812446282

[23] Rosdina, A.K. et al. Self-reported hearing loss among elderly Malaysians. Malaysian Family Phys. 2010;5(2);91–94.

[24] American Speech-Hearing-Language Association. Central auditory processing: current status of research and implications for clinical practice. ASHA. 1996;5;41–54.

[25] Fullgrabe, C., Moore, B.C.J., Stone, M.A. Age-group differences in speech identification despite matched audiometrically normal hearing: contributions from auditory temporal processing and cognition. Front. Aging Neurosci. 2014;6;1–25.

[26] Humes, L.E. Speech understanding in the elderly. J. Am. Acad. Audiol. 1996;7;161–167. DOI:10.3389/fnagi.2014.00347

[27] Humes, L.E., Christopherson, L. Speech identification difficulties of hearing- impaired elderly persons the contributions of auditory processing deficits. J. Speech Language Hearing Res. 1991;34;686–693. Available from: http://dx.doi.org/10.1044/jshr.3403.686

[28] Rajan, R., Cainer, E. Ageing without hearing loss or cognitive impairment causes a decrease in speech intelligibility only in informational maskers. Neuroscience. 2008;154;784–795. DOI:10.1016/j.neuroscience.2008.03.067

[29] Moore, D.R. Relation between speech-in-noise threshold, hearing loss and cognition from 40-69 years of age. PLoS One. 2014;9(9);107720. DOI: 10.1371/journal.pone.0107720

[30] Lunner, T. Cognitive function in relation to hearing aid use. Intl. J. Audiol. 2003;42;49–58. DOI:10.3109/14992020309074624

[31] Cardin, V. Effects of aging and adult-onset of hearing loss on cortical auditory regions. Front. Neurosci. 2016;10;1–12. DOI:10.3389/fnins.2016.60199

[32] Jerger, J., Oliver, T.A., Pirozzolo, F. Impact of central auditory processing disorder and cognitive deficit on the self-assessment of hearing handicap in the elderly. J. Am. Acad. Audiol. 1990;1;75–80.

[33] Cox, L.C. et al. Monotonic auditory processing disorders testes in the older adult population. J. Am. Acad. Audiol. 2008;19(4);293–308. Available from: http://dx.doi.org/10.3766/jaaa.19.4.3

[34] American Speech-Language-Hearing Association (ASHA). (Central) Auditory Processing Disorders [Technical Report]. 2005. Available from: http:// www.asha.org/docs/html/tr2005-00043.html.

[35] Bellis, T.J. Comprehensive central auditory assessment. In: BELLIS, T.J. Assessment and Management of central auditory processing disorders in the educational setting from science to practice. 2nd ed. NY: Delmar Thompsons Learning, 2003.

[36] Idrizbegovic, E. et al. Central auditory function in early Alzheimer's disease and in mild cognitive impairment. Age Ageing. 2011;40(2);249–254. DOI: 10.1093/ageing/afq168

[37] Roup, C.M., Wiley, T.L., Wilson, R.H. Dichotic word recognition in young and older adults. J. Am. Acad. Audiol. 2007;17(4);230–240. Available from: http://dx.doi.org/10.3766/jaaa.17.4.2

[38] Stewart, R., Wingfield, A. Hearing loss and cognitive effort in older adults' report accuracy for verbal materials. J. Am. Acad. Audiol. 2009;20(2);147–154. http://dx.doi.org/10.3766/jaaa.20.2.7

[39] Fitzgibbons, P.J., Gordon-Salant, S. Age-related differences in discrimination of temporal intervals in accented tone sequences. Hearing Res. 2010;264;41–47. DOI: 10.1016/j.heares.2009.11.008 DOI:10.1016%2Fj.heares.2009.11.008

[40] Gordon-Salant, S. Auditory temporal processing in elderly listeners. J. Am. Acad. Audiol. 1996;7;183–189.

[41] Gil, D., Iorio, M.C.M. Formal auditory training in adult hearing aid users. Clin. Sci. 2010;65(2);165–174. DOI:10.1590/S1807-59322010000200008

[42] Dubno, J.R. Benefits of auditory training for aided listening by older adults. Am. J. Audiol. 2013;22(2);335–338. DOI:10.1044/1059-0889(2013/12-0080)

[43] Pichora-Fuller, M.K., Singh, G. Effects of age on auditory and cognitive processing: implications for hearing aid fitting and audiologic rehabilitation. Trend. Amplif. 2006;10(1);29–59. DOI: 10.1177/108471380601000103

[44] Weinstein, B.E. Outcome measures in the hearing aid fitting. Trend. Amplif. 1997;2(4); 117–137. DOI: 10.1177/108471389700200402

[45] Ventry I., Weinsten, B.E. The hearing handicap inventory for the elderly: a new tool. Ear Hear. 1982;3;128–134. Available from: http://dx.doi.org/10.1097/00003446-198205000-00006

[46] Cox, R.M., Alexander, G.C. The abbreviated profile of hearing aid benefit. Ear Hear. 1995;16(2);176–183. Available from: http://dx.doi.org/10.1097/00003446-199504000-00005

[47] Dillon, H., James, A., Ginis, J. Client oriented scale of improvement (COSI) and its relationship to several other measures of benefit and satisfaction provided by hearing aids. J. Am. Acad. Audiol. 1996;8;27–43.

[48] Naylor, G., Elberling, C. Benefit from hearing aids in relation to the interaction between the user and the environment. Int. J. Audiol. 2003;42. DOI: http://dx.doi.org/10.3109/14992020309074627

[49] Mukrow, C.D., Tuley, M.R., Aguilar, C. Sustained benefits of hearing aids. J. Speech Language Hearing Res. 1992;35;1402–1405. DOI: 10.1044/jshr.3506.1402

[50] Humes, L.E., Wilson, D.L., Barlow, N.N., Garner, C. Chances in hearing aid benefit following 1 or 2 years of hearing aid use by older adults. J. Speech Language Hearing Res. 2002;445;772–782. DOI:10.1044/1092-4388

[51] Newman, C.W., Weinstein, B.E. The hearing handicap inventory for the elderly as a measure: of hearing aid benefit. Ear Hearing. 1988. Available from: https://doi.org/10.1097/00003446-198804000-00006

[52] Chmiel, R, Jerger, J. Hearing aid use, central auditory disorders and hearing handicap in elderly persons. J. Am. Acad. Audiol. 1996;7;190–202.

5

Sudden Sensorineural Hearing Loss

Harun Acıpayam, Hasan Emre Koçak and
Mustafa Suphi Elbistanlı

Abstract

Sudden hearing loss (SHL) is a common disease in the daily practice of ear-nose-throat (ENT) and audiology clinics. It is usually defined as a sensorineural type hearing loss of 30 dB or greater in three contiguous frequencies. Although several factors were suggested for the etiology of SHL, in most of the cases, no cause could be detected and they were diagnosed as idiopathic cases. Although certain specific treatments might be applied in patients with known etiology, corticosteroids are the main component in the treatment of idiopathic SHL. Many experts and centers have developed different treatment protocols with similar approaches. SHL is considered as an emergency in ENT, as it may cause a permanent loss in hair cells, if it is not treated or the treatment is not initiated at the right time. For patients, who did not or partially benefit from the initial treatment, different salvage treatment protocols had been developed. As SHL severely affects the patient's quality of life, its diagnosis and treatment should be thoroughly deliberated.

Keywords: idiopathic hearing loss, salvage treatment, sudden deafness, sudden hearing loss, treatment

1. Definition

Sudden hearing loss (SHL) is an ear-nose-throat (ENT) emergency and as sensorineural hearing loss of 30 dB or greater in three contiguous audiometric frequencies occurring over 72 h. SHL was first described by Dekleyn in [1] (**Figure 1A**). Although the definition mentioned above involves the widely accepted diagnostic criteria of SHL, it actually develops within hours or minutes and is usually noticed by the patient early in the morning or during a telephone conversation. With an approach from a broader perspective, we may consider all identifiable and measurable hearing losses, which are noticed within minutes or within few days, as SHL. Patients usually visit an ENT specialist in a great panic, thinking they became deaf.

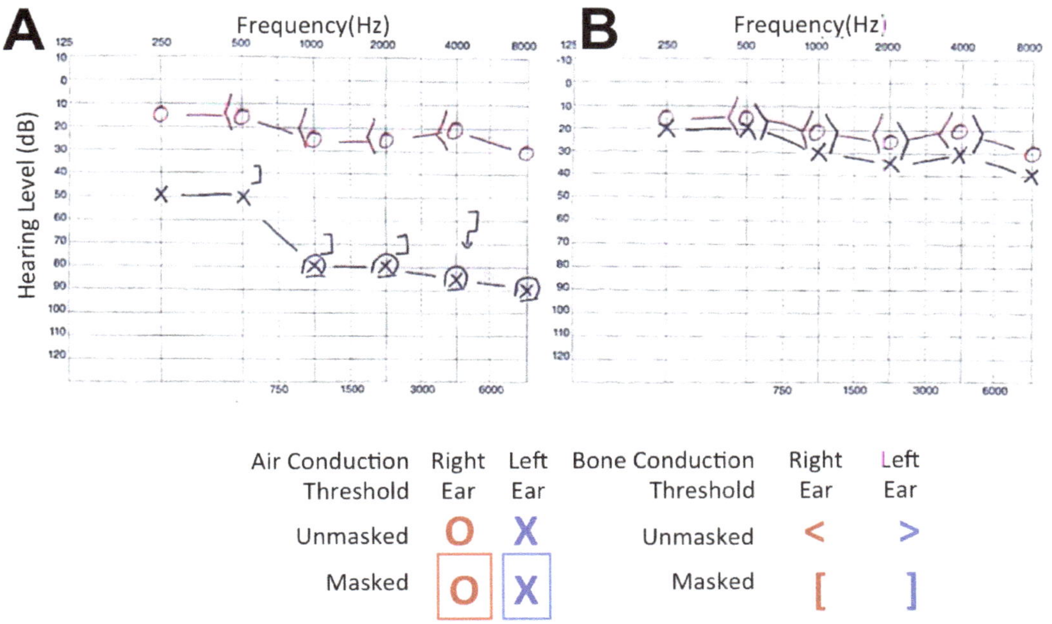

Figure 1. A: Sudden hearing loss sample audiogram. B: After treatment normal hearing level.

The physician, first of all, should calm the patient and then examine his/her medical condition, proceed immediately with the diagnostic procedures, identify—if possible—the etiology and initiate without delay the proper treatment.

2. Epidemiology

Although SHL constitutes approx. 1% of all sensorineural hearing losses, its incidence changes between 5 and 20/100,000 in different sources [2]. However, high rates such as 160/100,000 had also been reported in the literature and 40,000 new cases were diagnosed every year in the USA [3]. The incidence and prevalence of SHL are probably slightly higher than the calculated values, because of the rapid development of SHL and the high rate of spontaneous regression. Many studies reported that SHL had no correlation with gender and that the female/male ratio was equal or insignificantly different. In this regard, it seems safe to say that gender is not a risk factor. Similarly, no significant left/right ear distinction was detected. Although SHL is usually unilateral, bilateral involvement is emerging in a small percentage of patients (1–2%) [4]. Nevertheless, bilateral SHL is a more serious condition compared to the unilateral form and is often related to systemic disorders and has a relatively worse prognosis [5, 6].

3. Physiopathology

Among the mechanisms causing SHL, in particular, intracochlear hypoxia and/or inflammation in the inner ear play a major role. Several causes, which were suggested regarding the pathogenesis of SHL, can be classified into four main groups. Vascular factors, viral infections, autoimmune processes, and intracochlear membrane rupture.

3.1. Vascular factors

As it is well known, the cochlea is an end-organ perfused by the labyrinthine artery, which is a branch of the basilar artery and does not have collateral circulation [7]. The labyrinthine artery divides into two branches (vestibular and cochlear arteries) after entering through the internal acoustic meatus. The cochlear artery enters the cochlea after the division of its branch the vestibulocochlear artery [8]. Therefore, factors such as thrombi, emboli, atherosclerosis, vasospasm, and decreased blood flow may end up with vascular insufficiency and consequently a loss of function in the cochlea. A sudden interruption of the blood flow to the cochlea may induce the development of SHL, which will cause a complete restriction of the oxygen supply.

The obstructions in the vertebrobasilar system may also cause SHL. Here, it should be noticed that a bilateral SHL emerges, in these cases, as the basilar artery, which is the only artery supplying that region. Kim et al. [9] detected a thrombus in the bilateral distal vertebral artery in a patient with bilateral SHL and observed improvement after the restoration of the circulation with a stent. In his experimental study, Perlman [10] stated that the occlusion of the internal auditory artery caused changes in the cochlea secondary to the ischemia and some of these changes were irreversible. The difference of this study from SHL patients is that the findings in SHL are reversible. In a recent study similar to these studies, Chung [11] found out a relation between increased arterial stiffness and SHL development and the response to the treatment and drew attention to the development of SHL with vascular causes. Subclinical atherosclerosis has also been reported in the literature, as a cause of SHL [12].

It is understandable that the temporary and permanent problems in the cochlear microcirculation may cause SHL depending on the damage in the cochlear hair cells [13]. Also, in cases of hypercoagulopathy, a possible intravascular obstruction may cause damage to the inner ear in the same way. Bernhard [14] investigated the effects of experimental hyperfibrinogenemia on the development of SHL and stated that although they did not respond to corticosteroids, intravenous defibrinogenation (ancrod) improved the process markedly. He suggested that defibrinogenation therapy should be considered in non-responding SHL patients. Similarly, the relation of SHL to the factors capable of intravenous obstruction such as sickle cell anemia, Waldenström's macroglobulinemia or contraceptive drugs have been reported in the literature [15]. Although, some studies have suggested that there is a relationship between Factor V Leiden mutation and SHL, it was shown with a meta-analysis that there is no clear relationship between these two pathologies [16]. It is clear that these diseases will not respond to corticosteroids and the main treatment should be targeted to the underlying cause. Cochlear damage may emerge due to the acute emboli after the cardiopulmonary bypass or non-otological, non-coronary operations and may result consequently in SHL [17]. Any obstruction due to any reason in the cochlear microcirculation will manifest itself with the symptoms corresponding to the level of the obstructed artery. For example, although hearing loss is the only finding in the presence of the cochlear artery obstructions, vestibular symptoms like vertigo and tinnitus will also emerge in the labyrinthine artery obstructions along with hearing loss.

Cappacio [18] suggested that dyslipidemia may be associated with SHL pathogenesis and that impaired serum lipid profile might be an important factor in the development of SHL. There are also other studies in the literature linking serum lipid levels with SHL [19]. However, Chang [20] reported in his meta-analysis that serum lipid profile did not have any correlation with the SHL development and its prognosis.

3.2. Viral infections

Viral infections are the most common factor worldwide in the etiology of SHL in the world [21]. In 1954, Lindsay and Hemenway [22] detected degeneration in the tectorial membrane, corti organ, and stria vascularis during their cochlear histopathological examination and determined findings of measles virus in the cochlea in the same study. Shortly thereafter, Lindsay [23] found that the mumps virus could also do similar damage to the inner ear. So, the relationship between hearing loss and viral infections is well known. In a meta-analysis, it has been reported that 40% of the congenital hearing loss is associated with viruses and the most common responsible agent is cytomegalovirus (CMV) along with some other viral in utero infections [24]. Similarly, Van Dishoeck [25] suggested that there might be a link between upper airway infections and SHL and those upper airway viruses, which might penetrate the inner ear through neighborhood or blood circulation, might cause an immune response and an eventual damage in the inner ear. Especially, the herpes family of viruses, influenza, and enteroviruses are frequently blamed viral agents in the SHL etiology [26]. In a study conducted by Wilson [27], he found out that viral serology titration in SHL patients was two times higher than in the control group. It is believed that the penetration of the virus itself or the viral antigens to the membranous labyrinth cause an immune response and the resulting inflammation the formation of SHL. As the emerged cochleitis causes hearing loss, it is believed that the presence of vertigo, which is considered as a sign of bad prognosis for SHL, depends on the labyrinthitis emerging concomitantly.

In addition to the viral infections, bacteria can also cause the formation of SHL. In the USA, the two most common bacterial diseases causing SHL are Lyme disease and syphilis [28]. Lyme disease is caused by Borrelia burgdorferi and in long-term it may involve neurologic structures, especially the seventh nerve, which may cause facial paralysis. It may also cause hearing loss due to the involvement of the eighth nerve [28]. Although some studies showed that the incidence of Lyme disease is relatively high in SHL (up to 20%), some other reported very low rates [29, 30]. Syphilis is a systemic infection caused by *Treponema pallidum* and may present diverse clinical manifestations. Especially at the stage of neurosyphilis, if the neuritis of eighth nerve and cochleitis are added to the picture, it is called as otosyphilis. Otosyphilis may be encountered in different forms such as SHL, progressive hearing loss, fluctuating hearing loss or Meniere's syndrome [31].

In fact, viral infection hypothesis depends on three possible mechanisms considering its relation to the hearing loss [32]. The first of them, as mentioned above, is that the virus itself or its antigens, which may induce an immune response, penetrate the inner ear, and may cause cochleitis and neuritis in the cochlear nerve. The path may be hematogenous, but it may also spread directly through the neighborhood. The cerebrospinal fluid may be also a vehicle for the spread of the virus. The second hypothesis is that the latent virus infection in the inner ear may reactivate due to several reasons and cause SHL. Especially, it is a fact that *Varicella zoster* and other neurotropic viruses may cause latent virus infections, which strengthens this hypothesis. The next hypothesis is more complicated than the first two hypotheses and is indirectly related to viruses as well. As follows: the antibodies found in the systemic circulation and secreted against the viral antigens outside the inner ear may cause the development of a cross-reaction against the structural antigens in the inner ear, which may damage the inner ear and consequently cause hearing loss. In one respect, this last theory is an example of the relation between SHL and autoimmunity.

These findings, clinical, and histopathological studies eventually give the impression that viral etiology is one of the main etiologies in SHL. Nevertheless, it is also believed that the corticosteroids, which constitute the main therapeutic approach to SHL, have an anti-inflammatory effect in the inner ear, cures the emerged cochleitis, and enable healing through these mechanisms.

3.3. Autoimmunity

Autoimmunity theory is based on the main principle of the cross-reaction of the circulating antibodies or activated-cytotoxic T cells with the inner ear antigens [33]. The antibodies in the systemic circulation may be formed not only against a virus or bacterium, but also against several allergens. Eventually, these antibodies may become sensitive to the target antigens in the inner ear such as Type 2 collagen, tectorin, and beta-actin. The best documented among these antigens is the choline transporters like protein 2 (CTL-2) an inner ear glycoprotein [34–38]. In a study, antibodies formed against CLK-2 were detected in the systemic circulation in 9 of 20 patients [39]. In an experimental study on mice with Cogan syndrome, it was shown that the antibodies, which were formed against some supportive cells called CD148 and against connexin 26 (a well-known gap-junction protein), caused hearing loss [40].

In some SHL patients, antibodies against some cochlear proteins (p30, p80) and against some antigens such as Type 2 collagen and cardiolipin in the membranous labyrinth [41–43]. In some studies, it was also found out that the levels of some T-lymphocyte substances like C3b were increased in SHL [44]. Anti-endothelial antibodies (AECA) present another example. These antibodies are a group of heterogeneous autoantibodies that develop against endothelial cells and cause damage to the vessel walls. These antibodies may cause inflammation in the vascular endothelial cells in many different regions of the body via the immune system. They were also associated with many connective tissue disorders and systemic vasculitis; therewith, they got specific terminological naming [45]. The relationship between AECA and SHL was demonstrated with several studies [46, 47]. Harris reported that the relationship between circulating antibodies and bilateral, progressive, and fluctuating SHL was sufficiently evident [48]. In this study, although he detected antibodies against an antigen, which he thought was specific to the inner ear. He concluded that his further analyses revealed that this antigen was heat-shock protein 70 (Hsp-70) and that it existed not only in the inner ear, but also in different regions of the body. The relationship between the anti-Hsp70 antibodies and SHL were tried to be confirmed by further studies [49, 50].

It has also been reported in the literature that there is a relation between systemic lupus erythematosus (SLE) and SHL. It was reported that circulating autoantibodies might enter into the reaction directly with the inner ear antigens in SLE patients and the activated T cells might increase the levels of intracellular interferon gamma and some other cytokines and thus cause cellular damage [51]. Additionally, it is well known that in SLE, circulation antibodies such as anticardiolipin antibody, lupus anticoagulant, and anti-β2 GP1, antiphospholipid antibodies cause emboli and microinfarcts in the systemic circulation. As these antibodies may cause the same problems in the cochlear microcirculation, they may also cause SHL with the mechanism explained in the vascular hypothesis of SHL. Meanwhile, it was also stated in the literature that the SHL, which is believed to be developed due to SLE, might improve with a proper anticoagulant treatment [52, 53].

Hearing losses, which are believed that they develop in relationship with autoimmunity and manifest themselves with progressive, recurrent, and fluctuating clinical picture, are also called autoimmune hearing loss or autoimmune inner ear disease [54]. Yoo [41] created hearing loss in rats with Type 2 collagen immunization and showed the monoclonal antibodies, which were formed against the antigen related to the otic capsule, with radioimmunoassay. Harris [55] identified five antibodies formed against the inner ear antigens and suggested that the inner ear might have its own immunoreactive mechanism apart from the systemic immune response, but this was not supported by studies conducted after this hypothesis was introduced. Lymphocyte transformation and Western-blot tests are recommended for the diagnosis of the autoimmune hearing loss. Heywood [56] used infliximab in the treatment of fluctuating and progressive high-frequency recurrent hearing loss and reported that the patients benefited from this anti-TNF-alpha agent. Although all these findings might show the place of the autoimmunity in the etiology of SHL, there is still a need for further studies with larger samples size, as the sample sizes in the available studies are relatively small.

3.4. Intracochlear membrane rupture

Round- and oval-window membranes are two anatomical structures that separate the inner and middle ear from each other. These structures are responsible for restricting the endolymph to the inner ear and for preventing its penetration to the middle ear. There are other additional membranes in the inner ear that prevent the endolymph from interfering with the perilymph, and it is well known that their rupture will cause hearing loss. Goodhill [57] detected a perilymph fistula in three patients with SHL. Simmons [58] was one of the earliest authors, who suggested that the labyrinthine membrane damages might play a role in the etiology of SHL. Gussen [59] has identified healed Reissner membrane in the temporal bone dissections and succeeded to reveal membrane ruptures in the SHL etiology. Similarly, Kamerer [60] demonstrated microfissures between the posterior canal ampulla and the round-window niche during his temporal bone studies. Although there are other studies with small patient sizes, the main question is whether the hearing losses depending on membrane ruptures should be classified as SHL. Because, in that case, we have to assume that SHL arises from a mechanical problem and the treatment procedure should be based mainly on surgical or conservative procedures. But, the main thing that should be known about these patients is that they will not respond to standard SHL treatment protocols. However, if we look at the classic definition of SHL, they also conform to the SHL definition.

4. Histopathology

The histopathology of SHL is quite diverse because of the several factors blamed regarding its etiology. In the temporal bone studies, as mentioned above, along with the membrane ruptures, degenerative findings such as atrophy in the corti organ, loss of cochlear neurons, and neuron fibrils might be encountered in the viral etiology. On the other hand, histopathological findings such as labyrinthine fibrosis and new bone formation are the predominant histopathological findings in vascular events. Yood [61] observed certain changes in 7 of 11 temporal bones in his histopathological study. These changes include especially damage to the corti organ or loss of total corti organ; even it may differ according to the etiology. On the other hand, Vasama [62] determined in his study on 12 temporal bones degeneration and loss in the spiral ligament and stria vascularis. He also observed cochlear ossification in one patient. Since SHL's etiology is multifactorial, multiple histopathological findings are expected and it can be suggested that majority of these findings might be reversible regarding the spontaneous healing rates of SHL.

5. Etiology

Although an etiological factor could be determined only in a small number of SHL patients, a wide spectrum of etiologic factors and diseases were blamed. Among these, infectious cause being in the first place, vascular causes, endothelial dysfunctions, hyperlipidemia, hypercoagulopathy, increased oxidative stress, autoimmunity, trauma, neurological disorders, endocrinopathies, iron deficiency anemia, neoplastic causes, paraneoplastic causes, and toxic causes are the most important factors. The most blamed causes in the SHL etiology are shown in **Table 1**. But it should be emphasized that none of these factors has been confirmed as a cause of SHL and idiosyncrasy is still the most common category in SHL (**Table 1**).

Vascular Causes	**Trauma**
Hypercoagulopathy	Perilymph fistula
Vertebrobasilar Insufficiency	Round window rupture
Thrombo-embolism	Rupture of the oval window
Sickle Cell Anemia	Intralabyrinthine hemorrhage
Moyamoya disease	Temporal bone fractures
Polycythemia vera	Previous otological surgeries

Atherosclerotic disorders	Previous cardiopulmonary surgeries
Arteriovenous malformations	Acoustic trauma
Aneurysm	
Erythrocyte Deformities	**Neoplastic Causes**
Infection	Acoustic Schwannoma
Viral Causes	Multiple Myeloma
Herpes viridea family (HSV Type 1, 2; VZV, CMV, EBV)	Metastatic tumors
Mumps	Meningeal carcinomatosis
Rubella	
Rubeola	
HIV	**Endocrine Causes**
Influenza family	Hypothyroidism
Enteroviridea family	Iron deficiency anemia
Adenovirus	Diabetes mellitus
Human Spumaretrovirus	**Toxic Causes**
Bacteria-Parasite	Aminoglycosides
Treponema pallidum	Gold
Borrelia burgdorferi	Quinine
Toxoplasma gondii	Iron-containing drugs
Mycoplasma spp.	ACE inhibitors
Cryptococcus spp.	Loop Diuretics
Meningococci	Cisplatin
Enterobacteriae	Aspirin
Autoimmune Causes	Chemotherapeutic agents
Autoimmune inner ear disease	Phosphodiesterase Type-5 inhibitors
Crohn's Disease	Heroin
Ulcerative Colitis	Narcotic analgesics
SLE	Benzodiazepines
Small vessel vasculitis	**Neurological Causes**
Cogan syndrome	Multiple Sclerosis
Antiphospholipid Antibody Syndrome	**Psychiatric Causes**
Sarcoidosis	Histrionic (somatoform) deafness
Endolymphatic hydrops	**İdiosyncrasy** (most common cause)

Table 1. Etiology of sudden hearing loss.

6. Medical history and physical examination

Medical history is typical in SHL. Patients usually notice in the morning, during a telephone conversation, after exiting a noisy environment that their hearing sense is suddenly disappeared and generally they visit panicked the nearest physician with a fear of being deaf. In sudden hearing loss, as patients consult immediately a physician, early diagnosis and treatment are possible. During the physical examination, as no SHL-specific finding can be detected during the bilateral otomicroscopic examination, otoscopic examination is usually normal. In some cases, there can be an obstructive ear plug, which may be removed with difficulty. At the same time, in patients with otological disorders like chronic otitis media and tympanic membrane retraction, previous audiometry reports might be needed for the diagnosis and especially in patients with presbyacusis and missing audiometry reports, diagnosing is relatively difficult. In such cases, we have to depend only on the anamnesis. In the anamnesis, the important points are the presence of tinnitus and ringing, the presence of concomitant vertigo, and presence of a similar event in the past. Questioning of these aspects will provide useful information regarding the differential diagnosis. The patients should also be evaluated for the known chronic diseases and used medication. Especially autoimmune disorders, coagulation disorders, cardiovascular diseases, previous infectious diseases, and trauma should be questioned. Following the physical examination, hearing examination (Weber, Rinne) should be carried out in order to evaluate the type and severity of the hearing loss. Afterwards, the diagnosis should be confirmed with pure-tone audiometry.

7. Diagnosis

7.1. Audiology

The audiological examination is the most important process regarding the diagnosis. Pure-tone audiometry may enable a definitive diagnosis and also provide information about the severity of the hearing loss and the type of the audiological curve with additional data related to both differential diagnosis and prognosis. In addition to the pure-tone audiometry, tympanometric examination, acoustic reflex, speech audiometry may support the diagnosis. Such additional tests are not always needed. They are only recommended if there is a clinical necessity. In patients who cannot comply with the audiometry process ABR might be useful for the diagnosis. A definitive diagnosis of SHL can be made, if a hearing loss of 30 dB or greater is observed in three contiguous frequencies.

7.2. Laboratory analysis

As several different causes were suggested in respect of SHL etiology, the necessity of routine laboratory examination is still disputable regarding the diagnosis. The general consensus is that laboratory examination should be carried out only for the suspected etiological factors. If a viral involvement is suspected, viral antigen titration; if an autoimmune mechanism is suspected, levels of the relevant auto-antibodies; thyroid function tests, homocysteine, PT, APTT, INR or markers like specific factor levels, Elisa for HIV, HCV viruses, fasting blood sugar level, HbA1C, lipid profile, VDRL, RPR for syphilis, Lyme titration, serum iron levels can be checked. The control of all these parameters in each patient is not reasonable and also not always possible so that it is much more appropriate to make these analyses only in suspected etiological cases.

7.3. Radiology

In SHL, unlike the laboratory examinations, a radiological examination should be definitely performed considering the differential diagnosis. Approximately in 1% of patients diagnosed with SHL, a tumor was identified in the cerebellopontine angle. Therefore, a contrast-enhanced, thin-sectioned temporal MRI must be carried out regarding the differential diagnosis and to determine the etiological factor. In MRI examination, we may observe a space-occupying mass lesion and also in SHL cases with vascular pattern, we may also observe hyperintensity in the pre-contrast examinations depending on the methemoglobin accumulated in the inner ear. In the presence of inflammation, hyperintensity might be observed in the 3D-flair sequence depending on the accumulation of the proteinous materials in the dense exudation [63]. Regarding the literature, the rate of the patients with MRI findings related to SHL was between 27 and 53% [64, 65]. In addition, MRI may also enable the identification of AICA aneurysms and vertebrobasilar system anomalies.

8. Treatment

As the etiological factor is mostly not identifiable in SHL, its treatment is arranged in certain protocols. Several therapeutic modalities clinically different but similar in respect of main aspects have been developed. Systemic corticosteroids are beyond dispute the main therapeutic agents and they are also considered as the golden standard in the literature. Moreover, multiple medical agents can be used in the treatment. In patients, who did not respond or partially respond to the primary treatment, salvage treatment should be implemented. Although these treatments may change according to the patient and physician's algorithm, it should be initiated with the primary treatment. In SHL cases with identified etiology, treatment should be targeted to the underlying disorder. Hereinafter, the treatment protocols especially for the idiopathic SHL will be discussed.

8.1. Medical treatment

8.1.1. Systemic corticosteroids

They are currently the main therapeutic agents (**Figure 1B**). They should be included in the treatment protocols of SHL cases with unknown etiology. Although the mechanism of action of the corticosteroids considering the SHL pathogenesis is not fully elucidated, it is believed that they decrease the inflammation in the inner ear and accelerate the regeneration. An early initiation of the systemic corticosteroid therapy enables a relatively better respond to the treatment [66]. Wilson [66], in his randomized double-blind placebo-controlled study, showed clearly the positive effect of the corticosteroids on the SHL. The following numerous studies confirmed these findings. Although there are few studies in the literature reporting that corticosteroids are ineffective, we observed in our clinical practice, that they are highly effective and included them in our routine treatment protocol. Systemic corticosteroid therapy is a short-term treatment, which is initiated with a dose of 1 mg/kg and continued with a gradual dose reduction. This treatment with gradually declining dosage enables that the suppressed adrenal glands have enough time to produce steroids again. The SHL treatment guideline, which was published by the American Otolaryngology Academia in 2012, indicated the corticosteroids as the first-line therapy. It was stated that a dose of 1 mg/kg for approx. 10–14 days is sufficient for the treatment of SHL [67]. Systemic corticosteroids have diverse side effects. The most common side effects are acne, blurred vision, cataract or glaucoma, sleeping problems, hypertension, increased appetite, hypertrichosis, insomnia, immunosuppression, muscle weakness, irritability, uneasiness, osteoporosis, increase of insulin need in diabetic patients, diffuse edema due to the water and salt retention in kidneys, aseptic necrosis in the femur head. Steroids should be used carefully particularly in patients with comorbidity and in the pregnant and the risk-benefit of the therapy should be thoroughly evaluated. If in these patients corticosteroid use is risky, intratympanic corticosteroid injection should be considered in the primary treatment [68, 69].

8.1.2. Antiviral agents

Antiviral agents were added to the treatment protocols in many clinics in respect of the findings related to the role of viruses in the etiology of SHL. Even though the responsible virus mostly cannot be isolated, they are used in combination with corticosteroids. Stookross created labyrinthitis with HSV-1 antigens in an experimental animal study and applied corticosteroids as monotherapy or in combination with acyclovir. He observed that the viral replication was suppressed in the 14th day of the treatment and discontinued the application. He concluded that acyclovir and corticosteroid combination provided better recovery compared to the corticosteroid monotherapy [70]. Park [71] conducted a study with 85 patients and administered a combination of steroid + antiviral + anticoagulant + stellar ganglion blockage to one group and corticosteroid monotherapy to another group. He observed better recovery in the combination group. In contrary, Westerlaken [72] conducted a placebo-controlled randomized study with 91 patients and administered acyclovir + corticosteroid combination in one group and corticosteroid alone in the other group. He concluded that antiviral agents did not provide additional benefit. Similarly, Tucci [73] concluded in his study conducted with 105 patients that the addition of valacyclovir to the corticosteroid therapy did not provide additional benefit and that antiviral treatment is ineffective in SHL. Antiviral agents like valacyclovir and famciclovir might be used instead acyclovir.

8.1.3. Vasodilators and plasma expanders

The goal of this treatment is to increase the blood perfusion in the inner ear and the oxygenation. In order to obtain this, either the arteries in the inner ear should be dilated or the viscosity of the blood should be decreased in order to increase its fluidity. Papaverine, histamine, and carbogen (mixture of 5% CO_2 and 95% O_2) were used for this purpose in the literature. In particular, agents such as histamine and papaverine have found effective as they reduced systemic vascular pressure [74]. Compared to these agents, carbogen treatment is more effective and provides a safer treatment option, which means that the oxygenation of the perilymph changes depending on the blood concentration of O_2 and CO_2 and systemic vascular resistance. Especially, the partial CO_2 level in the peripheral blood is an important stimulator of the perilymphatic oxygenation. Kallinen demonstrated that carbogen treatment increased the perilymphatic oxygenation more than 100% O_2 [75]. There are plenty of studies conducted with piracetam, prostaglandin E1, dextran (plasma expander) and various rheological agents. These agents are not used alone in the idiopathic SHL but added to the systemic corticosteroid therapy protocol as adjuvant agents [76].

8.1.4. Diuretics

If endolymphatic hydrops is responsible for SHL, diuretics may be used in the treatment. Besides this, they are not included in the standard treatment protocols.

8.1.5. Magnesium

Nageris [77] showed that corticosteroid and magnesium combination is more effective in SHL compared to the corticosteroid and placebo combination. Similarly, Gordin [78] determined also that magnesium treatment had positive effects on the recovery in SHL via antioxidant effects and recommended the addition of magnesium to the treatment regimes as an antioxidant.

8.1.6. Low-density lipoprotein apheresis

Low-density lipoproteins may cause the development of SHL, if their elevated concentrations increase the plasma viscosity. In a study with a large sample size, it was reported that the treatment with low-density lipoprotein apheresis and fibrinogen increased the recovery rate in SHL although the result was not statistically significant [79].

8.1.7. Ozone therapy

Ragab [92] conducted a study with 45 patients and reinjected the 100 ml blood, which he had taken from the patients and exposed to a 1:1 gas mixture of oxygen and ozone. After the implementation of this treatment protocol for a total of 10 sessions twice a week, he compared the ozone group with the placebo group. He concluded that a significant recovery was observed in the ozone group.

8.2. Salvage therapies

If known treatment protocols provided no or limited response in SHL patients, salvage treatments should be considered. The efficacy of the salvage treatments, which became popular in the recent years, was shown in different studies with control groups. Hyperbaric O_2 and intratympanic steroid treatment can be mentioned among these treatment principles.

8.2.1. Intratympanic steroid therapy (ITS)

We already mentioned that corticosteroids had a well-established efficacy in the treatment of SHL. In patients, in whom corticosteroids have limited use or efficacy, they may be administered intratympanically with different methods. Thus corticosteroids penetrate through the middle ear membranes to the inner ear and achieve high concentrations, which consequently increased the recovery rate [80]. ITS is a treatment method, which has an ongoing increase in popularity, minimizes the side effects of corticosteroids and enables achievement of therapeutic steroid concentrations with low doses. ITS is not only effective as a salvage therapy, but it also enables good results if it is combined with systemic corticosteroids during the primary treatment or administered as the primary treatment agent in patients, who cannot tolerate systemic steroids [81–84].

8.2.2. Hyperbaric oxygen therapy

Hyperbaric O_2 therapy (HBO) is another salvage therapy method and investigated with a large number of studies. The basic principle is to increase the partial O_2 pressure, which is decreased in the perilymph and cochlea in patients with SHL. Experimental studies have demonstrated that HBO increased the partial O_2 pressure in the inner ear [85]. The increased partial O_2 pressure in the inner ear supplies the needed O_2 even if the blood flow is decreased and stimulates the cells. It decreases the platelet aggregation and increases the flexibility of the erythrocytes which positively affects the nutrition of the inner ear. Several recent studies demonstrated that the combined use of HBO therapy and corticosteroids or the use of HBO as a salvage therapy had positive effects on SHL [86–91]. The basic principle of the HBO therapy is to apply 100% O_2 with a 2–3 atm pressure in repeated doses and to increase the O_2 pressure in the inner ear with a controlled process. During the application of this procedure, the possible damage of the free O_2 radicals should be taken into consideration.

8.3. Surgical treatment

Surgical treatment can only be carried out in a subgroup of patients with a known etiology. Cases with membrane ruptures, intracochlear membrane ruptures, endolymphatic hydrops, and acoustic neuroma can be treated with surgical interventions.

9. Prognosis

As SHL has a multifactorial etiology, the prognosis is variable. Considering all SHL cases, spontaneous regression rate is over 60%. In addition, some factors, which have positive or negative effects on the prognosis, have been described. Even though these factors do not change the treatment, they provide useful information about the course of the disease.

The most important criterion is the time between the emergence of the symptoms and the initiation of the treatment. The prognosis is much better in patients started treatment early. Another factor is the age of the patient. An age less than 15 or greater than 65 years indicates a bad prognosis. The prognosis worsens with the severity of the hearing loss. Although the prognosis is relatively better in the low-frequency hearing loss compared to the high-frequency hearing loss, an ascendant type audiometric curve promises a better prognosis than the descendant type audiometric curve. The presence of vertigo and nystagmus, which shows that vestibular system is also affected, is a sign of bad prognosis. In contrary, tinnitus indicates a good prognosis in SHL, because tinnitus is considered as a sign that the hair cells in the inner ear are not completely destroyed. Bilateral SHL has a relatively worse prognosis. Increased sedimentation rate and an increase in the high sensitive CRP levels are related to the severity of the inflammation and thus to the bad prognosis. In SHL, recovery can be observed within 6 months to 1 year, it is wise to arrange the pre-rehabilitation follow-up plan according to this duration. In SHL patients, who did not show any recovery after 1 year, hearing rehabilitation can be planned upon the patient's request and according to the severity of the hearing loss.

10. Conclusion

As we have seen, SHL preserves its darkness as an enigma of ENT world. There are several already-published and a large number of ongoing studies on the etiology and treatment of SHL in the literature. Although certain diagnosis and treatment algorithms developed for SHL are already available, they cannot be implemented in all SHL cases. If corticosteroids cannot deliver sufficient results, there are not much treatment choices. Further studies for a full elucidation of the physiopathology, etiology, and treatment of SHL are required.

Abbreviations

SHL	Sudden hearing loss
ENT	Ear-nose-throat
CMV	Cytomegalovirus
CTL-2	Choline transporters like protein 2
AECA	Anti-endothelial antibodies
Hsp-70	Heat-shock protein 70
SLE	Systemic lupus erythematosus
ITS	Intratympanic steroid therapy
HBO	Hyperbaric O_2 therapy

Author details

Harun Acıpayam[1]*, Hasan Emre Koçak[2] and Mustafa Suphi Elbistanlı[2]

*Address all correspondence to: harunacipayam@gmail.com

1 Department of Otolaryngology, Kanuni Sultan Süleyman Training and Research Hospital-Beylikdüzü Campus, İstanbul, Turkey

2 Department of Otolaryngology, Bakırköy Sadi Konuk Training and Research Hospital, İstanbul, Turkey

References

[1] Kleyn AD. Sudden complete or partial loss of function of the octavus-system in apparently normal persons. Acta Oto-Laryngologica. 1944;**32**(5):407-429

[2] Oiticica J, Bittar RSM. Metabolic disorders prevalence in sudden deafness. Clinics. 2010;**65**(11):1149-1153

[3] Stachler RJ, Chandrasekhar SS, Archer SM, Rosenfeld RM, Schwartz SR, Barrs DM, et al. Clinical practice guideline: Sudden hearing loss. Otolaryngology and Head and Neck Surgery. 2012;**146**(3):1-35

[4] Sara SA, Teh BM, Friedland P. Bilateral sudden sensorineural hearing loss. The Journal of Laryngology & Otology. 2014 Jan;**128**(S1):8-15

[5] Fetterman BL, Luxford WM, Saunders JE. Sudden bilateral sensorineural hearing loss. Laryngoscope. 1996;**106**:1347-1350

[6] JH O, Park K, Lee SJ, Shin YR, Choung YH. Bilateral versus unilateral sudden sensorineural hearing loss. Otolaryngology and Head and Neck Surgery. 2007;**136**:87-91

[7] Lister RJ, Rhoton AL Jr, Matsushima T, Peace DA. Microsurgical anatomy of the posterior inferior cerebellar artery. Neurosurgery. 1982;**10**(2):170-199

[8] Çelik O. Otoloji-Nörootoloji. Manisa, Türkiye: Elit Ofset; 2013

[9] Kim JH, Roh KJ, Suh SH, Lee KY. Improvement of sudden bilateral hearing loss after vertebral artery stenting. Journal of Neurointerventional Surgery. 2016;**8**(3):12-13

[10] Perlman HB, Kimura R, Fernandez C. Experiments on temporary obstruction of the internal auditory artery. The Laryngoscope. 1959;**69**(6):591-613

[11] Chung JH, Lee SH, Park CW, Kim C, Park JK, Shin JH. Clinical significance of arterial stiffness in idiopathic sudden sensorineural hearing loss. The Laryngoscope. 2016;**126**(8):1918-1922

[12] Rajati M, Azarpajooh MR, Mouhebati M, Nasrollahi M, Salehi M, Khadivi E, Nourizadeh N, Hashemi F, Bakhshaee M. Is sudden hearing loss associated with atherosclerosis? Iranian Journal of Otorhinolaryngology. 2016;**28**(86):189

[13] Koçak HE, Filiz Acıpayam AŞ, Acıpayam H, Çakıl Erdoğan B, Alakhras WM, Kıral MN, Kayhan FT. Microvascular dysfunction affects the development and prognosis of sudden idiopathic hearing loss. Clinical Otolaryngology. 2017;**42**(3):602-607

[14] Weiss BG, Bertlich M, Bettag SA, Desinger H, Ihler F, Canis M. Drug-induced defibrinogenation as new treatment approach of acute hearing loss in an animal model for inner ear vascular impairment. Otology & Neurotology. 2017;**38**(5):648-654

[15] Hanna GS. Sudden deafness and the contraceptive pill. The Journal of Laryngology and Otology. 1986;**100**(6):701-706

[16] Shu J, Si Y, Yin S, He M. Association between the V Leiden G1691A mutation and sudden sensorineural hearing loss in Italian population: A meta-analysis. European Archives of Oto-Rhino-Laryngology. 2016;**273**(9):2467-2472

[17] Sargent EW. Sudden sensorineural hearing loss following nonotologic, noncardiopulmonary bypass surgery. Archives of Otolaryngology – Head & Neck Surgery. 1997;**123**(9):994-998

[18] Capaccio P, Ottaviani F, Cuccarini V, Bottero A, Schindler A, Cesana BM, et al. Genetic and acquired prothrombotic risk factors and sudden hearing loss. Laryngoscope. 2007;**117**:547-551

[19] Cadoni G, Scipione S, Agostino S, Addolorato G, Cianfrone F, Leggio L, Paludetti G, Lippa S. Coenzyme Q 10 and cardiovascular risk factors in idiopathic sudden sensorineural hearing loss patients. Otology & Neurotology. 2007;**28**(7):878-883

[20] Chang IJ, Kang CJ, Yueh CY, Fang KH, Yeh RM, Te Tsai Y. The relationship between serum lipids and sudden sensorineural hearing loss: A systematic review and meta-analysis. PLoS One. 2015;**10**(4):e0121025

[21] Linthicum FH Jr, Doherty J, Berliner KI. Idiopathic sudden sensorineural hearing loss: Vascular or viral? Otolaryngology – Head and Neck Surgery. 2013;**149**(6):914-917

[22] Lindsay JR, Hemenway WG. LIV inner ear pathology due to measles. Annals of Otology, Rhinology and Laryngology. 1954;**63**(3):754-771

[23] Lindsay JR, Davey PR, Ward PH. Inner ear pathology in deafness due to mumps. The Annals of Otology, Rhinology, and Laryngology. 1960;**69**:918-935

[24] Cohen BE, Durstenfeld A, Roehm PC. Viral causes of hearing loss: A review for hearing health professionals. Trends in Hearing. 2014;**18**:2331216514541361

[25] Van Dishoeck HAE, Bierman TA. Sudden perceptive deafness and viral infection: Report of the first one hundred patients. Annals of Otology, Rhinology and Laryngology. 1957;**66**(4):963-980

[26] Chau JK, Lin JR, Atashband S, Irvine RA, Westerberg BD. Systematic review of the evidence for the etiology of adult sudden sensorineural hearing loss. The Laryngoscope. 2010;**120**(5):1011-1021

[27] Wilson WR, Veltri RW, Laird N, Sprinkle PM. Viral and epidemiologic studies of idiopathic sudden hearing loss. Otolaryngology – Head and Neck Surgery. 1983;**91**(6):653-658

[28] Kuhn M, Heman-Ackah SE, Shaikh JA, Roehm PC. Sudden sensorineural hearing loss: A review of diagnosis, treatment, and prognosis. Trends in Amplification. 2011;**15**(3):91-105

[29] Lorenzi MC, Bittar RS, Pedalini ME, Zerati F, Yoshinari NH, Bento RF. Sudden deafness and Lyme disease. The Laryngoscope. 2003;**113**(2):312-315

[30] Walther LE, Hentschel H, Oehme A, Gudziol H, Beleites E. Lyme disease—A reason for sudden sensorineural hearing loss and vestibular neuronitis? Laryngo-Rhino-Otologie. 2003;**82**(4):249-257

[31] Marra CM. Update on neurosyphilis. Current Infectious Disease Reports. 2009;**11**(2):127

[32] Wilson WR. The relationship of the herpesvirus family to sudden hearing loss: A prospective clinical study and literature review. The Laryngoscope. 1986;**96**(8):870-877

[33] Greco A, Fusconi M, Gallo A, Marinelli C, Macri GF, De Vincentiis M. Sudden sensorineural hearing loss: An autoimmune disease? Autoimmunity Reviews. 2011;**10**(12):756-761

[34] Garcia Berrocal JR, Ramirez-Camacho R. Sudden sensorineural hearing loss: Supporting the immunologic theory. The Annals of Otology, Rhinology, and Laryngology. 2002;**111**:989-997

[35] Yoo TJ, Tomoda H, Hernandez AD. Type II collagen-induced autoimmune inner ear lesions in guinea pigs. The Annals of Otology, Rhinology, and Laryngology. 1984;**113**:3-5

[36] Solares CA, Edling AE, Johnson JM, Baek MJ, Hirose K, Hughes GB, et al. Murine autoimmune hearing loss mediated by CD4+ T cells specific for inner ear peptides. The Journal of Clinical Investigation. 2004;**113**:1210-1217

[37] Boulassel MR, Deggouj N, Tomasi JP, Gersdorff M. Inner ear autoantibodies and their targets in patients with autoimmune inner ear diseases. Acta Oto-Laryngologica. 2001;**121**:28-34

[38] Boulassel MR, Tomasi JP, Deggouj N, Gersdorff M. Identification of beta-actin as a candidate autoantigen in autoimmune inner ear disease. Clinical Otolaryngology and Allied Sciences. 2000;**25**:535-541

[39] Disher MJ, Ramakrishan A, Nair TS, Miller JM, Telian SA, Arts HA, et al. Human autoantibodies and monoclonal antibody KHRI-3 bind to a phylogenetically conserved inner-ear-supporting cell antigen. Annals of the New York Academy of Sciences. 1997;**830**:253-265

[40] Lunardi C, Bason C, Leandri M, et al. Autoantibodies to inner ear and endothelial antigens in Cogan's syndrome. Lancet. 2002;**360**:915-921

[41] Yoo TJ, Tomoda K, Stuart JM, Cremer MA, Townes AS, Kang AH. Type II collagen induced autoimmune sensorineural hearing loss and vestibular dysfunction in rats. Annals of Otology, Rhinology and Laryngology. 1983;**92**:267-271

[42] Toubi E, Ben-David J, Kessel A, Podoshin L, Golan TD. Autoimmune aberration in sudden sensorineural hearing loss: Association with anti-cardiolipin antibodies. Lupus. 1997;**6**:540-542

[43] Joliat T, Seyer J, Bernstein J, et al. Antibodies against a 30kDA cochlear protein and type II and type IX collagens in the serum of patients with inner ear disease. The Annals of Otology, Rhinology, and Laryngology. 1992;**101**:1000-1006

[44] Nordang L, Laurent C, Mollnes TE. Complement activation in sudden deafness. Archives of Otolaryngology – Head & Neck Surgery. 1998;**124**:633-636

[45] Meroni PL, D'Cruz D, Khamashta M, Youinou O, Hughes GRV. Anti-endothelial cell antibodies: Only for scientists or for clinicians too ? Clinical and Experimental Immunology. 1996;**104**:199-202

[46] McCabe BF. Autoimmune sensorineural hearing loss. The Annals of Otology, Rhinology, and Laryngology. 1979;**88**:585-589

[47] Ottaviani F, Cadoni G, Marinelli M, et al. Anti-endothelial autoantibodies in patients with sudden hearing loss. Laryngoscope. 1999;**109**:1084-1087

[48] Harris JP, Sharp PA. Inner ear autoantibodies in patients with rapidly progressive sensorineural hearing loss. Laryngoscope. 1990;**100**:516-524

[49] Garcia Berrocal JR, Ramirez-Camacho R, Arellano B, Vargas JA. Validity of the western blot immunoassay for heat shock protein-70 in associated and isolated immunorelated inner ear disease. Laryngoscope. 2002;**112**:304-309

[50] Samuelsson AK, Hyden D, Roberg M, Skogh T. Evaluation of anti-hsp 70 antibody screening in sudden deafness. Ear and Hearing. 2003;**24**:233-235

[51] Chawki S, Aouizerate J, Trad S, Prinseau J, Hanslik T. Bilateral sudden sensorineural hearing loss as a presenting feature of systemic lupus erythematosus: Case report and brief review of other published cases. Medicine. 2016;**95**(36):e4345

[52] Compadretti GC, Brandolini C, Tasca I. Sudden SNHL in lupus erythematosus associated with antiphospholipid syndrome. The Annals of Otology, Rhinology, and Laryngology. 2005;**114**:214-218

[53] Naarendrop M, Spiera H. Sudden SNHL in patients with SLE and antiphospholipid antibodies. The Journal of Rheumatology. 1998;**25**:589-592

[54] Harris JP, Sharp PA. Inner ear autoantibodies in patients with rapidly progressive sensorineural hearing loss. The Laryngoscope. 1990;**100**(5):516-524

[55] Stearns GS, Keithley EM, Harris JP. Development of high endothelial venule-like characteristics in the spiral modiolar vein induced by viral labyrinthitis. The Laryngoscope. 1993;**103**(8):890-898

[56] Heywood RL, Hadavi S, Donnelly S, Patel N. Infliximab for autoimmune inner ear disease: Case report and literature review. The Journal of Laryngology & Otology. 2013;**127**(11):1145-1147

[57] Goodhill V, Harris I. Sudden hearing loss syndrome. In: Ear Diseases, Deafness, and Dizziness. New York: Harper-Collins; 1979. pp. 664-681

[58] Simmons FB. Theory of membrane breaks in sudden hearing loss. Archives of Otolaryngology. 1968;**88**(1, 1):41-48

[59] Gussen R. Sudden hearing loss associated with cochlear membrane rupture: Two human temporal bone reports. Archives of Otolaryngology. 1981;**107**(10):598-600

[60] Kamerer DB, Sando I, Hirsch B, Takagi A. Perilymph fistula resulting from microfissures. Otology & Neurotology. 1987;**8**(6):489-494

[61] Yood TH, Paparella MM, Schacern PA, Alleva M. Histopathology of sudden hearing loss. The Laryngoscope. 1990;**100**(7):707-715

[62] Vasama JP, Linthicum FH Jr. Idiopathic sudden sensorineural hearing loss: Temporal bone histopathologic study. Annals of Otology, Rhinology and Laryngology. 2000;**109**(6):527-532

[63] Conte G, Di Berardino F, Sina C, Zanetti D, Scola E, Gavagna C, Gaini L, Palumbo G, Capaccio P, Triulzi F. MR imaging in sudden sensorineural hearing loss. Time to talk. AJNR – American Journal of Neuroradiology. 2017 Aug;**38**(8):1475-1479

[64] Lee JI, Yoon RG, Lee JH, et al. Prognostic value of labyrinthine 3DFLAIR abnormalities in idiopathic sudden sensorineural hearing loss. AJNR. American Journal of Neuroradiology. 2016;**37**:2317-2322

[65] Ryu IS, Yoon TH, Ahn JH, et al. Three-dimensional fluid-attenuated inversion recovery magnetic resonance imaging in sudden sensorineural hearing loss: Correlations with audiologic and vestibular testing. Otology & Neurotology. 2011;**32**:1205-1209

[66] Wilson WR, Byl FM, Laird N. The efficacy of steroids in the treatment of idiopathic sudden hearing loss: A double-blind clinical study. Archives of Otolaryngology. 1980;**106**(12):772-776

[67] Stachler RJ, Chandrasekhar SS, Archer SM, Rosenfeld RM, Schwartz SR, Barrs DM, Brown SR, Fife TD, Ford P, Ganiats TG, Hollingsworth DB. Clinical practice guideline: Sudden hearing loss. Otolaryngology – Head and Neck Surgery. 2012;**146**(3_suppl):S1-35

[68] Goh AY, Hussain SS. Sudden hearing loss and pregnancy: A review. The Journal of Laryngology & Otology. 2012;**126**(4):337-339

[69] Rauch SD, Halpin CF, Antonelli PJ, Babu S, Carey JP, Gantz BJ, Goebel JA, Hammerschlag PE, Harris JP, Isaacson B, Lee D. Oral vs. intratympanic corticosteroid therapy for idiopathic sudden sensorineural hearing loss: A randomized trial. Journal of the American Medical Association. 2011;**305**(20):2071-2079

[70] Stokroos RJ, Albers FWJ, Schirm J. The etiology of idiopathic sudden sensorineural hearing loss. Experimental herpes simplex virus infection of the inner ear. The American Journal of Otology. 1998;**19**:447-452

[71] Park KH, Lee CK, Lee JD, Park MK, Lee BD. Combination therapy with systemic steroids, an antiviral agent, anticoagulants, and stellate ganglion block for treatment of sudden sensorineural hearing loss. Korean Journal of Audiology. 2012;**16**(2):71-74

[72] Westerlaken BO, Stokroos RJ, Wit HP, Dhooge IJ, Albers FW. Treatment of idiopathic sudden sensorineural hearing loss with antiviral therapy: A prospective, randomized, double-blind clinical trial. Annals of Otology, Rhinology and Laryngology. 2003;**112**(11):993-1000

[73] Tucci DL, Farmer JC Jr, Kitch RD, Witsell DL. Treatment of sudden sensorineural hearing loss with systemic steroids and valacyclovir. Otology & Neurotology. 2002;**23**(3):301-308

[74] Kronenberg J, Almagor M, Bendet E, Kushnir D. Vasoactive therapy versus placebo in the treatment of sudden hearing loss: A double-blind clinical study. The Laryngoscope. 1992;**102**(1, 1):65-68

[75] Kallinen J, Laippala P, Laurikainen E, Grénman R. Sudden deafness: A comparison of anticoagulant therapy and carbogen inhalation therapy. Annals of Otology, Rhinology and Laryngology. 1997;**106**(1):22-26

[76] Probst R, Tschopp K, Lodin E, Kellerhals B, Podvinec M, Pfaltz CR. A randomized, double-blind, placebo-controlled study of dextran/pentoxifylline medication in acute acoustic trauma and sudden hearing loss. Acta Oto-Laryngologica. 1992;**112**(3):435-443

[77] Nageris BI, Ulanovski D, Attias J. Magnesium treatment for sudden hearing loss. Annals of Otology, Rhinology and Laryngology. 2004;**113**(8):672-675

[78] Gordin A, Goldenberg D, Golz A, Netzer A, Joachims HZ. Magnesium: A new therapy for idiopathic sudden sensorineural hearing loss. Otology & Neurotology. 2002;**23**(4): 447-451

[79] Suckfüll M. Hearing loss study group. Fibrinogen and LDL apheresis in treatment of sudden hearing loss: A randomised multicentre trial. The Lancet. 2002;**360**(9348):1811-1817

[80] Slattery WH, Fisher LM, Iqbal Z, Friedman RA, Liu N. Intratympanic steroid injection for treatment of idiopathic sudden hearing loss. Otolaryngology – Head and Neck Surgery. 2005;**133**(2):251-259

[81] Xenellis J, Papadimitriou N, Nikolopoulos T, Maragoudakis P, Segas J, Tzagaroulakis A, Ferekidis E. Intratympanic steroid treatment in idiopathic sudden sensorineural hearing loss: A control study. Otolaryngology – Head and Neck Surgery. 2006;**134**(6):940-945

[82] Herr BD, Marzo SJ. Intratympanic steroid perfusion for refractory sudden sensorineural hearing loss. Otolaryngology – Head and Neck Surgery. 2005;**132**(4):527-531

[83] Battaglia A, Burchette R, Cueva R. Combination therapy (intratympanic dexamethasone+ high-dose prednisone taper) for the treatment of idiopathic sudden sensorineural hearing loss. Otology & Neurotology. 2008;**29**(4):453-460

[84] Gülüstan F, Yazıcı ZM, Alakhras WM, Erdur O, Acipayam H, Kufeciler L, Kayhan FT. Intratympanic steroid injection and hyperbaric oxygen therapy for the treatment of refractory sudden hearing loss. Brazilian Journal of Otorhinolaryngology. 2016

[85] Lamm K, Lamm C, Arnold W. Effect of isobaric oxygen versus hyperbaric oxygen on the normal and noise-damaged hypoxic and ischemic guinea pig inner ear. In: Yanagita N, Nakashima T, editors. Hyperbaric Oxygen Therapy in Otorhinolaryngology. Advances in Otorhinolaryngology. Vol. 54. Basel: Karger; 1998. pp. 59-85

[86] Fattori B, Berrettini S, Casani A, Nacci A, De Vito A, De Iaco G. Sudden hypoacusis treated with hyperbaric oxygen therapy: A controlled study. Ear, Nose, & Throat Journal. 2001;**80**:655-660

[87] Pilgramm M, Roth M, Fisher B. Der Einfluss der hyperbaren oxygenation auf rheologische parameter. Perfusion. 1988;**2**:79-82

[88] Racic G, Maslovara S, Roje Z, Dogas Z, Tafra R. Hyperbaric oxygen in the treatment of sudden hearing loss. ORL. 2003;**65**(6):317-320

[89] Bennett MH, Kertesz T, Yeung P. Hyperbaric oxygen for idiopathic sudden sensorineural hearing loss and tinnitus. Cochrane Database of Systematic Reviews. 2007 Jan 24;(1):CD004739

[90] Fujimura T, Suzuki H, Shiomori T, Udaka T, Mori T. Hyperbaric oxygen and steroid therapy for idiopathic sudden sensorineural hearing loss. European Archives of Oto-Rhino-Laryngology. 2007;**264**(8):861-866

[91] Horn CE, Himel HN, Selesnick SH. Hyperbaric oxygen therapy for sudden sensorineural hearing loss: A prospective trial of patients failing steroid and antiviral treatment. Otology & Neurotology. 2005;**26**(5):882-889

[92] Ragab A, Shreef E, Behiry E, Zalat S, Noaman M. Randomised, double-blinded, placebo-controlled, clinical trial of ozone therapy as treatment of sudden sensorineural hearing loss. The Journal of Laryngology & Otology. 2009;**123**(1):54-60

6

Controlling the Biocompatibility and Mechanical Effects of Implantable Microelectrodes to Improve Chronic Neural Recordings in the Auditory Nervous System

Payton Lin, Yu Tsao and Li-Wei Kuo

Abstract

Implantable microelectrodes are useful for monitoring neural response patterns in the auditory cortex, however chronic neural recordings can often deteriorate with time (e.g. impedance measures across electrode arrays generally increase monotonically over the first 7 days post-implant). This problem is caused by the increasing spatial distribution of reactive tissue responses (corresponding to changes in impedance spectra along the electrode-tissue-interface). Therefore, the design of microelectrode probes must ensure that the neuronal ensembles lie within a cylindrical radius of the recording electrodes. In this chapter, chronic neural recording failure is examined via cortical spike patterns, histological analyses, indentation experiments, and finite element models. Next, the microfabrication of the "Utah" electrode array and the "Michigan" probe is compared to determine how their size, shape, and geometry address: (1) the spatial distribution of neurons (as related to recording quality); (2) the initial penetrating profile (as related to insertion killzones); (3) the reactive cell responses (as related to glial encapsulation); (4) the anchoring of the probe's position in the tissue (as related to micromotions) and (5) the embedding of various bioactive reagents (ex: growth factors, anti-inflammatory drugs, etc.). Finally, a novel hydrogel "Dropping Method" is proposed for controlling the biocompatibility and mechanical properties at the electrode-tissue-interface.

Keywords: auditory cortex, implantable microelectrode array, chronic neural recording, neural probe, brain machine interface, inflammatory response, biocompatibility, insertion killzone, glial encapsulation, micromotion, finite element model, hydrogel

1. Introduction

Brain machine interfaces connect the human brain to electronic devices and computer software [1]. Machine intelligence can offer the inherent advantages of greater processing speeds, computing power, memory capabilities, and even unrestricted sensory perception (e.g. infrared, ultra violet, X-ray, and ultrasonic spectra). With the emergence of deep brain stimulation, neuroprosthesis, neurofeedback, and exoskeleton technologies, science fiction is being bridged into a modern reality. However, the ultimate realization of a brain machine interface is to have a computer system that can chronically interface with the neural tissues. This neurotechnology will require neuroscientists and engineers to work together to address the technical challenges of accessing neural communication channels (for data routing and transmission), preserving the *biocompatibility* (to interface electronic components within the biological neural tissues), and maintaining the bio-signal processing (for selecting the appropriate control signals).

This chapter will focus on the *microelectrode*: a neural probe used in neurophysiology for either recording neural representations in the brain or for electrically stimulating the nervous tissue. Micromachined electrodes and microwires are often used to monitor the neuronal activities by characterizing extracellular field potentials of multiple active neurons. These neural interfaces are artificially-engineered extensions of the nervous system that must coexist in the precise connections of supporting glial cells, oligodendrocytes, astrocytes, and microglia (**Figure 1A**).

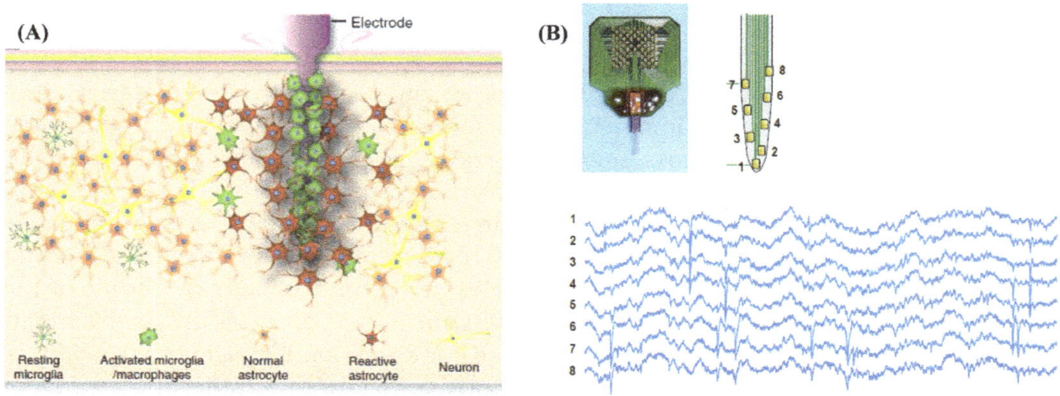

Figure 1. (A) Depiction of cellular changes induced by an implanted electrode and (B) multichannel neural recordings.

Multichannel microelectrodes (**Figure 1B**) can be used to monitor the activity in the *auditory cortex* and to investigate the functional organization of the auditory system [2–4]. For example, a chronic microelectrode investigation of the human auditory cortex [5] revealed a "tonotopic" pattern where the sound-driven units had excitatory receptive fields with sharply tuned best-frequency response over a range of frequencies. These micro-machined devices are currently being developed to control brain machine interfaces [6–8] and can benefit many applications in medicine, communication, entertainment, military, and education. However, there has been one limiting factor that has obstructed their reliability as a fully-implantable neural prosthesis: *chronic neural recordings* have been shown to deteriorate [9, 10] with time (**Figure 2**).

In Section 2, chronic neural recording failure is examined by reviewing cortical spike patterns, histological analyses, indentation experiments, and *finite element models* (FEM). For instance, probe impedance measures have been shown to increase, histological analyses have indicated that changes in the impedance spectra along the electrode-tissue interface are caused by the increasing spatial distribution of the reactive tissue responses, indentation experiments have shown persistent *inflammatory reactions* on the indwelling microelectrodes, and FEMs have simulated that surrounding tissues are compressed by the large stiffness mismatch of the implanted substrates (with pressure profiles revealing extensive tension at the probe tip).

In Section 3, the microfabrication of the *"Utah" electrode array* and the *"Michigan" neural probe* is compared by reviewing how their different sizes, shapes, and geometries can be redesigned to address: (1) the spatial distribution of neurons (as related to improving the recording quality); (2) the initial penetrating profile (as related to minimizing the *insertion killzone*); (3) the reactive cell responses (as related to preventing *glial encapsulation*); (4) the anchoring of a neural probe's position in the tissue (as related to reducing *electrode micromotion*) and (5) the embedding of various bioactive reagents (as related to eluting growth factors, anti-inflammatory drugs, etc.).

In Section 4, a *hydrogel coating* layer is proposed for improving the mechanical properties and *biocompatibility* at the electrode-tissue interface. Hydrogel coatings can be tailored to provide a buffer layer (for reducing stiffness mismatch), and to control the swelling properties to anchor the position of the probe in the tissue. In addition, a novel hydrogel coating method called the *"Dropping Method"* is proposed to control the mechanical properties at the electrode-tissue-interface. The Dropping Method will be compared versus the traditional *"Dipping Method."*

2. Chronic neural recording failure

2.1. Deterioration of neural recordings over time

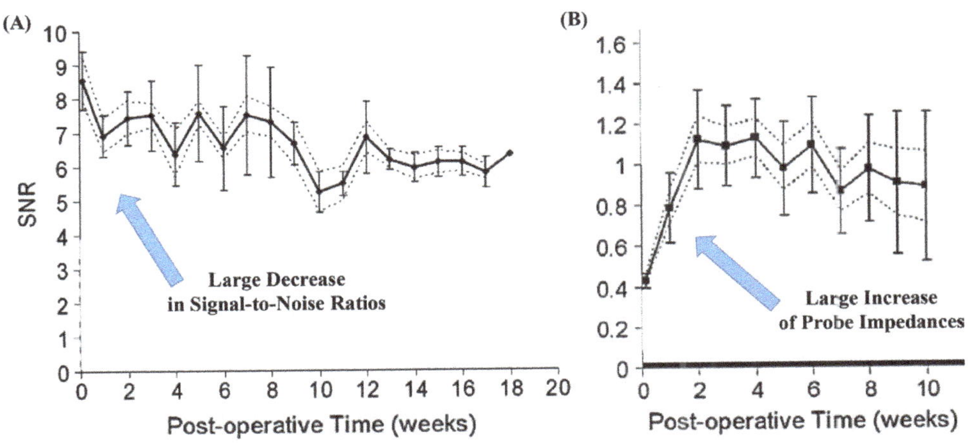

Figure 2. (A) Mean SNR across implanted probes over time and (B) mean impedance values. Reproduced from [10].

Silicon-substrate micromachined probes can provide high-quality multichannel spike activity recordings and local field potentials in the auditory cortex. For acute neural recordings, these measurements are generally stable. However, chronic long-term recordings are limited by the foreign body responses that occur during the wound healing process [9]. Previous research showed signal-to-noise-ratios (SNR) decreased as a function of postoperative time (**Figure 2A**) [10]. Impedance measures across electrode arrays were also shown to increase monotonically over the first 2 weeks (**Figure 2B**). This problem (of electrical signals gradually decreasing over time post-implant) must be solved to improve the chronic recording of neural activity.

Histological analyses have revealed tissue reactions to the implanted probe shanks during the assessment periods. For instance, confocal microscopy and immunohistochemistry protocols were used to measure the cellular density around the implanted electrodes and confirmed that a region of extensive reactive responses occurs around each individual electrode track [11]. By differentiating the spatial distribution of reactive tissue responses corresponding to changes in impedance spectra along the electrode-tissue interface, these findings confirm that reactive tissue responses directly influence the impedance spectra over time.

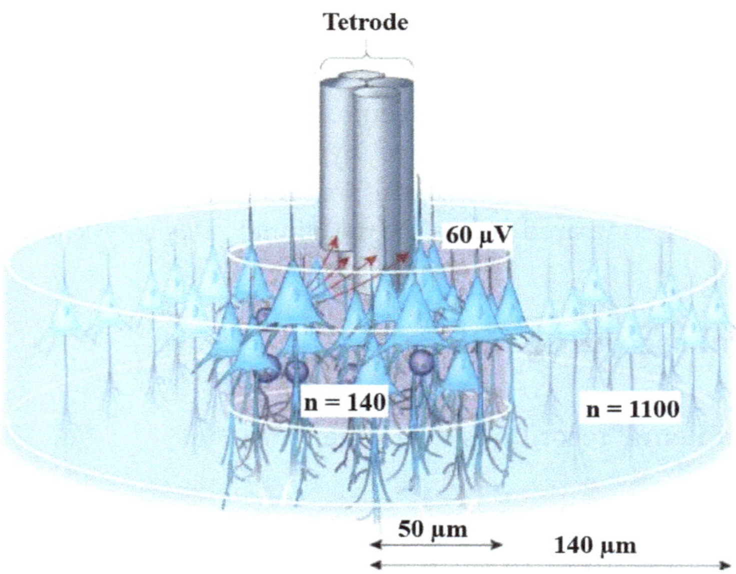

Figure 3. Unit isolation quality varies as a function of distance from the electrode. The spike amplitudes of the neuronal ensembles must lie within a cylindrical radius (n = 140 μm) to be detected. Reproduced from [12].

The recorded spike amplitudes were also measured as a function of the distance between the neuron and the electrode (by making comparisons from a multisite tetrode wire [12]). **Figure 3** shows that the extracellularly recorded spike amplitudes decreased rapidly with distance (a finding that indicates that the neuronal ensembles must lie within a cylindrical radius of ~140 μm of the recording electrode to effectively monitor the extracellular spike amplitudes). These *"cylindrical radius"* distances will be important to consider since previous studies have shown that the inflammatory responses can extend to ~100 μm.

2.2. Insertion killzone

When inserting a microelectrode, the microshaft must penetrate through arteries, veins, tight junction cells, collagen, and smaller vessels in the pia. The shaft must then penetrate through tissues composed of neurons, glial cells, capillaries, arterioles, and venules. The tip of the shaft must be sharp enough to puncture through the microtubules and the fibrous structures within the neurofilaments. This electrode insertion process inevitably causes death and degeneration of its neighboring neurons and capillaries during the surgical implantation [13]. The *insertion killzone* is defined as the region around the shaft where the local neuron density is lower than the expected neuron density by a 90% confidence interval (**Figure 4A**). The tearing of neurons will cause the temporary loss of action potential capability and cell death due to the influx of calcium. The cutting of vessels and capillaries will cause microhemorrhages that can displace the neural tissue. If the neural tissue is compressed or stretched, the leakage of ions can lead to the loss of cellular homeostasis. Therefore, the penetrating shafts should be carefully fixed to a manipulator to prevent significant misalignment and to minimize the killzone (**Figure 4B**).

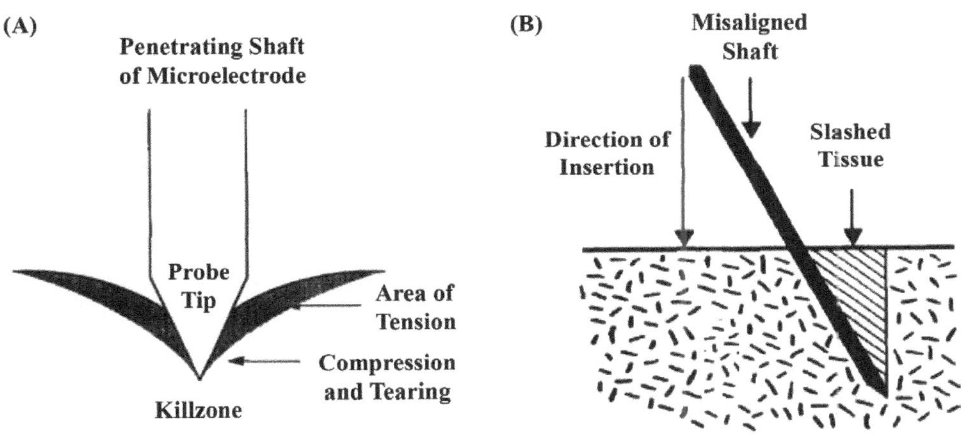

Figure 4. (A) Damage during insertion of a sharp microelectrode (where the shaft stretches the tissue beyond its elastic limits while passing through) and (B) significant axial misalignment of a shaft creates a swath of damage during insertion.

Penetrating shafts should be designed to minimize the initial mechanical trauma, to preserve the neuronal density in a local area around the implanted array, and to minimize the early reactive responses caused by the pathway of tissue damage. Indentation experiments have shown that immediate vascular and brain damage results in the recruitment of cells from the peripheral immune system and the activation of resident astrocytes or microglia. The reactive responses can be compared by immunochemically labelling for glial fibrillary acidic protein (GFAP), vimentin (for astrocytes), or ED1 (for microglia). When devices of different size were inserted, it was found that the volume of the reactive tissue responses was proportional to the cross-sectional area [14]. For instance, the smallest device (smallest cross-sectional area) with smooth surfaces and rounded corners caused less damage to the tissue, produced a smaller volume of reactive tissue, and left a smaller hole when removed from the tissue 1 week later.

2.3. Prolonged injury response

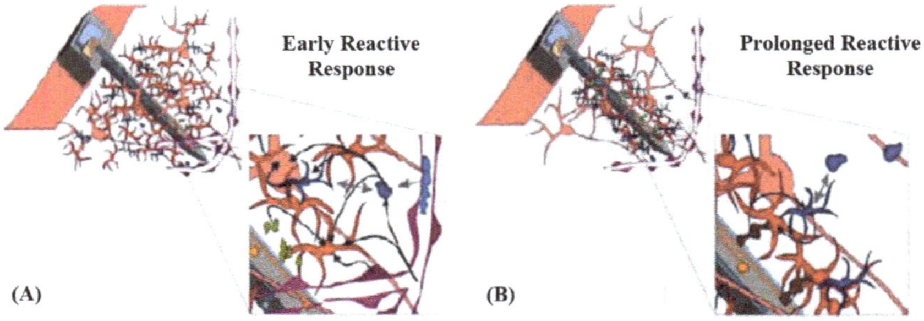

Figure 5. (A) Early reactive responses and (B) prolonged reactive responses to a chronically implant. Reproduced from [14].

An immunohistochemistry experiment [14] showed that the early reactive response (within 1 week (**Figure 5A**)) was associated with the amount of damage generated during the insertion (which depends on the device size or shape). However, this same study also showed that the prolonged reactive responses (after 4 weeks (**Figure 5B**)) eventually became similar (ultimately resulting in a compact cellular sheath containing astrocytes and microglia). While it is always better to minimize the insertion killzone, these results clearly indicate that a second sustained response occurs that is related to the tissue-device interactions. For instance, a long-term study [15] showed that the persistent ED1 up-regulation and neuronal loss (associated with the foreign body responses) were not observed in microelectrode stab controls (which indicates that the phenotype did not result from the initial mechanical trauma of the electrode implantation). Moreover, chronically-implanted electrodes were also covered in ED1/MAC-1 immunoreactive cells and released the pro-inflammatory cytokines MCP-1 and TNF-α (which are only characteristics of chronic inflammatory reactions). **Figure 6** shows that the zones of astrocytosis and connective tissue vary in proportion to an implant's reactivity [16]. Although the normal long-term response to an indwelling microelectrode is to develop a reactive glial tissue (that eventually forms into a fibrotic encapsulation layer or a glial scar), this sustained injury response has also been associated with chronic recording failure since the encapsulation (from persistent inflammatory reactions) isolates the electrodes from the surrounding neurons and decreases the stability and quality of the neural recordings.

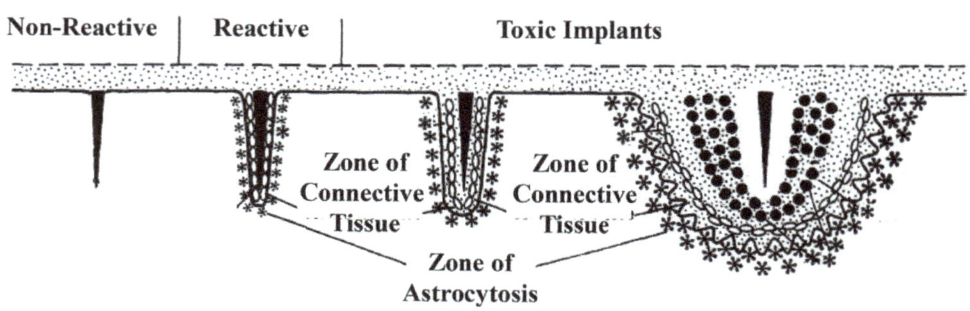

Figure 6. Histopathological changes that occur around a non-reactive implant, a reactive implant, and toxic implants.

2.4. Micromotion

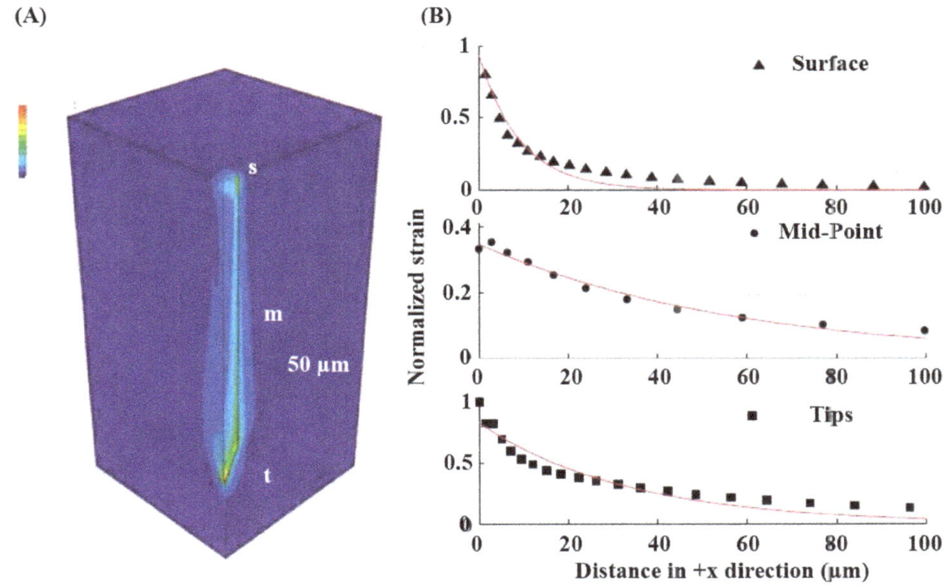

Figure 7. (A) Finite element model (FEM) strain profile of the radial tethering forces in the brain tissue that results from a 1 µm displacement of a silicon probe extended to 100 µm from the interface (s = surface, m = midpoint, t = tip). (B) Normalized strain values decreased exponentially as a function of distance in the brain tissue. Reproduced from [18].

The mechanical properties of the brain can be researched by mathematical simulation models that faithfully represent the geometry, material properties, and boundary or load conditions. For instance, an in-vivo indentation experiment [17] described the soft tissue deformation with a three-dimensional non-linear finite element model (FEM) of geometric information from the brain (obtained via magnetic resonance imaging techniques). Another FEM study measured the effects of tethering forces, probe-tissue adhesion, and the stiffness of the probe substrate on the interfacial strains induced around the implant site [18]. The results indicated that the interfacial strains were created by *micromotions* of the chronically implanted electrode, and that these mechanical strains around the implant site are likely responsible for the sustained tissue responses in chronic implants. In addition, the elevated strains at the probe tip were shown to cause poor probe-tissue adhesion and delamination of the tissue from the probe. The simulated probes also induced strain fields that displayed high radial tethering forces, with pressure profiles revealing extensive tension and maximum frictional shear stress at the tips of the arrays (**Figure 7**). Therefore, these findings indicate that softer substrates should be used to reduce the strain at the probe-tissue interface (to reduce tissue responses in chronic implants). Specifically, the magnitude of the micromotions should be reduced at the microelectrode's tip position to ensure the stability of the recordings at the cortical surface since gliosis is typically observed at the probe tips [13] (with up to a three-fold increase in the size of the surrounding glial sheath compared to at other areas of the arrays [19]). Micromotions and cortical surface displacements can also result from respiratory pulsations [20], behavioral sources [21], and the translational movements of the electrode's tethering lead wire [22] (which can occur due to the rotational acceleration of the head [23]).

3. Comparing "Utah" electrode arrays versus "Michigan" neural probes

Implantable probe designs have primarily focused on modifying the size, shape, or geometry to minimize reactive cell responses. For the *"Utah" electrode array* [24] and the *"Michigan" neural probe* [25], Section 3.1 compares the spatial distribution of neurons (as related to improving recording quality), Section 3.2 compares the initial penetrating profile (as related to minimizing the insertion kill-zone), Section 3.3 compares the reactive responses (as related to preventing glial encapsulation), Section 3.4 compares the anchoring of the probe's position in the tissue (as related to reducing electrode micromotion), Section 3.5 compares the embedding of bioactive reagents (as related to eluting growth factors, anti-inflammatory drugs, etc.).

3.1. Spatial distribution of neurons

3.1.1. Utah electrode array

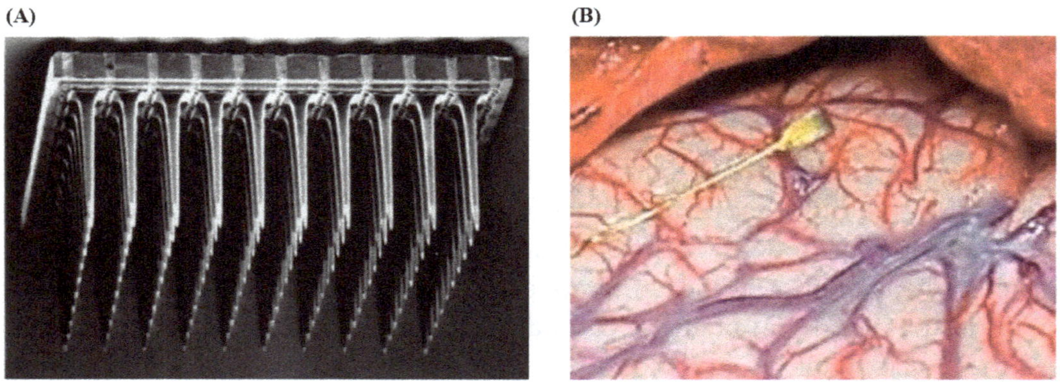

Figure 8. (A) The 100 microelectrode Utah electrode array and (B) the electrode probe tips implanted into the cortex.

The Utah array was designed from the ground up (with new manufacturing techniques [26]) to meet the specific needs of a multichannel neural interface [24]. Psychophysical experiments usually require evoking discriminable patterned percepts from many electrodes. Therefore, the Utah array (**Figure 8A**) was designed to possess a large number (~100) of large electrodes (~1.5 mm) that are typically in a square grid that projects out from a thin (~0.2 mm) substrate. **Figure 8B** shows the tapered electrodes suspended in a "sea of glass" substrate (that isolates each of the individual electrodes in the array from each other (~0.4 mm separation) to form a very effective dielectric insulating layer between the adjacent electrodes). The electrode probe tips are coated with platinum, gold, or iridium to facilitate the electronic to ionic transduction. The array's substrate was designed to be thick enough to prevent breaking upon insertion, but thin enough to rest on the cortical surface without producing a constant downward force on the array that could push it further into the cortex.

3.1.2. Michigan neural probe

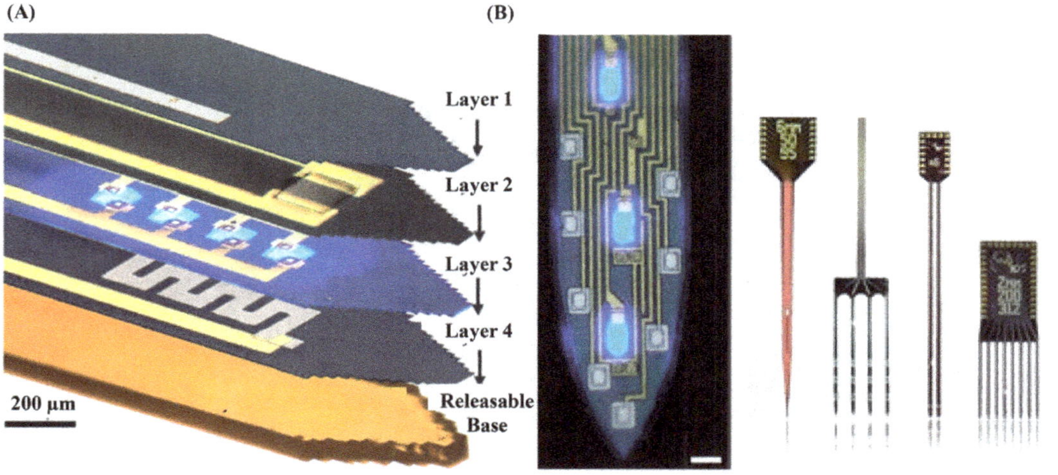

Figure 9. (A) Silicon-substrate Michigan probe and (B) microfabrication borrows semiconductors manufacturing methods.

Unlike the Utah electrode array [23], the planar Michigan probe [27] was only designed to take advantage of photolithographic manufacturing techniques from the semiconductor industry (**Figure 9A**). The extensibility of this platform technology enables these micromachined probes to be built with batch fabrication, easy customization of recording site placements or substrate shape, high reproducibility of geometrical/electrical characteristics, and the ability to integrate with ribbon cables or to incorporate on-chip electronics for signal conditioning (**Figure 9B**).

Unfortunately, the Michigan probes are known to induce a chronic breach of the blood–brain barrier [28] which leads to more chronic inflammation and culminates in neurodegeneration and ultimately to electrode failure (as described in Section 2). For instance, Michigan probes showed a significantly higher breach and worse wound-healing in comparison to microwires.

Since there is a trade-off between the size (spatial selectivity) and quality of signal recordings (sensitivity) in a neural microelectrode, previous research have altered the electrical properties by synthesizing biocompatible conducting polymers (**Figure 10A**) such as polypyrrole (PPy) and poly(3,4-ethylenedioxythiophene) (PEDOT) directly onto the electrode. Electrochemical deposition (**Figure 10B**) allows polymer films to be formed in a one-step process with a high degree of control over the film thickness and surface properties (e.g. with nanotubes in [27]).

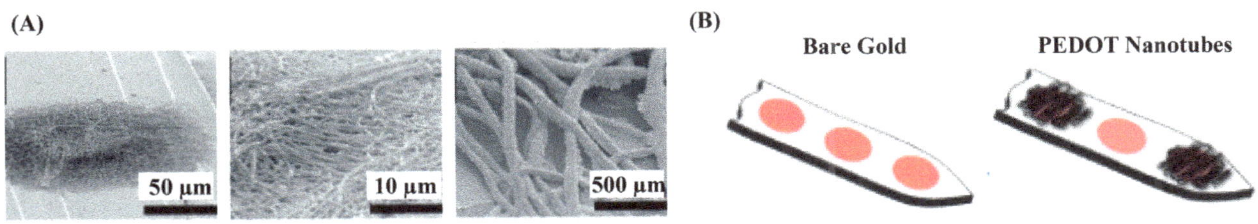

Figure 10. (A) Scanning electron microscope of deposited polymer and (B) uncoated vs. PEDOT nanotube (NT) electrodes.

3.2. Initial penetrating profile

3.2.1. Utah electrode array

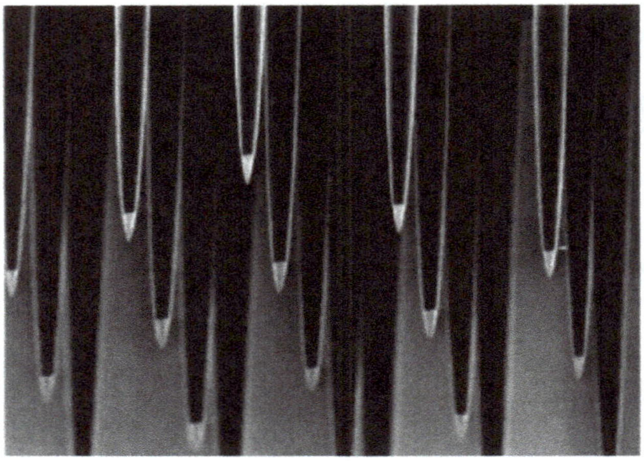

Figure 11. Penetrating shafts of the Utah electrode array with probe tips coated with platinum, gold, or iridium.

The penetrating electrodes of the Utah array (**Figure 11**) were designed to be slender enough to retain sufficient strength for withstanding the implantation procedure, yet to compromise as little cortical volume as possible (only 80 μm in diameter at the base). The needles were intentionally designed to have a cylindrical/conical geometry (rather than a planar geometry) to displace the tissues they are inserted (rather than cutting their way through). In addition, an "Impact Insertion" technique was designed to inject the array into the cortex at a high velocity [26]. This momentum transfer tool preserves uniformity and prevents dimpling of the cortex.

3.2.2. Michigan neural probe

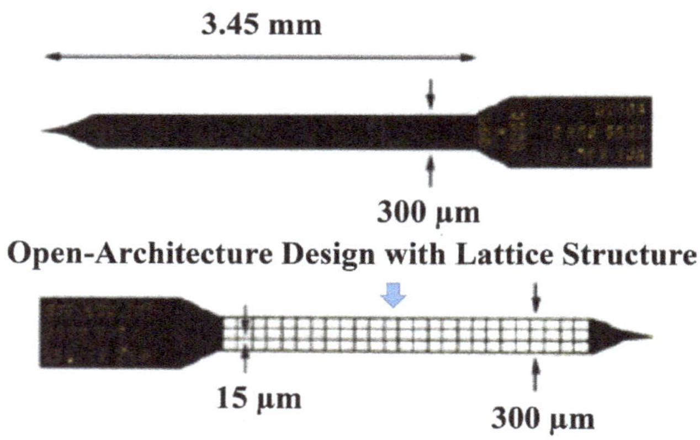

Figure 12. Comparison of a solid shank vs. the open-architecture design with a lattice structure. Reproduced from [25].

Despite evidence that smaller implants can increase the survival of neurons [29], the research direction for Michigan probes has been primarily guided by the *critical surface area model* [25]. This theory is supported by results showing microelectrodes with lattice structures (**Figure 12**) exhibited less inflammation-related biomarker distribution in tissues compared to the solid shanks (even though both have identical penetrating profiles). However, Section 3.4.2 will show the alternative theory of *mechanical property differences* [30] can also explain these results.

3.3. Reactive processes

3.3.1. Utah electrode array

The electrodes are built from biocompatible materials such as silicon, silicon nitride, silicon dioxide, platinum, titanium, tungsten, and silicone. Histological analyses show the neuronal cell bodies remain in close apposition to the electrode tracks (especially in sections where the tracks are similar in diameter to blood vessels). The benign tissue response showed that a thin capsule (~2–5 microns) forms around each electrode track. Histological samples also revealed gliosis, fibrotic-tissue buildup between the array and the meninges, bleeding in some tracks, and some array displacement through the cortex. Despite these reactive responses, electrodes were shown to be able to record single- and multi-unit responses in the cortex for over 3 years (the longest intervals studied). Therefore, the stability of these units over periods of months provides the most compelling evidence for the biocompatibility [23].

3.3.2. Michigan neural probe

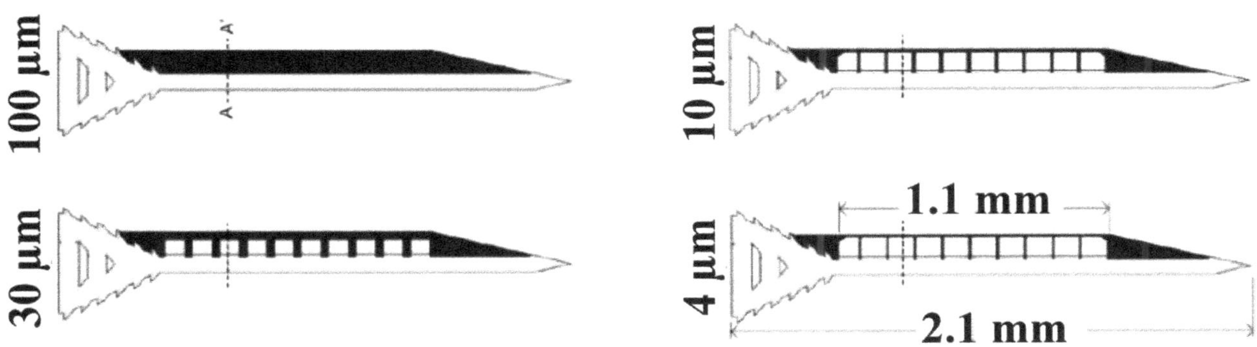

Figure 13. Comparison of a solid shank vs. open-architecture designs with varying lattice sizes. Reproduced from [30].

Glial sheaths (consisting of activated microglia and hypertrophied astrocytes, meningeal cells, and oligodendrocyte precursors that produce extracellular proteins that hinder local nerve regeneration) have been shown to form around the probe tract. As mentioned in Section 2, this tissue encapsulation is concomitant with a decrease in signal quality for neural recordings. Therefore, probe geometry has been investigated as a parameter for reducing chronic tissue encapsulation. Open-architectures (**Figure 13**) can reduce tissue encapsulation by presenting a narrow edge of surface area to prevent the prototypical attachment and spreading of foreign body responses (as cells would theoretically be unable to attach or create cytoskeleton tension below a certain dimension [30]). The tissue reactivity around the smallest lattice structure was expected to induce the least encapsulation. However, the comparison between probe designs indicated that the differences in encapsulation and neuronal loss was insignificant. Qualitative histology also showed similar responses inside the lattice region and around the shank. This has led to the *mechanical property differences* theory (which is discussed further in Section 3.4.2).

3.4. Anchoring of the probe's position

3.4.1. Utah electrode array

The large number of penetrating electrodes presents a very large surface area to the cortex and the implanted array tends to self-anchor to the cortical tissues. More importantly, the "sea of glass" allows the array to float in the cortical tissues as the cortex moves due to respiration, blood pumping, and skeletal displacements. This design feature produces an extremely stable interface with the surrounding neurons as it moves with the cortex and thereby produces very little micromotion between the electrode tips and the neurons near its active tips. In addition, GFAP staining showed that a fixation mode that un-tethers the implant from the skull elicits a smaller tissue reaction and results in the survival of a larger number of neurons in the region closest to the tissue interface [29].

3.4.2. Michigan neural probe

In Sections 3.2.2 and 3.3.2, the *critical surface model* was used to explain the benefits of open-architecture designs [25, 30]. However, an alternative theory [30] was offered to explain how the open-architecture designs reduce tissue encapsulations compared to the solid shanks. The theory of *mechanical property differences* assumes that lattice structures reduce the induced strain from relative movements (e.g. micromotion) between the probe and the tissue (occurring from the continual pulsations of vascular and respiratory oscillations). In other words, the adjoining lattice structure is assumed to present a more flexible mechanical interface that can improve the mechanical surface properties (relative to the solid probe shank). This competing theory of *mechanical property differences* is supported by FEM results that demonstrate that the shape of the electrode substantially influences the local pattern and the magnitude of strain around the electrode (especially at the electrode tip where the shank has a spear-head shape or at regions that have discontinuous or sharp edges [31]).

The theory of *mechanical property differences* is also supported by electrophysiological data [28] showing the Michigan electrode's recording performance failed faster relative to a microwire electrode. Since persistent micromotions are known to trigger a complex cascade of events, it was hypothesized that the different material properties and design of the Michigan electrode was the cause for the diminished wound healing response, the increased inflammation, the enhanced blood–brain barrier permeability, and the infiltration of inflammatory myeloid cells. For instance, a genomic analysis revealed an upregulation of MMP-2 (for facilitating wound healing and promoting neuronal regeneration) and blood–brain barrier stabilizing proteins in microwire electrodes (indicating enhanced stability and reduced micromotions compared to Michigan electrodes). Despite these findings, the *critical surface area model* theory is preferred over the theory of *mechanical property differences* because of previous results that have shown negligible differences in glial encapsulation between the soft and flexible parylene/SU-8-based structures in [30] and the silicon-based arrays (that are orders of magnitude stiffer) in [25].

3.5. Embedding of bioactive reagents

3.5.1. Utah electrode array

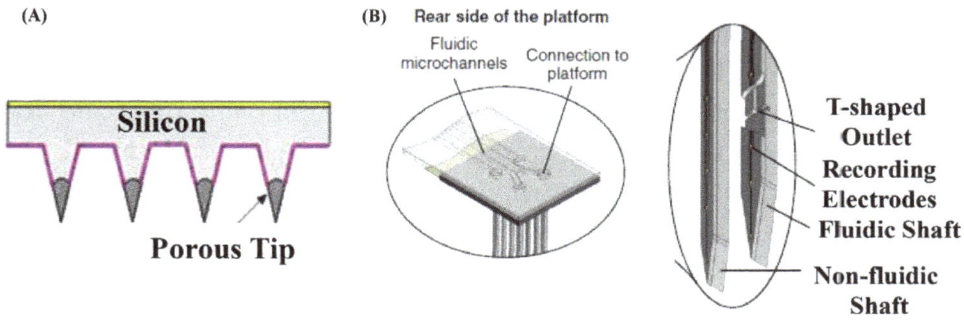

Figure 14. Platinum coated tips of the Utah electrode. Scale bar = 0.5 mm. Reproduced from [32, 33].

The microneedle array can be fabricated with porous tips that can be loaded with drugs that have a high molecular weight [32]. These porous tips are nano-structured silicon (**Figure 14A**), a material that is biocompatible, bioactive, biodegradable, and appropriate for the cultivation of adherent cells in-vivo without noticeable toxicity for biological applications. Drug delivery is also possible in the 3D floating silicon array by using a silicon platform that has microfluidic cables with adapters used for liquid supply [33]. Selected shafts can be equipped with fluidic integration (**Figure 14B**) with either one independent fluidic channel (to maximize the volume coverage) or two independent microchannels (to infuse both a drug and a buffer reference at the same location) when combining drug delivery within the array of recording electrodes.

3.5.2. Michigan neural probe

Planar microelectrodes can directly utilize innovations from micro-fabrication technology and lab-on-a-chip delivery devices. For instance, aerosol jet printing technology can be utilized to directly construct a patterned neural interface with anti-inflammatory nanocarriers [34]. 3D probe structures with microfluidic channels can also be fabricated via surface micromachining and deep reactive ion etching (DRIE) [35]. Neural probe designs (**Figure 15**) can also be bulk-microfabricated to include microchannels along the shanks for microscale and controlled fluid delivery through the blood–brain barrier [36].

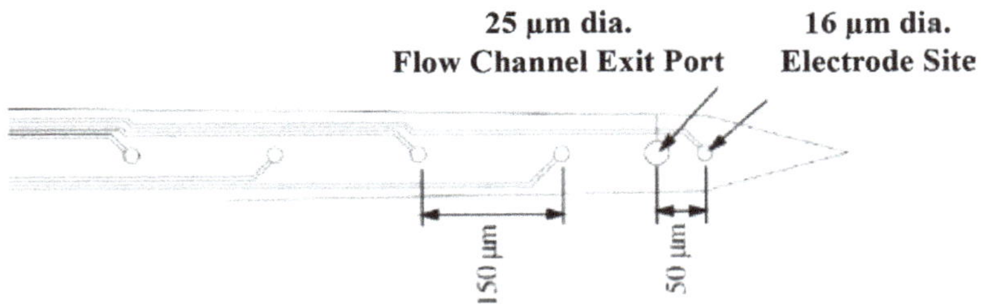

Figure 15. Probe design with microchannels along the shanks for controlled fluid delivery. Reproduced from [36].

4. Hydrogel improves biocompatibility and mechanical properties

4.1. Improved biocompatibility

Hydrogels such as Alginate are naturally occurring polysaccharides that are typically obtained from brown algae seaweed (**Figure 16**). These water-soluble biomaterials have many versatile properties such as gelling and film-forming. Hydrogels are biocompatible and are commonly used in biomedical or tissue engineering applications. Hydrogels are formed by cross-linking hydrophilic organic components and can respond to specific environmental changes [37]. This makes hydrogels the ideal polymer matrix for controlling the delivery of drugs and bioactive components into a complex biologic system.

Alginate hydrogels have been successfully applied as a coating on the Michigan probes. One study [38] showed that biodegradable neurotrophin-eluting hydrogels can be applied on the microelectrode arrays to attract neurites to the surface of the electrodes (for improved neuron-electrode proximity). Hydrogels can also be loaded with nanoparticles of anti-inflammatory agent dexamethasone (DEX) for drug delivery [39]. In-vitro drug release kinetics has revealed that 90% of the DEX can be successfully released from entrapped nanoparticles over 2 weeks. In addition, the impedance of the nanoparticle-loaded hydrogel coatings on microfabricated neural probes were equivalent to the unmodified/uncoated probes controls (indicating that the loaded-nanoparticles do not hinder electrical transport). Most importantly, the chronically implanted electrodes loaded with DEX were shown to maintain impedances in-vivo (unlike the control electrodes that showed increases after 2 weeks of implantation). This improvement in chronic neural recordings indicates the DEX-modified neural probes reduced the amount of glial inflammation via local administration of therapeutic agents. Hydrogels can also be used as a scaffold to encapsulate drug-incorporated biodegradable nanofibers for a more sustained and slower release (to reduce the burst effect [40]).

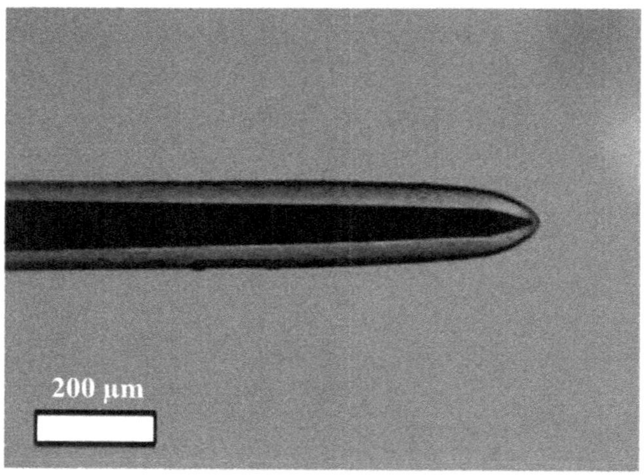

Figure 16. Optical microscopy image of an Alginate hydrogel coating on a Michigan probe. Reproduced from [41].

4.2. Improved mechanical properties

Hydrogels have also been proposed to improve the mechanical properties of the implantable microelectrodes. First, hydrogel coatings can be dehydrated to minimize the initial penetrating profile [41]. Second, the degree of reswelling can be controlled by using different cross-linking molecules to better anchor the position of the probe in the tissue after the implantation [42]. Third, the shear moduli of a hydrogel can be tightly regulated by controlling the cross-linking densities to reduce the stiffness mismatch between the hard silicon-based probes (~100 GPa) and the soft tissue (~10 kPa). Fourth, the uniformity of the hydrogel coating can be controlled by changing the concentration of the solution. Lastly, the hydrogel thickness can be controlled by quickly drying the coated surfaces in air and then overlaying additional layers on top.

Despite the many advantages of hydrogels, the spatial distribution of neurons (as it relates to recording quality) has been a barrier to the practical implementation of hydrogel coatings on microelectrodes. For instance, neural recordings in the auditory cortex showed a significant loss in functionality (as determined by the number of clearly detectable units and the average signal-to-noise ratios [43]). In fact, in-vivo experiments showed that only 30% of the electrode sites (with 80 μm thick hydrogel coatings) could record detectable signals from surrounding neurons and that the average signal-to-noise ratio dramatically decreased (even for 5 μm thick coatings). The loss in neural recording quality is hypothesized to be caused by the reswelling properties of the dehydrated hydrogel coatings (which can affect the spatial distribution of the target neurons around the implanted electrode). In other words, the low signal detection is hypothesized to be caused by the post-implantation water absorption which pushes the target neurons away from the electrode surfaces as they rehydrate (and beyond the *cylindrical radius* distances in [12] that are required for effective electrode recording, as illustrated in **Figure 3**).

To solve the hydrogel swelling problem, [44] proposed to modify the electrode design to place the recording sites in closer proximity to the hydrogel's surface (**Figure 17**). The deposition of conducting polymer PEDOT has also been shown to restore some of the lost functionality of electrode sites with thicker hydrogel coatings [43]. Alternatively, fibrin can be selected (rather than Alginate) to be reabsorbed in the surrounding tissues 7 days after the implantation [45].

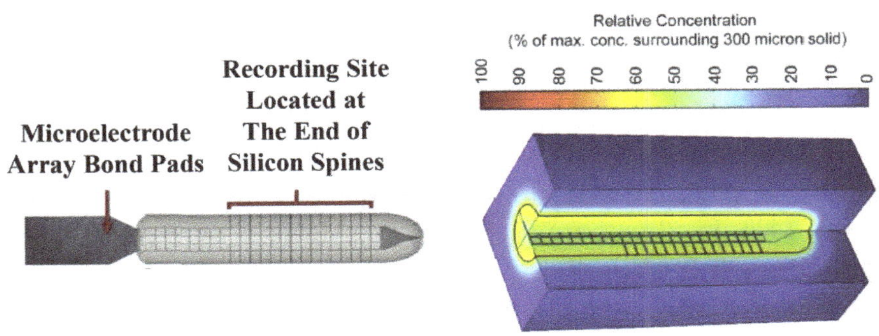

Figure 17. Electrode design with recording sites in closer proximity to the hydrogel's surface. Reproduced from [44].

4.3. The "Dipping Method"

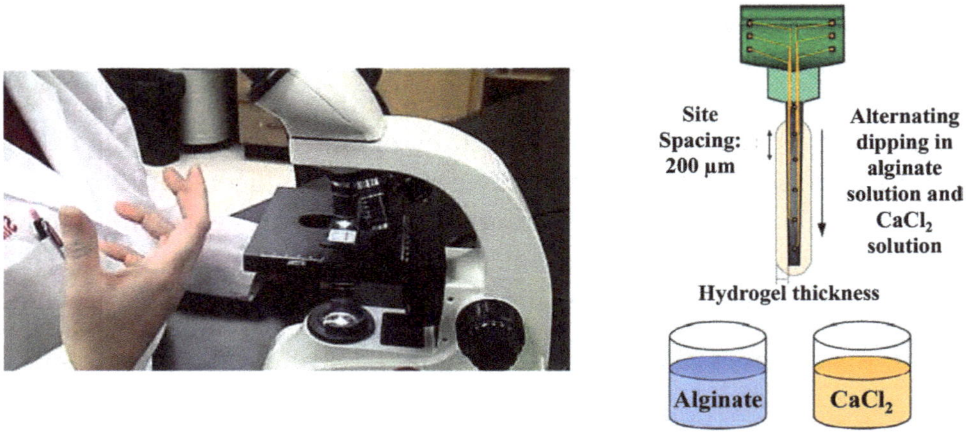

Figure 18. Dipping Method for hydrogel coating of neural electrodes with optical microscopy. Reproduced from [43].

While previous solutions to the hydrogel swelling problem have mostly proposed physical changes to the actual microelectrode or the hydrogel [39–45], most attempts still rely on the "*Dipping Method*" for depositing the hydrogel coatings onto the microelectrodes (as proposed in [41]). **Figure 18** shows the Dipping Method involves the repetitive dipping of electrodes (e.g. via an inverted fine-tooth syringe pump [44]) into an alginate solution followed by immersion in a $CaCl_2$ solution until a desired coating thickness is achieved. The thickness of the hydrogel coating is roughly controlled by monitoring the sample as a function of the number of dips with an optical microscope [43]. For instance, 1 dip is sufficient for a thin coating, and roughly 20 dips are needed to obtain a thick diameter coating. The hydrogel-coated electrodes are then dried in a laminar hood [43] or by exchanging ethanol and drying in an air stream [40].

In practice, the Dipping Method has several problems. First, lateral movements of the neural electrode effect the reproducibility of the alginate coating around the shank of the probe [40]. Second, it is impossible to control the average thickness by just approximating the number of dipping cycles (as verified by ellipsometry data in Figure 4B of [44]). Third, it is impossible to control the maximum radial thickness by just altering the number of dips (as demonstrated in Figure 2C of [45]). Fourth, the speed of dipping effects the uniformity of the alginate coating around the shank of the probe [40]. These limitations of the Dipping Method are confounding and counter-productive when considering that the entire rationale for using hydrogel coatings was to control the mechanical properties of the electrodes in [41]. Furthermore, the Dipping Method requires a human observer to subjectively monitor the entire dipping process with an optical microscope [43]. Therefore, this proposed Dipping Method essentially eliminates one of the primary advantage of the Michigan probes: exploiting semiconductor manufacturing techniques to allow batch fabrication for the high reproducibility of geometrical/electrical characteristics (as highlighted in Section 3.1.2).

4.4. The "Dropping Method"

Techniques for coating hydrogels onto microelectrodes include spray coating, brush coating, Dipping Methods [39–45], and micropipetting [38]. Unfortunately, none of these methods can produce uniform coatings in a reproducible manner [46]. Therefore, novel strategies such as the Molding Method (which involves the photopolymerization of hydrogels in a polyethylene tube) have been proposed to provide hydrogel coatings that are more reproducible and have a means to control coating uniformity and thickness (e.g. by varying the polyethylene tubing).

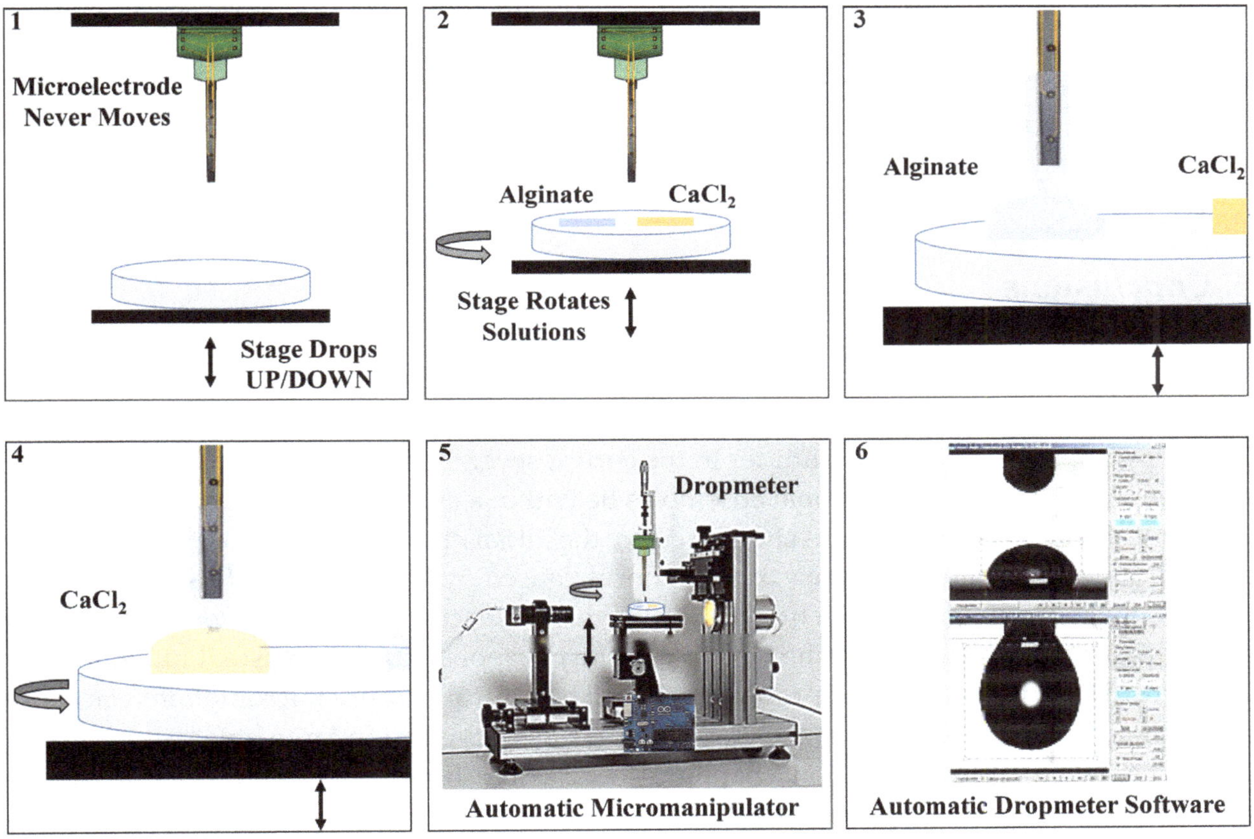

Figure 19. Dropping Method for hydrogel coating of neural electrodes with a fully-automated procedure.

Figure 19 proposes a novel procedure called the "Dropping Method" to address the reported limitations of the Dipping Method. First, the microelectrode is permanently attached in one location to eliminate lateral movements (to improve reproducibility [40]). Second, a stage that contains solutions is automatically revolved to eliminate the requirement of approximating movements (to improve the average thickness [44]). Third, the stage is dropped downward to allow gravity to align the droplets and to evenly pull down the edges (to improve the radial thickness [45]). Fourth, the speed of dropping is automated by a digital micromanipulator (to improve the uniformity of the alginate coating around the shank of the probe [40]). Finally, the optimal contact angle is automated on a Dropmeter stage via programmable software (instead of relying on subjective interpretations of a human observer via optical microscopy as in [43]).

FEM and histological analyses have shown that elevated local strains correspond to increases in gliosis (with a three-fold increase in gliosis at the probe tips compared to other areas of the explanted arrays [19]). In addition, FEM pressure profiles predict that the strain at the tip can be reduced by utilizing more flexible or softer substrates, reducing the opening angle of the probe face, and by promoting tissue integration to reduce excessive adhesion. Therefore, the Dropping Method is recommended for coating hydrogel at the tips of the microelectrodes to optimize the mechanical effects for improved chronic recording stability. Applying hydrogel coatings on the probe tips should stabilize the mechanical interface and lower the interfacial tension with the surrounding biological environment. Constraining hydrogel coating depths to just the tips will also avoid the electrode coverage issue [12]. Finally, the initial penetrating profile should be reduced since only the dehydrated probe tips will reswell in thickness upon water absorption (unlike previous studies that coated the hydrogel layers along the entire length of the neural electrode shanks in efforts to reduce the sustained injury responses).

5. Conclusions

This chapter reviewed how controlling the biocompatibility and mechanical properties of a microelectrode is critical when implanting deeper within the auditory system. To effectively monitor extracellular spike amplitudes in the cortex, several design considerations should be factored to ensure that the neuronal ensembles lie within a cylindrical radius of the recording electrode. First, penetrating shafts should reduce the initial mechanical trauma during surgical implantation (to minimize the reactive responses caused by the pathway of tissue damage). Second, the indwelling microelectrodes should embed bioactive reagents since chronic neural recording failure is associated with sustained injury responses from persistent inflammatory reactions. Third, the mechanical properties should be controlled since micromotions can cause shearing and compression to the surrounding tissues (due to the large stiffness mismatch of the implanted substrates). This chapter also describes how hydrogels can minimize the cross-sectional area while ensuring the neuronal density is maintained in local areas surrounding the implant. A novel hydrogel coating "Dropping Method" is proposed instead of the Dipping Method to eliminate the problems of lateral movements, approximated cycles, and uniformity.

Acknowledgements

In this chapter, some parts of this work was performed when the first author was with the Centre for Biosystems, Neuroscience, and Nanotechnology, City University of Hong Kong, Hong Kong, with Stella Pang. The author is now working at the Center for Information Technology Innovation (CITI), Academia Sinica, Taipei, Taiwan with Yu Tsao.

Glossary

Auditory cortex: region of the temporal lobe that is responsible for processing auditory information.

Biocompatibility: ability of a biomaterial to perform with an appropriate host response in the body.

Brain machine interface: technology that allows direct communication pathways between the brain.

Chronic neural recordings: long-term neural recordings by implantable (e.g. intracortical) electrodes.

Critical surface area model: theory of minimizing electrode surfaces to reduce tissue encapsulations.

Cylindrical radius: neuronal ensembles must lie within ~140 μm of the recording electrode [12].

Dipping method: hydrogel coating as a function of the number of dips (via optical microscopy).

Dropping Method: hydrogel coating automated on Dropmeter stage (via programmable software).

Electrode micromotion: induced strain from relative movements between the probe and the tissue.

Finite element model: numerical analysis that can approximate the behavior of mechanical systems.

Glial encapsulation: formation of a fibrotic encapsulation layer or a glial scar surrounding an implant.

Hydrogel coating: biomaterials with many versatile properties such as gelling and film-forming.

Inflammatory reactions: complex biological responses of tissues that protect from harmful stimuli.

Insertion killzone: region around the shaft where the local neuron density is lower than expected.

Utah electrode array: 3D arrays consisting of conductive needles (designed at University of Utah).

Mechanical property difference: theory of minimizing micromotions to reduce tissue encapsulation.

Michigan probe: planar shanks from semiconductor platforms (designed at University of Michigan).

Microelectrode: electrical conductor used for recording neural representations in the brain.

Author details

Payton Lin[1,2]*, Yu Tsao[2] and Li-Wei Kuo[3]

*Address all correspondence to: paytonlin20@gmail.com

1 Centre for Biosystems, Neuroscience, and Nanotechnology (CBNN), City University of Hong Kong, Hong Kong SAR

2 Academia Sinica, Center for Information Technology Innovation, Taipei, Taiwan

3 National Health Research Institute, Institute of Biomedical Engineering and Nanomedicine, Taiwan

References

[1] Kennedy PR, Bakay RAE, Moore MM, Adams K, Goldwaith J. Direct control of a computer from the human nervous system. IEEE Transactions on Rehabilitation Engineering. 2000;**8**:198-202

[2] Merzenich MM, Brugge JF. Representation of the cochlear partition on the superior temporal plane of the macaque monkey. Brain Research. 1973;**50**(2):275-296

[3] Rauschecker JP, Tian B, Hauser M. Processing of complex sounds in the macaque nonprimary auditory cortex. Science. 1995;**268**:111-114

[4] Kaas JH, Hacket TA. Subdivisions of auditory cortex and processing streams in primates. Proceedings of the National Academy of Sciences. 2000;**97**(22):11793-11799

[5] Howard MA, Volkov IO, Abbas PJ, Damasio H, Ollendieck MC, Granner MA. A chronic microelectrode investigation of the tonotopic organization of the human auditory cortex. Brain Research. 1996;**724**(2):260-264

[6] Sanchez JC, Principe JC, Nishida T, Bashirullah R, Harris JG, Fortes JA. Technology and signal processing for brain-machine interfaces. IEEE Signal Processing Magazine. 2008; **25**(1):29-40

[7] Moxon KA, Kalkhoran NM, Markert M, Sambito MA, McKenzie JL, Webster JT. Nanostructured surface modification of ceramic-based microelectrodes to enhance biocompatibility for a direct brain-machine interface. IEEE Transactions on Biomedical Engineering. 2004;**51**(6):881-889

[8] Polikov VS, Tresco PA, Reichert WM. Response of brain tissue to chronically implanted neural electrodes. Journal of Neuroscience Methods. 2005;**148**(1):1-18

[9] Kim GB, Fattahi P, Abidian MR. Electrode–neural tissue interactions: Immune responses, current technologies, and future directions. In: Taubert A, Mano JF, Rodríguez-Cabello JC, editors. Biomaterials Surface Science. Weinheim, Germany: Wiley-VCH Verlag GmbH & Co. KGaA; 2013. p. 539-565

[10] Vetter RJ, Williams JC, Hetke JF, Nunamaker EA, Kipke DR. Chronic neural recording using silicon-substrate microelectrode arrays implanted in cerebral cortex. IEEE Transactions on Biomedical Engineering. 2004;**51**(6):896-904

[11] Williams JC, Hippensteel JA, Dilgen J, Shain W, Kipke DR. Complex impedance spectroscopy for monitoring tissue responses to inserted neural implants. Journal of Neural Engineering. 2007;**4**(4):410

[12] Buzsáki G. Large-scale recording of neuronal ensembles. Nature Neuroscience. 2004;**7**(5): 446

[13] Edell DJ, Toi VV, Mcneil VM, Clark LD. Factors influencing the biocompatibility of insertable silicon microshafts in cerebral cortex. IEEE Transactions on Biomedical Engineering. 1992;**39**(6):635-643

[14] Szarowski DH, Andersen MD, Retterer S, Spence AJ, Isaacson M, Craighead HG, Turner JN, Shain W. Brain responses to micro-machined silicon devices. Brain Research. 2003;**983**(1):23-35

[15] Biran R, Martin DC, Tresco PA. Neuronal cell loss accompanies the brain tissue response to chronically implanted silicon microelectrode arrays. Experimental Neurology. 2005;**195**(1): 115-126

[16] Stensaas SS, Stensaas LJ. Histopathological evaluation of materials implanted in the cerebral cortex. Acta Neuropathologica. 1978;**41**(2):145-155

[17] Miller K, Chinzei K, Orssengo G, Bednarz P. Mechanical properties of brain tissue in-vivo: Experiment and computer simulation. Journal of Biomechanics. 2000;**33**(11):1369-1376

[18] Subbaroyan J, Martin DC, Kipke DR. A finite-element model of the mechanical effects of implantable microelectrodes in the cerebral cortex. Journal of Neural Engineering. 2005;**2**(4):103

[19] Hoogerwerf AC, Wise KD. A three-dimensional microelectrode array for chronic neural recording. IEEE Transactions on Biomedical Engineering. 1994;**41**(12):1136-1146

[20] Britt RH, Rossi GT. Quantitative analysis of methods for reducing physiological brain pulsations. Journal of Neuroscience Methods. 1982;**6**(3):219-229

[21] Fee MS. Active stabilization of electrodes for intracellular recording in awake behaving animals. Neuron. 2000;**27**(3):461-468

[22] Gilletti A, Muthuswamy J. Brain micromotion around implants in the rodent somatosensory cortex. Journal of Neural Engineering. 2006;**3**(3):189

[23] Goldstein SR, Salcman M. Mechanical factors in the design of chronic recording intracortical microelectrodes. IEEE Transactions on Biomedical Engineering. 1973;**4**:260-269

[24] Normann RA, Maynard EM, Rousche PJ, Warren DJ. A neural interface for a cortical vision prosthesis. Vision Research. 1999;**39**(15):2577-2587

[25] Skousen JL, Merriam SM, Srivannavit O, Perlin G, Wise KD, Tresco PA. Reducing surface area while maintaining implant penetrating profile lowers the brain foreign body response to chronically implanted planar silicon microelectrode arrays. Progress in Brain Reserach. 2011;**194**:167-180

[26] Jones KE, Campbell PK, Normann RA. A glass/silicon composite intracortical electrode array. Annals of Biomedical Engineering. 1992;**20**(4):423-437

[27] Seymour JP, Wu F, Wise KD, Yoon E. State-of-the-art MEMS and microsystem tools for brain research. Microsystems & Nanoengineering. 2017;**3**:16066

[28] Saxena T, Karumbaiah L, Gaupp EA, Patkar R, Patil K, Betancur M, Garrett B, Bellamkonda RV. The impact of chronic blood–brain barrier breach on intracortical electrode function. Biomaterials. 2013;**34**(20):4703-4713

[29] Thelin J, Jörntell H, Psouni E, Garwicz M, Schouenborg J, Danielsen N, Linsmeier CE. Implant size and fixation mode strongly influence tissue reactions in the CNS. PLoS One. 2011;**6**(1):e16267

[30] Seymour JP, Kipke DR. Neural probe design for reduced tissue encapsulation in CNS. Biomaterials. 2007;**28**(25):3594-3607

[31] Lee H, Bellamkonda RV, Sun W, Levenston ME. Biomechanical analysis of silicon micro-electrode-induced strain in the brain. Journal of Neural Engineering. 2005;**2**(4):81

[32] Ji J, Tay FE, Miao J, Iliescu C. Microfabricated microneedle with porous tip for drug delivery. Journal of Micromechanics and Microengineering. 2006;**16**(5):958

[33] Spieth S, Brett O, Seidl K, Aarts AAA, Erismis MA, Herwik S, Trenkle F, Tatzner S, Auber J, Daub M, Neves HP, Puers R, Paul O, Ruthner P, Zengerle R. A floating 3D silicon micro-probe array for neural drug delivery compatible with electrical recording. Journal of Micromechanics and Microengineering. 2011;**21**(12):125001

[34] Huang WC, Lai HY, Kuo LW, Liao CH, Chang PH, Liu TC, Chen SY, Chen YY. Multi-functional 3D patternable drug-embedded nanocarrier-based interfaces to enhance signal recording and reduce neuron degeneration in neural implantation. Advanced Materials. 2015;**27**(28):4186-4193

[35] Retterer ST, Smith KL, Bjornsson CS, Neeves KB, Spence AJ, Turner JN, Shain W, Isaacson MS. Model neural prostheses with integrated microfluidics: A potential inter-vention strategy for controlling reactive cell and tissue responses. IEEE Transactions on Biomedical Engineering. 2004;**51**(11):2063-2073

[36] Rathnasingham R, Kipke DR, Bledsoe SC, McLaren JD. Characterization of implantable microfabricated fluid delivery devices. IEEE Transactions on Biomedical Engineering. 2004;**51**(1):138-145

[37] Gong C, Wong KL, Lam MH. Photoresponsive molecularly imprinted hydrogels for the photoregulated release and uptake of pharmaceuticals in the aqueous media. Chemistry of Materials. 2008;**20**(4):1353-1358

[38] Winter JO, Cogan SF, Rizzo JF. Neurotrophin-eluting hydrogel coatings for neural stimu-lating electrodes. Journal of Biomedical Materials Research Part B: Applied Biomaterials. 2007;**81**(2):551-563

[39] Kim DH, Martin DC. Sustained release of dexamethasone from hydrophilic matrices using PLGA nanoparticles for neural drug delivery. Biomaterials. 2006;**27**(15):3031-3037

[40] Abidian MR, Martin DC. Multifunctional nanobiomaterials for neural interfaces. Advanced Functional Materials. 2009;**19**(4):573-585

[41] Kim DH, Abidian M, Martin DC. Conducting polymers grown in hydrogel scaffolds coated on neural prosthetic devices. Journal of Biomedical Materials Research Part A. 2004;**71**(4):577-585

[42] Lee KY, Rowley JA, Eiselt P, Moy EM, Bouhadir KH, Mooney DJ. Controlling mechanical and swelling properties of alginate hydrogels independently by cross-linker type and cross-linking density. Macromolecules. 2000;**33**(11):4291-4294

[43] Kim DH, Wiler JA, Anderson DJ, Kipke DR, Martin DC. Conducting polymers on hydrogel-coated neural electrode provide sensitive neural recordings in auditory cortex. Acta Biomaterialia. 2010;**6**(1):57-62

[44] Skousen JL, Bridge MJ, Tresco PA. A strategy to passively reduce neuroinflammation surrounding devices implanted chronically in brain tissue by manipulating device surface permeability. Biomaterials. 2015;**36**:33-43

[45] De Faveri S, Maggiolini E, Miele E, De Angelis F, Cesca F, Benfenati F, Fadiga L. Bio-inspired hybrid microelectrodes: A hybrid solution to improve long-term performance of chronic intracortical implants. Frontiers in Neuroengineering. 2014;**7**(7):1-12

[46] Jhaveri SJ, Hynd MR, Dowell-Mesfin N, Turner JN, Shain W, Ober CK. Release of nerve growth factor from HEMA hydrogel-coated substrates and its effect on the differentiation of neural cells. Biomacromolecules. 2008;**10**(1):174-183

7

Hearing Loss in Congenital Microtia

Kenichi Takano

Abstract

Congenital microtia occurs in approximately one in 10,000–20,000 live births as a result of the aberrant development of the first and second branchial arches. However, the exact pathogenesis of microtia remains unknown; it is considered a multifactorial disease where both environmental and genetic factors play a role. Microtia and aural atresia are known to be associated with conductive or mixed hearing loss caused by the developmental failure of the auricle, the external auditory canal (EAC), and middle ear structures. Cholesteatoma and mandibular dysplasia are also known to occur in microtia and atresia, as well as rare conditions, such as facial nerve paralysis, chorda tympani dysfunction, and inner ear deformity. The first branchial arch is the origin of the malleus head and the incus body as well as of the mandible, and the second arch derivatives include the stapes bone, the long process of the incus, and the manubrium of the malleus. It has been reported that the grade of microtia and the severity of middle ear abnormalities are correlated, and it is thought that better development indicates more developed middle ear structures. The existence of additional structural anomalies is suggestive of a broader developmental problem in most patients with microtia. This chapter will focus on hearing loss and structural anomalies in congenital microtia.

Keywords: microtia, atresia, facial nerve, taste disorder, hearing

1. Introduction

Congenital microtia occurs in approximately one in 10,000–20,000 live births as a result of aberrant development of the first and second branchial arches [1]. The exact pathogenesis of microtia remains unclear, but it is considered to be a multifactorial disease in which both environmental and genetic factors are thought to be associated with its pathogenesis. Microtia and aural atresia are known to be associated with conductive or mixed hearing loss and are caused by developmental failure of the auricle, the external auditory canal (EAC), and structures of the middle ear [2, 3]. Other complications, such as cholesteatoma and mandibular dysplasia, are also known to occur in microtia and atresia, as well as rare conditions such as inner ear deformity, facial nerve paralysis, and chorda tympani dysfunction [4, 5]. It is well known that the first branchial arch is the origin of the head of the malleus, body of the incus, and the mandible, and the derivatives of the second arch include the stapes bone, the long process of the incus, and the manubrium of the malleus [2, 3]. Developmental abnormalities of the first and second branchial arches can give rise to congenital microtia and atresia, which have a significant effect on the development of the ear, including the course of the facial nerve.

Most children with congenital microtia are identified by an obvious anomaly at birth; however, they do not always receive the necessary medical care. Although otolaryngologists frequently examine only the hearing level of patients with microtia, those born with both microtia and aural atresia have a complex craniofacial condition that may affect all aspects of their lives, requiring up-to-date and unbiased patient information.

Patients with microtia are unable to undergo corrective plastic surgery until they are in their early teens since their rib bones need to be of a sufficient size for harvesting in order to create an adequately sized graft. Otolaryngologists are responsible for providing care and support to them throughout their lives.

In this chapter, we present the clinical characteristics of congenital microtia and atresia and associated complications observed at our hospital for the benefit of medical staff involved in the care of patients with these conditions.

2. Clinical characteristics and embryology of congenital microtia

The grade of microtia and the severity of middle ear abnormalities are correlated, and it is thought that better development indicates more developed middle ear structures. We investigated 172 patients (191 ears) who underwent reconstructive surgery for their external ear malformations at our university. Consistent with a previous study [1], there was a predominance of right-sided microtia (62%) and boys (64%) (**Table 1**). Although the basis for the sex discrepancy in microtia incidence has not been determined, the difference appears to be more common in Asia. Only 11% of patients had bilateral involvement. **Figure 1** shows the distribution of microtia according to severity using the Marx system proposed by Marx in 1926 [6]. Briefly, grade I microtia corresponds to a normal-shaped but small pinna, grade II to a residual vertical ridge of the tissue, and grade III to the complete absence of the pinna or the presence of only rudimentary soft tissue. The distribution was as follows: 3% was classified as grade I, 27% as grade II, and 78% as grade III (**Table 1**). It has been reported that 74% of cases of microtia are complicated with narrow external auditory atresia [2, 3], and one in five cases with congenital external auditory stenosis are complicated with ear canal cholesteatoma [6]. In our patients, narrow external auditory atresia described as complete atresia was present in approximately 70%, and external auditory stenosis affected 30%.

Careful observation is required to detect external auditory stenosis patients with ear canal cholesteatoma.

Embryologically, the auricle is formed from several protuberances in the first and second branchial arches. These protuberances, known as auricular hillocks, surround the first branchial cleft, which is the space between the first and second branchial arches [8]. Each of the hillocks contributes to a specific component of the auricle, and those in the second branchial arch form most of the ear structure. The external auditory canal and lateral tympanic membrane are derived from the ectoderm of the first branchial cleft and the epithelium of the middle ear cavity, which is derived from the endoderm of the first pharyngeal pouch. The ossicles develop from the mesenchyme of the proximal area of the branchial arches, and the malleus and incus both derive from the first branchial arch (mandibular area and maxillary area, respectively), while the stapes is formed from the second branchial arch.

Marx's classification	%
Grade I	3
Grade II	27
Grade III	78
Sex	
Male	64
Female	36
Laterally	
Right	62
Left	27
Bilateral	11

Table 1. Characteristics of patients with congenital microtia.

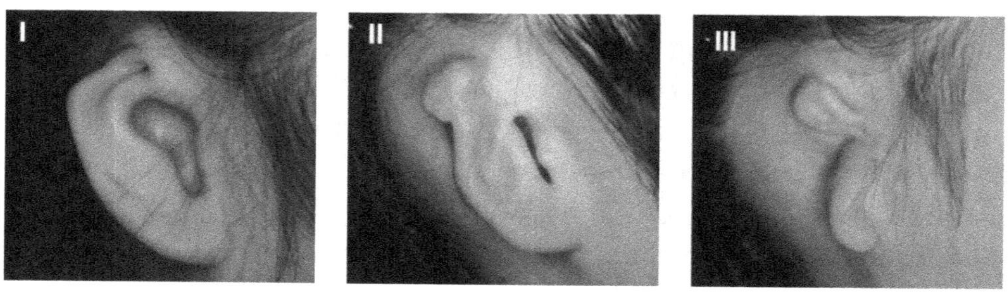

Figure 1. Marx system. Grade I: A normal-shaped but small pinna. Grade II: A residual vertical ridge of the tissue. Grade III: Complete absence of the pinna or the presence of only rudimentary soft tissue.

3. Hearing level

The pure-tone hearing average (average air conduction threshold at 0.5, 1, and 2 kHz) is used as a representative value for the hearing level, and the normal hearing range is generally defined as greater than 20 dB with an air-bone gap within 15 dB. We investigated the hearing levels for our patients with congenital microtia and compared these hearing levels with Marx's classification results (**Table 2**). Marx's classification scores did not show a correlation with the pure-tone hearing level. A previous report also found that the hearing level in microtic ears does not correlate with the degree of microtia [7].

Marx's classification	Air conduction threshold (dB)	Bone conduction threshold (dB)	Air-bone gap (dB)
Grade I	27.5	5.8	21.7
Grade II	60.9	12.8	48.1
Grade III	76.8	11.9	64.9

Table 2. Average hearing level in patients with microtia.

4. Facial nerve and chorda tympani nerve palsy

Facial nerve palsy and chorda tympani are also known to occur in some cases of congenital microtia. In our study [5], facial nerve paralysis (House-Brackmann grade more than III) and change in taste detection threshold due to chorda tympani nerve dysfunction were found in 8 and 10% of patients with microtia, respectively. We found that chorda tympani nerve dysfunction did not correlate significantly with the anatomic structure of the ear anomalies based on Jahrsdoerfer scores. On the other hand, facial nerve paralysis was significantly correlated with the presence of a malleus-incus complex, a pneumatized mastoid, an incus-stapes connection, and an external auditory canal, and facial nerve paralysis patients had a higher Jahrsdoerfer score than the chorda tympani nerve dysfunction patients.

The facial nerve canal arises initially as a sulcus in the cartilaginous otic capsule, and ossification begins from two distinct sites, such as anteriorly near the apex of the cochlea and posteriorly at the pyramidal eminence, at 20 and 25 weeks' gestation, respectively. The bone progressively covers the facial nerve, and the process is usually complete by 3 months after birth. Since the mastoid process and tympanic ring grow after birth, they displace the nerve medially. Therefore, the development of the facial nerve is closely related to the development of the middle ear and the mastoid process. Meanwhile, the chorda tympani branches from the facial nerve at 5 weeks' gestation and subsequently separates the stapes primordium and the incus primordium from the hyoid visceral bar. Unlike the facial nerve, the chorda tympani in the middle ear is not encased by a bony wall. This early branching and development of the chorda tympani may be one of the reasons why our study did not show a significant correlation between chorda tympani nerve dysfunction and facial nerve paralysis; 83% of patients with chorda tympani nerve dysfunction did not have facial nerve paralysis. In addition, there was no significant difference in Jahrsdoerfer scores for the facial nerve between those with and without chorda tympani nerve dysfunction [5]. It is speculated that facial nerve paralysis, probably including chorda tympani nerve dysfunction, does not always correspond to an anatomic abnormality of the nerve tract.

5. Management of patients with congenital microtia

Because approximately 20–60% of patients with congenital microtia are known to have associated anomalies or an identifiable syndrome [8], patients with microtia should be examined for other dysmorphic features. In our patients, although there were no cases complicated by anomalies in the kidney and spine, there were some children complicated by esophageal atresia, ventricular septal defect, funnel chest, and cleft lip and palate. Especially, symptomatic microtia, which includes Goldenhar syndrome, hemifacial microsomia, trisomy 21, trisomy 18, and Treacher Collins syndrome, may have additional associated congenital anomalies.

Gorlin et al. [9] proposed an encompassing term "oculo-auriculo-vertebral spectrum (OAVS)," which is characterized by facial asymmetry, microtia, ear and facial tags, epibulbar dermoids, microphthalmia, and macrostomia. Hemifacial microsomia, Goldenhar syndrome, and all of its associated anomalies and variations are thought to be included in this spectrum. Extracranial features include renal, cardiac, and vertebral anomalies; at present, there is no consensus on the minimal diagnostic criteria for OAVS [10]. OAVS and microtia share the following characteristics: (1) variable phenotypic expression, (2) asymmetric involvement of facial structures, (3) right-side preponderance, (4) male predilection, and (5) familial occurrence of microtia or related anomalies, such as preauricular tags and pits [10]. Thus, isolated microtia represents a milder phenotype of OAVS.

The clinical expression of congenital microtia and OAVS overlap; hence, clinicians should consider multiple medical assessments when examining patients with microtia. First, all patients with microtia should have a diagnostic ear-specific hearing assessment within the first 6 months of age, to identify hearing loss and to assess the type and severity of hearing impairment. In children with conductive hearing loss, high-resolution CT examination of the temporal bone is useful for evaluating the middle and inner ear structures when the child is of preschool or school age. Renal ultrasound, cardiovascular examination at diagnosis, and cervical spine films at the age of 3 years are also recommended [11]. Treatment for atresia should be considered in the context of hearing, speech and language development, and reconstructive surgery at approximately 10 years of age.

Since lack of landmarks, abnormal anatomies of the facial nerve and middle ear structures, and limited space for sound reconstruction, surgical correction of hearing improvement is sometimes difficult and challenging. Therefore, not only surgery but also hearing acquisition through the use of a device should be considered. To date, osseointegrated implants known as bone-anchored hearing aids (BAHA® by Cochlear) and active middle ear implants known as Vibrant Soundbridge® (VSB by Med-El) have been the most reliable method of hearing habilitation. These devices have been shown to improve hearing outcomes and quality of life in patients with microtia who might not otherwise benefit from traditional hearing aids. However, in order to use these implants, patients need to underwent surgery, and the portion of the implant exposed to open air has a risk of infection.

More recently, a new hearing device utilizing cartilage conduction has been developed [12]. Since the transducer is not necessarily fixed with pressure, the attachment causes no pain, unlike conventional bone conduction. Moreover, this cartilage conduction device does not require surgery. Cartilage conduction hearing aids have a potential as a useful amplification device for patients with congenital microtia and aural atresia.

6. Conclusion

We conclude that longitudinal care is required for patients with congenital microtia. This care involves the precise and regular evaluation of hearing levels from birth and investigation of malformations of the external auditory canal, middle ear, and inner ear, as well as cholesteatoma and abnormal occlusions occurring at predictable times in relationship with craniofacial growth and development. Microtia can be associated with other congenital abnormalities that are not obvious at birth. Furthermore, the external surface malformations frequently cause adverse psychosocial effects during children's growth process. Patients and their families should be supported in an unbiased manner when making decisions regarding which treatments are the most appropriate for the patient at a particular point of development, and this support must continue throughout the patients' life. In addition, means of hearing improvement should not simply be a difficult operation and instead involve careful consideration of the patient's interests and careful selection among the various options.

Terminology index

Atresia: The absence or closure of the external auditory canal

Auricular hillocks: Six (three-paired) mesenchymal condensations around the first pharyngeal cleft

Branchial arch: Paired structures associated with the pharynx that contribute greatly to the formation of the head and neck

Branchial cleft: The slit-like openings in the gills of fish between the branchial arches

Ectoderm: One of the three primary germ layers in the early embryo

Goldenhar syndrome: A complex congenital anomaly characterized by abnormal development of the eye, ear, and spine

Hemifacial microsomia: A congenital condition in which one or more parts of the face are underdeveloped

Pharyngeal pouch: Saclike diverticula that formed on the endodermal side between the pharyngeal arches

Primordium: An organ or part in the earliest recognizable stage of development

Mesenchyme: A type of undifferentiated connective tissue comprised of loose cells embedded in the extracellular matrix

Microtia: A congenital malformation of variable severity of the ear

Otic capsule: The cartilage that surrounds the developing otic vesicle and develops into the bony labyrinth of the internal ear

Author details

Kenichi Takano

Address all correspondence to: kent@sapmed.ac.jp

Department of Otolaryngology, Sapporo Medical University, School of Medicine, Sapporo, Hokkaido, Japan

References

[1] Luquetti DV, Leoncini E, Mastroiacovo P. Microtia-anotia: A global review of prevalence rates. Birth Defects Research Part A: Clinical and Molecular Teratology. 2011;**91**:813-822

[2] Harris J, Kallen B, Robert E. The epidemiology of anotia and microtia. Journal of Medical Genetics. 1996;**33**:809-813

[3] Okajima H, Takeichi Y, Umeda K, Baba S. Clinical analysis of 592 patients with microtia. Acta Oto-Laryngologica. Supplementum. 1996;**525**:18-24

[4] Takano K, Takahashi N, Ogasawara N, Himi T. The association of external and middle ear anomaly and mandibular morphology in congenital microtia. Otology & Neurotology. 2016;**37**:889-894

[5] Takano K, Takahashi N, Ogasawara N, Yotsuyanagi T, Himi T. Chorda tympani nerve dysfunction associated with congenital microtia. Acta Otorrinolaringológica. 2017;**137**:686-689

[6] Jahrsdoerfer RA, Yeakly JW, Guilar EA, Cole RR, Gray LC. Grading system for the selection of patients with congenital aural atresia. The American Journal of Otology. 1992;**13**:6-12

[7] Ishimoto S, Ito K, Karino S, Takegoshi H, Kaga K, Yamasoba T. Hearing levels in patients with microtia: Correlation with temporal bone malformation. The Laryngoscope. 2007;**117**:461-465

[8] Luquetti DV, Heike CL, Hing AV, Cunningham ML, Cox TC. Microtia: Epidemiology and genetics. American Journal of Medical Genetics. Part A. 2012;**158**:124-139

[9] Gorlin RJ, Cohen MM, Hennekam RCM. Syndromes of the Head and Neck. 4th ed. New York: Oxford University Press; 2001. p. 1344

[10] Shonka DC Jr, Livingston 3rd WJ, Kesser BW. The Jahrsdoerfer grading scale in surgery to repair congenital aural atresia. Archives of Otolaryngology – Head & Neck Surgery 2008;**134**:873-877

[11] Heike CL, Hing AV, Aspinall CA, Bartlett SP, Birgfeld CB, Drake AF, Pimenta LA, Sie KC, Urata MM, Vivaldi D, Luquetti DV. Clinical care in craniofacial microsomia: A review of current management recommendations and opportunities to advance research. American Journal of Medical Genetics. Part C, Seminars in Medical Genetics. 2013;**163**:271-282

[12] Nishimura T, Hosoi H, Saito O, Miyamae R, Shimokura R, Matsui T, Iwakura T. Benefit of a new hearing device utilizing cartilage conduction. Auris, Nasus, Larynx. 2013;**40**: 440-446

8

Characterization of Hearing Loss in Children with Mucopolysaccharidosis

Diego Zanetti, Margherita Vezzani,
Federica Di Berardino, Serena Gasperini and
Rossella Parini

Abstract

Hearing impairment is common in patients with mucopolysaccharidoses (MPS) in the preschool age. Conductive or mixed hearing loss is the most frequent occurrence while the involvement of the inner ear or central auditory pathways may occur in more severe forms. A retrospective review of 82 children with MPS admitted at the Pediatric Department of the University of Milano Bicocca was performed to determine the incidence of otological symptoms. We focused particularly on audiological investigations in a subgroup of 47 children diagnosed before 6 years of age (MPS I, n = 11 patients; MPS II, n = 10; MPS III, n = 7; MPS IV, n = 14; MPS VI, n = 5). In 37 children, a magnetic resonance imaging (MRI) of the brain and cervical spine was also performed in order to correlate the audiological findings with the imaging of the middle and inner ear. A total of 40 out of 47 children (86%) showed some degree of hearing impairment: sensorineural or mixed hearing loss in 23 cases (48.93%) and retrocochlear in 4 (8.51%). MRI ascertained multiple CNS abnormalities in 13 (35.3%): dilated perivascular spaces in 5 (38.5%); dilated ventricular cavities in 5 (38.5%); demyelinated and gliotic areas in 3 (23.0%). Conversely, one-fourth of the children's inner ears showed some morphological anomaly (24.3%).

Keywords: mucopolysaccharidoses, hearing loss, auditory brainstem responses (ABR), transient-evoked otoacoustic emissions (TEOAE), MRI

1. Introduction

Mucopolysaccharidoses (MPSs) are a group of rare inherited metabolic disorders resulting from deficiencies of enzymes involved in the breakdown of glycosaminoglycans (GAGs).

MPS disorders have an overall incidence reported of 1.53 per 100,000 live births ranging from 1 in 150,000 to as high as 1 in 10,000 live births [1]. The highest birth prevalence was 0.84 for MPS II, accounting for 55% of all MPS. MPS I, III, and IV accounted for 15, 16, and 10%, respectively. MPS VI and VII were more rare and accounted for 1.7 and 1.3%, respectively.

The majority are characterized by an autosomal recessive pattern (except for X-linked MPS II type). The deficiency of one of the enzymes participating in the GAGs degradation pathway causes progressive storage in the lysosomes, leading to cellular, tissues and organs dysfunction. The damage is both direct or by activation of secondary and tertiary pathways among which a role is played by inflammation.

Nowadays 11 different enzyme deficiencies are known to be involved in MPSs producing seven distinct clinical phenotypes. In contrast to a recent past when there was only palliative treatment for these diseases, now many specific treatments like hematopoietic stem cell transplantation (HSCT) in selected cases (severe MPS I) and enzyme replacement therapy (ERT) for MPS I, II, IV and VI are available.

MPSs can manifest as severe or attenuated clinical picture. The "severe" forms frequently appear in the first 2–3 years of life with skeletal abnormalities often accompanied by dysmorphic facies, organomegaly, multiple hernias (inguinal, umbilical), abnormally frequent and severe upper airways infections, otitis media and chronic rhinitis. In the "attenuated" forms of the disease instead, the progression of signs and symptoms is much slower [2, 3].

These patients may show the prevalent involvement of a single organ and are often seen by one or two specialists for years before reaching the diagnosis [2, 3].

The most frequent signs of presentation are cardiac valve disease, eye disease, hearing loss, carpal tunnel syndrome and functional limitation of major joints [4–6].

In both forms, the disease invariably progresses with time. MRI of the brain and cervical spine is recommended at the time of diagnosis and at regular intervals thereafter [7].

Surgery to stabilize the spine by posterior fusion can be life-saving. Both central and peripheral nervous systems are affected in the MPSs. Prominent perivascular spaces, hydrocephalus, brain atrophy, gliosis and white matter changes are common [8, 9].

The communicating hydrocephalus that occurs in MPSs is usually slowly progressive, with mild or absent clinical symptoms. Corneal clouding in MPS I, IV, VI and VII may lead to significant visual disability. Glaucoma and cataracts have been reported in MPS I and MPS VI and in MPS III and IV respectively [10].

In the ENT field, these patients often present obstructive sleep apnea/hypopnea (OSAHS), noisy breathing, upper respiratory tract infections, chronic rhinitis, frequent middle ear infections and mixed (conductive + sensorineural) hearing loss. The conductive component is explained by Eustachian tube obstruction or insufficiency by macroglossia, pharyngeal and soft palate mucosal swelling, hyperplasia of adenoids and tonsils. Occasionally, congenital deformities of the middle ear ossicles are observed. Treatments with continuous positive airways pressure (CPAP) during the night sleep, adenotonsillectomy, grommets insertion and hearing aids may be needed [11]. The sporadic finding of sensorineural hearing loss is related to the central and peripheral nervous systems involvement; in some instances it is retrocochlear in nature [12], and it slowly worsens over time [13]. In this study, we reviewed the clinical data of a consecutive series of patients with MPSs, focusing on the early involvement of the auditory pathways.

2. Materials and methods

A retrospective chart review was undertaken to document the otological clinical features and the hearing status of a group of 82 children affected by MPS who were consecutively admitted at the Department of Pediatrics of the San Gerardo Hospital, University of Milano-Bicocca, Monza, Italy, for diagnostic purposes. The young patients were included in the study at the end of the diagnostic process, when the disease had been already characterized by its enzymatic and genetic substrate. Thus, the diagnosis was definite in all cases. We then selected to restrict the investigation to a subgroup of 47 younger children, aged less than 6 years, in order to define audiological profiles with an early prognostic value and early treatment.

We classified the 47 children according to the known MPS types (**Table 1**).

All children underwent an ENT examination during their in-hospital admission, including fiberoptic endoscopy of the upper airways and otomicroscopy. The audiological workup included:

1. Either behavioral audiometry (children <4 years of age) or pure-tone audiometry (children >4 years of age): they were conducted in a soundproof booth, with procedures adequate for the child's age: (a) infants: conditioned oriented responses—COR; (b) toddlers: play audiometry; (c) older children: air (AC) and bone conducted (BC) six frequencies pure tone threshold determination with conventional procedures
2. Middle ear impedance testing: tympanograms and contralateral stapedial reflexes
3. Auditory brainstem responses (ABR): responses elicited by 0.1 ms alternated polarity clicks at intensities decreasing by 10 dB-steps starting from 120 dB p.e.SPL, via ER3A inserts; the electrodes setup was A1/A2-Cz-Fpz; the electrodes impedance <5 kOhm; threshold estimation was obtained by visually checking the wave V latencies and by a test/retest procedure of the lowest amplitude recognizable of the Vth peak. In younger children the procedure was performed during spontaneous sleep; in selected instances, it was obtained during the sedation required for the MR imaging.

   Criteria for labeling a response as "abnormal" were the following:

- Absence of any of the III main wave peaks
- Increased latency of any peak, compared with the normative data for the corresponding age groups at the Audiology Service

- Increased interpeak latency (IPI) compared with the normative data
- Interaural latency difference greater than 0.20 ms

A test/retest procedure was applied at 120 dB SPL stimulation and at the wave V threshold tracing.

A control group of 20 normally hearing children aged 1 year (*normative 1*), 20 children aged 18–24 months (*normative 2*) and 20 aged 3–6 years (*normative 3*) provided the ABR waves latencies normative data.

Therefore, we selected to restrict the investigation to a subgroup of younger children, aged less than 6 years. A full set of audiological data was then gathered for these 47 younger children; among them, 37 (80.43%) underwent also an MRI of the brain and ear. It was therefore possible to cross-check the outcomes of the hearing test and neuroradiological imaging in this subgroup of 37 children. They were 21 males and 16 females with a median age at admission of 3.2 years, ranging between 12 months and 6 years. **Figure 1** shows the flowchart of the study protocol.

In the majority of cases the MRIs of the brain and ear were performed under slight sedation (infants, toddlers and uncooperative children). The MRIs were obtained by a basic protocol

Disease	Number of observed cases	Defective enzyme	GAG storage material	Estimated incidence
MPS-I (Hurler, Hurler/Scheie Scheie)	11	α-L-Iduronidase	Dermatan sulfate, heparan sulfate	1:84,000
MPS-II (Hunter)	10	Iduronate-2-sulfatase	Dermatan sulfate, heparan sulfate	1:196,000
MPS-IIIa (Sanfilippo A)	7	Heparan N-sulfatase	Heparan sulfate	1:92,000
MPS-IIIb (Sanfilippo B)		N-Acetyl-α-glucosaminidase	Heparan sulfate	1:157,000
MPS-IIIc (Sanfilippo C)		Acetyl-CoA:α-glucosamide N-acetyltransferase	Heparan sulfate	1:714,000
MPS-IIId (Sanfilippo D)	0	N-Acetylglucosamine-6-sulfatase	Heparan sulfate	1:1,000,000
MPS-IVA (Morquio A)	14	Galactose-6-sulfatase	Keratan sulfate, chondroitin-6-sulfate	1:131,000
MPS-IVB (Morquio B)		Beta-galactoidase	Keratan sulfate	1:130,000
MPS-VI (Maroteaux-Lamy)	5	Arylsulfatase B	Dermatan sulfate	1:120,000

Table 1. Clinical types of mucopolysaccharidosis (MPSs) with their underlying enzyme deficiency, accumulated substrate, and relative incidence.

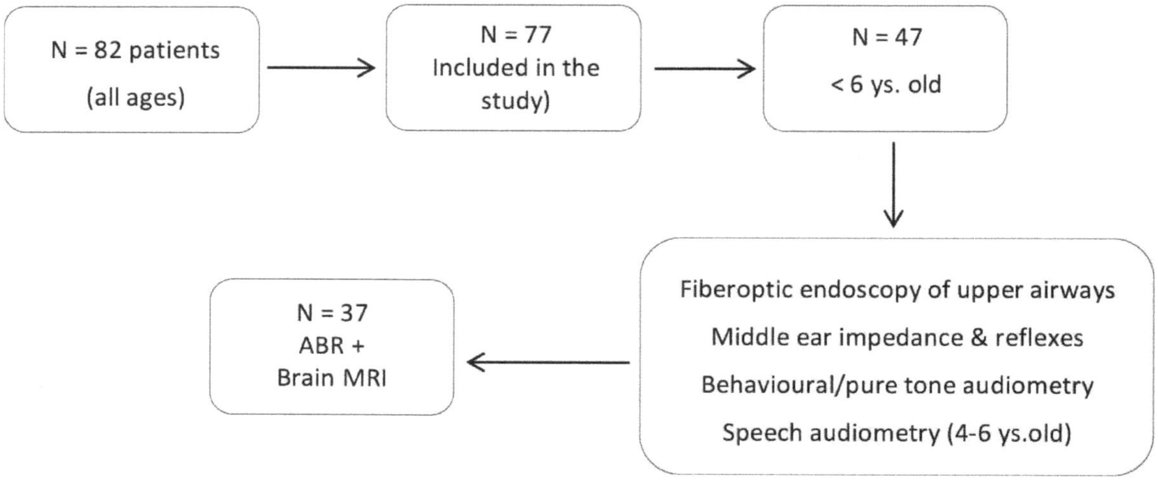

Figure 1. Flowchart showing the young patients' distribution according to the tests performed in the current study.

including axial, coronal and sagittal 3D–Steady-State Free Procession sequence (SSFP), T1-weighted Fast Spin-Echo (FSE) sequence, and T2-weighted 3D Fluid Attenuated Inversion Recovery (FLAIR) sequence. MRI scans were extended from top of the skull to C7. No intravenous injection of contrast medium was applied as a standard procedure. An expert senior Neuroradiologist categorized the findings according to the three most prevalent patterns: (a) dilated perivascular spaces; (b) dilated ventricular cavities; (c) demyelinated and gliotic areas.

After establishing an audiological diagnosis in terms of presence and type of hearing loss (conductive, mixed, sensorineural → cochlear or retrocochlear), degree of loss, laterality, and checking the eardrum morphology at otomicroscopy, these data were contrasted with the MRI findings.

Children were divided in two groups according to the type of hearing loss: "C" = purely conductive; "S" = sensorineural or mixed that is reported in **Figure 2**.

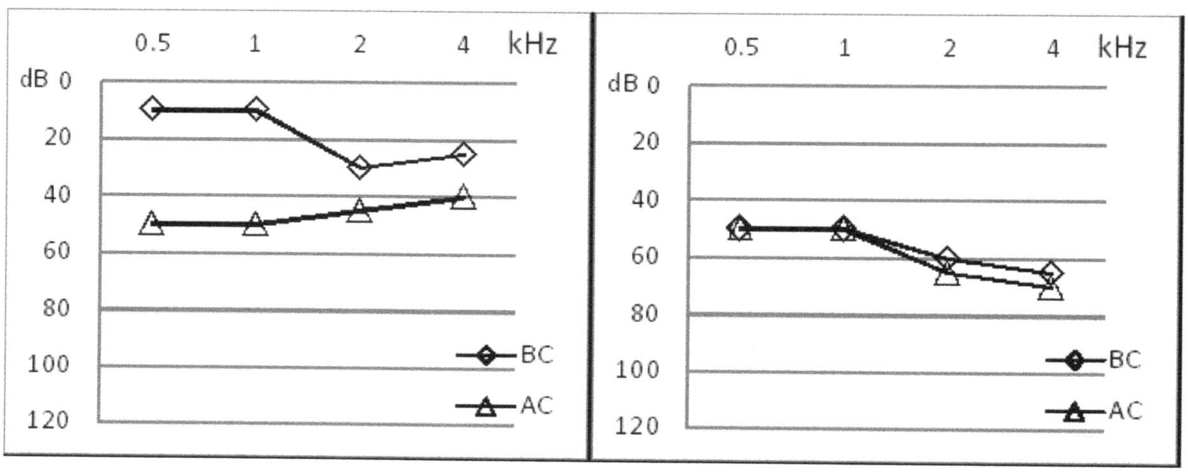

Figure 2. Mean hearing thresholds levels in the "mixed" (left panel) and in the "sensorineural" hearing loss group (right panel). n = 47.

3. Results

3.1. Audiological workup

Some degree of hearing impairment was present in 61 children (74.4%) of the whole cohort of 82 young patients (up to 14 years of age). A total of 21 children (25.6%) were normally hearing. Approximately the same rate of hearing impairment was found in 36 children of the cohort 47 under 6 years of age (76.6%) rather than at older ages; it was sensorineural or mixed in almost half of the ears (47.44%) and purely conductive in about one-third (27.02%). Hearing loss was always symmetrical in the two ears (within 10 dB differences between ears at same frequencies).

Five children presented with normal hearing at admission (mean PTA <20 dB HL bilaterally). The average AC threshold in the "C" group was 44 dB HL with an air-bone gap (ABG) of 21 dB HL; the "S" group showed an AC threshold PTA = 62.5 dB HL with an ABG of 2.3 dB HL. In 7 children (18.9%), the tympanograms were normal (type "A") at the time of the initial assessment and contralateral stapedial reflexes showed a normal threshold and morphology; in the other 30 (81.0%) they were pathological in both ears (Type "B" n = 14; type "C" n = 16).

Transient evoked otoacoustic emissions (TEOAE) were absent bilaterally in all children with a hearing threshold worse than 25 dB HL; normal otoacoustic emission responses were obtained in 9 out of 10 normally hearing ears.

Normative latencies for the three main ABR peaks in normally hearing children of different ages are reported in **Table 2**, and compared to those obtained in the MPS cohort stratified in the same three age groups. Statistical analysis was performed by means of Wilcoxon signed rank test; $p < 0.005$ was considered statistically significant.

In MPS children, ABRs to click stimuli were morphologically normal with peak latencies within normal limits (avg ± 1 SD) in 25 out of 47 subjects (53.2%), whereas 22 tracings showed abnormalities (46.8%). A typical waveform with the 3 main peaks was recognizable or only wave I was missing in 18 of these 22 cases at a stimulus intensity of 90 dB HL, but the amplitudes were reduced and all the latencies delayed ("cochlear" site of lesion); in 7 children no

Wave latencies	MPS 12 mo	Norm 1	p	MPS 18–24 mo	Norm 2	p	MPS 2–6 ys	Norm 3	p
Wave I	1.89 ± 0.21	1.62 ± 0.31	0.046	2.01 ± 0.18	1.88 ± 0.26	n.s.	2.18 ± 0.29	1.99 ± 0.48	n.s.
Wave III	4.30 ± 0.12	4.00 ± 0.34	n.s.	4.51 ± 0.25	4.12 ± 0.11	0.0001	4.45 ± 0.22	4.17 ± 0.3	0.0001
Wave V	6.39 ± 0.18	5.92 ± 0.25	0.0001	7.02 ± 0.2	5.96 ± 0.28	0.0001	7.39 ± 0.26	5.98 ± 0.11	0.0001
IPI I–III	2.40 ± 0.22	2.37 ± 0.21	n.s.	2.50 ± 0.31	2.24 ± 0.25	n.s.	2.27 ± 0.22	2.18 ± 0.21	n.s.
IPI I–V	4.33 ± 0.1	4.31 ± 0.16	n.s.	5.01 ± 0.18	4.98 ± 0.16	n.s.	5.21 ± 0.1	4.0 ± 0.26	0.0001

Latency values expressed in ms. Wilcoxon signed rank test, statistical significance at $p < 0.005$.

Table 2. ABR's absolute wave latencies (ms) and inter-peak intervals (IPI, ms) in the MPS cohort stratified by age and compared to those obtained in the normally hearing age-matched children (control groups Norm 1-2-3).

identifiable response was obtained: in 3 of them, the hearing threshold was severe enough to explain the absence of the response; in 4 cases a retrocochlear involvement was suspected. Overall, a retrocochlear involvement was likely in 8.5% of MPS children.

The relationship between the MPS types and the ABR findings is shown in **Table 3**: all children with MPS III demonstrated an altered ABR; the greatest majority of MPS II also proved pathological, as well as half of the MPS I. None of the patients affected by MPS IVA and VI revealed abnormal ABR tracings.

According to ABR response, the hearing loss was of the "cochlear" type in 83.3, 77.8 and 85.7% of MPS I, MPS II and MPS III, respectively. One case of absent wave I plus absent or delayed wave III and V were observed in MPS I and III, similarly to two cases of MPS II. In no instance an isolated delay of wave V was observed, thus excluding purely "central" site of lesions.

In most MPS children with hearing loss, the hearing threshold derived from the ABRs wave V thresholds ranged between 70 and 90 dB SPL (40–60 dB HL) with an average of 85.62 dB SPL.

3.2. Neuroimaging

Among the 37 MRI, 14 (37.84%) were normal, whereas 23 (62.16%) were pathologic. The most frequent abnormal neuroradiological findings were represented by dilated perivascular spaces (due to extracellular storage of GAGs) in = 12 (32.43%); dilated ventricular cavities n = 15 (40.54%); demyelinated and gliotic areas n = 9 (24.32%). The frequent observation of a J-shaped sella was considered a non-pathological anatomical variant.

We reviewed all MRI with a particular attention on the middle and inner ear findings, although imaging was a standard brain study, not addressing the ear morphology per se. We ascertained five cases of globose internal auditory canal (IAC), and one case of cystic cochlear

MPS type	Normal latencies (all peaks recognizable)	Abnormal ABR	Absent wave I or delayed wave I-III-V (cochlear hearing loss (IPI within normal range)	Absent wave I and absent or delayed wave III and V	Delayed wave V only
MPS-I (n = 11)	5 (46.5%)	6 (54.5%)	5	1	0
MPS-II (n = 10)	1 (10%)	9 (90%)	7	2	0
MPS III (n = 7)	0	7 (100%)	6	1	0
MPS IV (n = 14)	14	0	0	0	0
MPS VI (n = 5)	5	0	0	0	0
Total	25/47 (53.2%)	22/47 (46.8%)	18 (81.8%)	4 (8.5%)	0

Table 3. Distribution of abnormal ABR findings according to MPS type (n = 47).

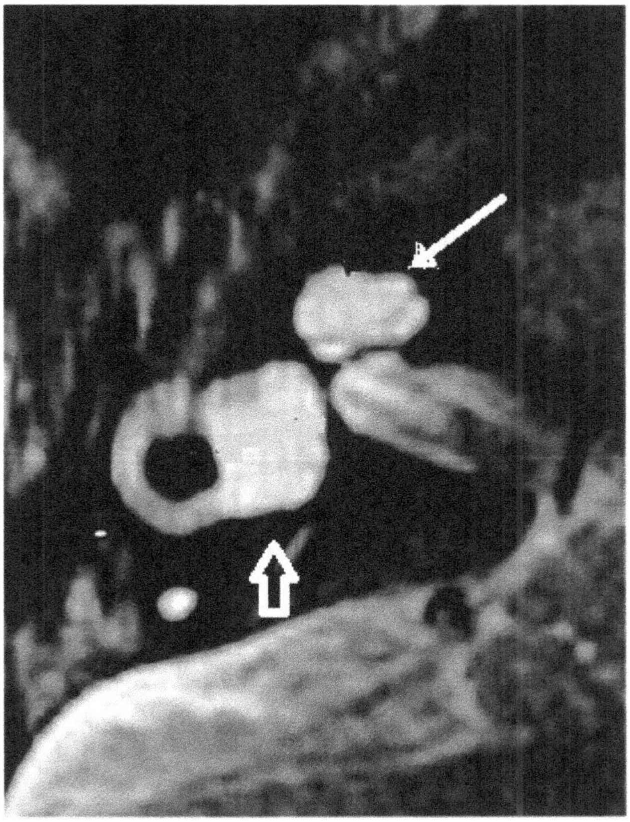

Figure 3. Detail of axial T2-weighted MRI scan of the right ear of patient #14, showing cystic cochlear apex (thin arrow) and enlarged vestibule (empty arrow).

apex and dilated vestibule, which is shown in **Figure 3**. All detected anomalies were bilateral except for the dilated vestibule (right ear, pt. # 14). The middle ear pathological findings consisted in 15 cases of sero-mucinous effusion in the mastoid cells and in the tympanic cavity, 9 bilateral and 4 unilateral (always the right side). In no instance an enlarged vestibular aqueduct was detected. Similarly, no pathological conditions were identified along the central auditory pathways in any young MPS patients.

We further stratified the 37 MR+ patients in 3 subgroups related to age: 5 (13.51%) patients were under 1 years old, only 2 children (5.4%) were between 1 and 2 years old and 30 children

Age	# of patients (%)	Rate of pathological ABRs	Rate of pathological brain MRIs
<1 year	5	2 (40%)	3 (60%)
1–2 years	2	2 (100%)	1 (100%)
2–6 years	30	23 (77.7%)	22 (72.2%)
Total	37	27 (72.9%)	26 (70.2%)

Table 4. Incidence of pathological ABRs and MRIs at different ages in the subgroup of 37 MPS patients who underwent both investigations.

(81.08%) were between 2 and 6 years old. By contrasting the rate of pathological ABR and the MRI findings according to the age layers we obtained the outcomes illustrated in **Table 4**. Noticeably, the majority of children underwent an ABR after 2 years of age, when, theoretically, the physiological maturation of the central auditory pathways should be completed.

4. Discussion

The MPSs are a group of monogenic disorders due to lysosomal storage of glycosaminoglycans (GAGs), previously called mucopolysaccharides [14]. The deficiency of one of the enzymes participating in the GAGs degradation pathway causes progressive storage in the lysosomes and cytoplasm, leading to cell swelling and multiple organs dysfunction. The damage is both direct or by activation of secondary and tertiary pathways among which a role is played by inflammation. [15] All MPSs have an autosomal recessive transmission with the exception of MPS type II (Hunter syndrome) which is X-linked [16].

The incidence of MPSs as a group is reported between 1:25,000 and 1:45,000 [17]. At present, 11 different enzyme deficiencies are involved in MPSs producing 7 distinct clinical phenotypes [14] (**Table 1**). Depending on the enzyme deficiency, the catabolism of dermatan sulfate, heparin sulfate, keratin sulfate, chondroitin sulfate, or hyaluronan may be impaired, singularly or in combination.

MPSs virtually affect all organs and tissues and show a progressive worsening with time. Diagnosis is suspected clinically on the basis of rather constant physical appearance (signs can be subtle or overt) such as: coarse facial features; short stature; "claw hand" and/or joint stiffness or ligamentous laxity (seen in MPS VI); corneal clouding (from very mild to severe), retinopathy, glaucoma; chronic nasal congestion, noisy breathing; abdominal protuberance owing to liver and spleen enlargement; spinal deformity (gibbus, scoliosis, kyphosis, lordosis); abnormal gait (e.g., toe walking); hearing deficits and brain involvement with progressive cognitive delay. In MPS III and II, mental retardation at 2–3 years may be the only, or most evident, presenting sign. Heart failure and severe valve disease in the first year of life are reported as the first presenting symptom in the *severe* forms [18–20]. In these patients, quality of life and life span are generally substantially reduced [21, 22].

The *attenuated* forms have widely variable clinical presentations with different presenting signs at different ages, often one or few organs only clinically manifest the disease [2, 3]. In these milder forms the progression of signs and symptoms is much slower than in the severe ones. These patients may have a presentation apparently limited to one organ only and are often seen by a specialist for years before reaching the diagnosis [2, 3], that is usually accomplished by means of biochemical, enzymatic and molecular tests.

Currently, specific treatments such as hematopoietic stem cell transplantation in selected cases of severe MPS I and enzyme replacement therapy for MPS I, II, IV and VI are available [23]. These treatments are able to improve the clinical course of the disease if started early. This brings along the responsibility for the clinician to recognize these diseases at the first signs to allow access to treatment before a severe damage has been established.

Although similar, each type of MPSs has a peculiar phenotypic expression [14]; besides, within the same type of MPSs, the phenotypic spectrum is largely variable, as a result of the different severity of mutations and overall genetic background of the single individual.

The otorhinolaryngological involvement is represented by otitis media with effusion, progressive mixed hearing loss, OSAHS, pathology of the Waldeyer lymphatic ring and difficulties during intubation [24].

In the *severe* forms, which most frequently present in the first 2–3 years of life with skeletal abnormalities dysmorphic facies, organomegaly and multiple hernias, children suffer abnormally frequent and severe upper airways infections, chronic rhinitis and otitis media. Hearing loss is a frequent feature of the more severe forms of MPS; therefore, it should be identified as early as possible in order to help assessing a correct diagnosis and provide an etiological treatment [33].

It occurs frequently in the early childhood, mainly as a consequence of recurrent episodes of otitis media. It is often discovered occasionally, during an otorhinolaryngological referral requested for the control of the upper airways. OME is the most frequent finding: if the clinical history is silent, it may be overlooked; its incidence in children affected by MPS is higher than in the general population [24].

A middle ear effusion can easily mask an underlying sensorineural hearing loss. The inner ear involvement has been generally neglected in the literature; the major pathologic alterations have been found in the Corti organ, tectorial and Reissner's membranes, ciliated cells and auditory nerve [13]. In the *attenuated* forms of MPS, hearing loss occurs more frequently at a later stage, but it sometimes develops already in first infancy. If correctly recognized, it can be effectively rehabilitated with hearing aids, reducing the already existing disability related with the multi-organ dysfunction.

In our series, 32% of the young patients were affected by mixed hearing loss, 28% by purely conductive, 16% by sensorineural type and 24% were normally hearing. This distribution is coherent with other reports [25, 26]. The degree of hearing loss in purely sensorineural involvement ranged between 40 and 60 dB (average 55.62 dB HL).

In our MPS children, auditory brainstem responses to click stimuli were morphologically normal with peak latencies within normal limits (avg ± 1 SD) in 25 out of 47 subjects (53.2%), whereas 22 tracings showed abnormalities (46.8%). At a stimulus intensity of 90 dB HL, the 3 main peaks of the typical ABR waveform were recognizable, or only wave I was missing, in 18 of these 22 cases. Reduced amplitudes and delayed latencies with regular interpeak latencies indicated a "cochlear" site of lesion; in 7 children no identifiable response was obtained: in 3 of them the hearing threshold was severe enough to explain the absence of the response; in 4 cases a retrocochlear involvement was suspected. Overall, a retrocochlear involvement was likely in 8.5% of MPS children.

The relationship between the MPS types and the ABR findings is shown in **Table 3**: all children with MPS III demonstrated an altered ABR; the greatest majority of MPS II also proved pathological, as well as half of the MPS I. None of the patients affected by MPS IVA and VI revealed abnormal ABR tracings. On a speculative basis, this might reflect a more severe compromise of the auditory periphery in MPS I-II and III.

Based on the ABR response, the hearing loss was of the "cochlear" type in 83.3, 77.8 and 85.7% of MPS I, MPS II and MPS III, respectively; purely "central" lesions were excluded.

The retrocochlear patterns of auditory evoked potentials observed in four of our patients with sensorineural hearing loss highlighted a conduction delay within the central auditory system, possibly related to progressive storage of GAGs.

Up to date, the reason for the sensorineural component of the hearing loss has not been fully ascertained: some alterations, such as the presence of lysosomal deposit in the outer and /or inner hair cells suggest a dysfunction of the cochlear sensorial structures; conversely, the findings of PAS+ material occupying the cytoplasm of the spiral and vestibular ganglion cells might indicate an altered neural transmission [27, 28]. Furthermore, animal studies also showed an alteration in the mechanical properties of the Reissner's and Basilar membranes [12].

The most characteristic modification in the CNS is the dilatation of the perivascular spaces, caused by extracellular storage of GAGs; it appears as a variable amount of tiny spot-like cystic lesions with CSF-like signal in all sequences. It is probably determined by large GAG inclusions between vascular adventitial cells, typically at basal ganglia, subcortical parietal and occipital white matter, and in the corpus callosum, with radial orientation along the vascular developmental lines [29]. Widening of liquoral spaces and hydrocephalus, secondary to pathologic leptomeningeal thickening with resorption deficit by the Pacchioni's granulations and/or obstruction of the CSF flow, can lead to severe neurologic compromise (requiring a shunt) or to neuronal loss and decrease of association fibers and atrophy [30]. The expression of white matter dystrophy in mucopolysaccharidoses, probably on a microvascular basis, is common also to several other diseases that share the same vulnerable areas, such as the peritrigonal white matter. Compared to dilated perivascular spaces, these lesions show brighter (hyperintense) signals both in T_2-weighted and FLAIR images.

In our series of 37 MPS children who underwent MRI, 14 (37.84%) were normal, whereas 23 (62.16%) showed some abnormalities such as dilated perivascular spaces in 12 (32.43%), dilated ventricular cavities in 15 (40.54%), demyelinated and gliotic areas in 9 (24.32%). A globose internal auditory canal was observed in five cases of IAC, and a cystic cochlear apex and dilated vestibule in 1 child. The middle ear pathological findings consisted in 15 cases of sero-mucinous effusion in the mastoid cells and in the tympanic cavity. The limited number of children tested under 2 years of age does not allow to draw general conclusions. Instead, within the group of 30 children aged 2–6 years, the rate of pathological ABRs (77.7%) and of pathological MRI of the brain (72.2%) showed a high degree of correlation. Assuming that the physiological maturation of the central auditory pathways is being completed during this age range, the ABR abnormalities would possibly be attributed no longer to a delayed myelinization. Therefore, the "retrocochlear" ABR findings might be a real expression of "central" auditory dysfunction, although the MRI abnormalities did not seem to involve directly the auditory pathways.

The interpretation of these neuroimaging findings is somehow challenging, because a clear relationship with cognitive insufficiency in MPS patients is lacking [30, 31], although mental retardation has been reported in the more severe forms of MPS 1 [32–37].

Similarly, the relationship with hearing loss is not clear. Nevertheless, a prompt recognition of the hearing difficulties, which can be among the first manifestations of the disease, might help assessing an earlier diagnosis and, therefore, provide a timely treatment.

5. Conclusions

Inner ear and retrocochlear involvement in MPS patients is more frequent than initially suspected. Observation of seromucinous effusion in the middle ear does not exclude the presence of a sensorineural hearing loss. An otological and audiological investigation should be warranted to all defined or suspected MPS patients. Inner ear or central auditory lesions detected by the audiological tests should be further investigated by specific MR imaging processing algorithms.

Early identification of hearing loss not only enables proper acoustic rehabilitation, but also supports the diagnosis of MPS, especially in its milder forms and/or initial stages.

Acknowledgements

The authors wish to thank Dr. Paolo Remida, M.D. for the Neuroradiological workup; Prof. Werner Garavello, M.D. for clinical advice; and Dr. Serena Costanzo, Ph.D., for audiological testing. No funding sources supported research.

Conflicts of interest

The authors report no financial interest in the subject matter, no actual/potential conflict of interest.

Abbreviations

ABR	auditory brainstem responses (acoustically evoked potentials)
AC	air conduction (pure tone audiometry)
avg.	average
BC	bone conduction (pure tone audiometry)
CNS	central nervous system
COR	conditioned oriented responses (test of hearing for babies)
CPAP	continuous positive airways pressure

dB	decibel
ENT	ear, nose and throat (otorhinolaryngology)
ERT	enzyme replacement therapy
FLAIR	fluid attenuated inversion recovery sequence
FSE	Fast Spin-Echo sequence
GAG	glycosaminoglycans
HL	hearing level
HSCT	hematopoietic stem cell transplantation
IAC	internal auditory canal
MPS	mucopolysaccharidoses
MRI	magnetic resonance imaging
MR+	positive at MRI
OME	otitis media with effusion
OSAHS	obstructive sleep apnea/hypopnea syndrome
p.e.SPL	peak-equivalent sound pressure level
PTA	pure tone average (average of thresholds to pure tone stimuli at 0.5–1–2-3 kHz; value expressed in dB HL)
SD	standard deviation
SSFP	3D–Steady-State Free Procession sequence
TEOAE	transient-evoked oto-acoustic emissions

Author details

Diego Zanetti[1]*, Margherita Vezzani[2,3], Federica Di Berardino[1], Serena Gasperini[4] and Rossella Parini[4]

*Address all correspondence to: diego.zanetti.bs@gmail.com

1 Audiology Unit, Department of Community Health and Clinical Sciences, Università degli Studi di Milano; Fondazione IRCCS Cà Granda, Ospedale Maggiore Policlinico Milano, Italy

2 Otorhinolaryngology Department, University of Milano-Bicocca, San Gerardo Hospital, Monza, Italy

3 Pediatric Otorhinolaryngology Department, Children's Hospital, Cincinnati, USA

4 Rare Metabolic Diseases Unit, Department of Pediatrics, University of Milano-Bicocca, San Gerardo Hospital, Monza, Italy

References

[1] Khan SA, Peracha H, Ballhausen D, Wiesbauer A, Rohrbach M, Gautschi M, Mason RW, Giugliani R, Suzuki Y, Orii KE, Orii T, Tomatsu S. Epidemiology of mucopolysaccharidoses. Molecular Genetics and Metabolism. 2017;**121**(3):227-240

[2] Thomas JA, Beck M, Clarke JTR, Cox GF. Childhood onset of Scheie syndrome, the attenuated form of mucopolysaccharidosis I. Journal of Inherited Metabolic Disease. 2010;**33**:421-427

[3] Munoz-Roja MV, Bay L, Sanchez L. Clinical manifestations and treatment of mucopolysaccharidosis type I patients in Latin America as compared with the rest of the world. Journal of Inherited Metabolic Disease. 2011;**34**:1029-1037

[4] Muenzer J, Beck M, Eng CM, Escolar ML, Giugliani R, Guffon NH, Harmatz P, Kamin W, Kampmann C, Koseoglu ST, Link B, Martin RA, Molter DW, Muñoz Rojas MV, Ogilvie JW, Parini R, Ramaswami U, Scarpa M, Schwartz IV, Wood RE, Wraith E. Multidisciplinary management of Hunter syndrome. Pediatrics. 2009;**124**(6):e1228-e1239

[5] Haddad FS, Jones DH, Vellodi A, Kane N, Pitt MC. Carpal tunnel syndrome in the mucopolysaccharidoses and mucolipidoses. Journal of Bone and Joint Surgery. British Volume (London). 1997;**79**(4):576-582

[6] Lin HY, Chuang CK, Chen MR, Lin SM, Hung CL, Chang CY, Chiu PC, Tsai WH, Niu DM, Tsai FJ, Lin SJ, Hwu WL, Lin JL, Lin SP. Cardiac structure and function and effects of enzyme replacement therapy in patients with mucopolysaccharidoses I, II, IVA and VI. Molecular Genetics and Metabolism. 2016;**117**(4):431-437

[7] Nestrasil I, Vedolin L. Quantitative neuroimaging in mucopolysaccharidoses clinical trials. Molecular Genetics and Metabolism. 2017 Sep 15. pii: S1096-7192(17)30340-2. DOI: 10.1016/j.ymgme.2017.09.006

[8] Rasalkar DD, Chu WCW, Hui J, et al. Pictorial review of mucopolysaccharidosis with emphasis on MRI features of brain and spine. The British Journal of Radiology. 2011; **84**:469-477

[9] Manara R, Priante E, Grimaldi M, et al. Brain and spine MRI features of Hunter disease: Frequency, natural evolution and response to therapy. Journal of Inherited Metabolic Disease. 2011;**34**:763-780

[10] Summers CG, Ashworth JL. Ocular manifestations as key features for diagnosing mucopolysaccharidoses. Rheumatology. 2011;**50**(Suppl 5):34-40

[11] Valayannopoulos V, Wijburg FA. Therapy for the mucopolysaccharidoses. Rheumatology (Oxford). 2011;**50**(Suppl 5):49-59

[12] Ohlemiller KK, Hennig AK, Lett JM, Heidbreder AF, Sands MS. Inner ear pathology in the mucopolysaccharidosis VII mouse. Hearing Research. 2002;**169**(1-2):69-84

[13] Netzloff ML, Elsea SH, Fisher RA. Genetic hearing loss associated with metabolic disorders. In: Toriello, Reardon, Gorlin, editors. Hereditary Hearing Loss and Its Syndromes. Oxford University Press; 2004. pp. 387-392

[14] Neufeld EF, Muenzer J. The mucopolysaccharidoses. In: Scriver CR et al., editors. The Metabolic and Molecular Bases of Inherited Disease. New York: McGraw Hill; 2001. pp. 3421-3452

[15] Clarke LA. Pathogenesis of skeletal and connective tissue involvement in the mucopolysaccharidoses: Glycosaminoglycan storage is merely the instigator. Rheumatology (Oxford, England). 2011;**50**(Suppl 5):13-18

[16] Hopwood JJ, Bunge S, Morris, et al. Molecular basis of mucopolysaccharidosis type II: Mutations in the iduronate-2-sulphatase gene. Human Mutation. 1993;**2**:435-442

[17] Nelson J, Crowhurst J, Carey B, Greed L. Incidence of the mucopolysaccharidoses in Western Australia. American Journal of Medical Genetics. 2003;**123A**:310-313

[18] Fesslová V, Corti P, Sersale G, Rovelli A, Russo P, Mannarino S, Butera G, Parini R. The natural course and the impact of therapies of cardiac involvement in the mucopolysaccharidoses. Cardiology in the Young. 2009;**19**(2):170-178

[19] Hirth A, Berg A, Greve G. Successful treatment of severe heart failure in an infant with Hurler syndrome. Journal of Inherited Metabolic Disease. 2007;**30**:820

[20] Hayflick S, Rowe S, Kavanaugh-McHugh A, Olson JL, Valle D. Acute infantile cardiomyopathy as a presenting feature of mucopolysaccharidosis VI. The Journal of Pediatrics. 1992;**120**(2 Pt 1):269-272

[21] Muenzer J. The mucopolysaccharidoses: A heterogeneous group of disorders with variable pediatric presentations. Journal of Pediatrics. 2004;**144**:527-534

[22] Muenzer J. Overview of the mucopolysaccharidoses. Rheumatology. 2011;**50**(Suppl 5):4-12

[23] Bradley LA, Haddow HRM, Palomaki GE. Treatment of mucopolysaccharidosis type II (Hunter syndrome): Results from a systematic evidence review. Genetics in Medicine. 2017;**19**(11):1187-1201

[24] Motamed M, Thorne S, Narula A. Treatment of otitis media with effusion in children with mucopolysaccharidosis. International Journal of Pediatric Otorhinolaryngology. 2000;**53**:121-124

[25] Simmons MA, Bruce IA, Penney S, Wraith E, Rothera MP. Otorhinolaryngological manifestations of the mucopolysaccharidoses. International Journal of Pediatric Otorhinolaryngology. 2005;**69**(5):589-595. Review

[26] Wold SM, Derkay CS, Darrow DH, Proud V. Role of the pediatric otolaryngologist in diagnosis and management of children with mucopolysaccharidoses. International Journal of Pediatric Otorhinolaryngology. 2010;**74**(1):27-31

[27] Zechner G, Moser M. Otosclerosis and mucopolysaccharidosis. Acta Oto-Laryngologica. 1987;**103**(5-6):384-386

[28] Friedmann I, Spellacy E, Crow J, Watts RW. Histopathological studies of the temporal bones in Hurler's disease [mucopolysaccharidosis (MPS) IH]. The Journal of Laryngology and Otology. 1985;**99**(1):29-41

[29] Van der Knaap MS, Valk J, Barth PG, Smit LM, van Engelen BG, Tortori Donati P. Leukoencephalopathy with swelling in children and adolescents: MRI patterns and differential diagnosis. Neuroradiology. 1995;**37**(8):679-686

[30] Matheus MG, Castillo M, Smith JK, Armao D, Towle D, Muenzer J. Brain MRI findings in patients with mucopolysaccharidosis types I and II and mild clinical presentation. Neuroradiology. 2004;**46**:666-672

[31] Gabrielli O, Polonara G, Regnicolo L, Petroni V, Scarabino T, Coppa GV, Salvolini U. Correlation between cerebral MRI abnormalities and mental retardation in patients with mucopolysaccharidoses. American Journal of Medical Genetics. 2004;**125**:224-231

[32] Arn P, Wraith JE, Underhill L. Characterization of surgical procedures in patients with mucopolysaccharidosis type I: findings from the MPS I Registry. Journal of Pediatrics. 2009;**154**(6):859-864.e3

[33] D'Aco K, Underhill L, Rangachari L, Arn P, Cox GF, Giugliani R, Okuyama T, Wijburg F, Kaplan P. Diagnosis and treatment trends in mucopolysaccharidosis I: Findings from the MPS I Registry. European Journal of Pediatrics. 2012;**171**(6):911-919

[34] Arn P, Whitley C, Wraith JE, Webb HW, Underhill L, Rangachari L, Cox GF. High rate of postoperative mortality in patients with mucopolysaccharidosis I: Findings from the MPS I Registry. Journal of Pediatric Surgery. 2012;**47**(3):477-484

[35] Beck M, Arn P, Giugliani R, Muenzer J, Okuyama T, Taylor J, Fallet S. The natural history of MPS I: Global perspectives from the MPS I Registry. Genetics in Medicine. 2014; **16**(10):759-765

[36] Arn P, Bruce IA, Wraith JE, Travers H, Fallet S. Airway-related symptoms and surgeries in patients with mucopolysaccharidosis I. The Annals of Otology, Rhinology, and Laryngology. 2015;**124**(3):198-205

[37] Mendelsohn NJ, Harmatz P, Bodamer O, Burton BK, Giugliani R, Jones SA, Lampe C, Malm G, Steiner RD, Parini R, Hunter Outcome Survey Investigators. Importance of surgical history in diagnosing mucopolysaccharidosis type II (Hunter syndrome): Data from the Hunter Outcome Survey. Genetics in Medicine. 2010;**12**(12):816-822

9

Hearing Aids

Ryota Shimokura

"Blindness cuts you off from things; deafness cuts you off from people."

Immanuel Kant (Philosopher, 1724–1804).

Abstract

This chapter presents an overview of the current state of a hearing aid tracing back through the history. The hearing aid, which was just a sound collector in the sixteenth century, has continued to develop until the current digital hearing aid for realizing the downsizing and digital signal processing, and this is the age of implanted hearing devices. However, currently popular implanted hearing devices are a fairly large burden for people soon after they become aware of their hearing loss, although auditory stimulation to the nerve in the early stage can avoid accelerated cognitive decline and an increased risk of incident all-cause dementia. For this reason, we tend to stick to wearable hearing aids that are easy to be put on and take off. Although the digital hearing aid has already reached the technical ceiling, the noninvasive hearing aids have some severe problems that are yet to be resolved. In the second half of this chapter, we discuss the scientific and technical solutions to broaden the range of permissible users of hearing aids.

Keywords: dementia, EuroTrak, bone-conducted ultrasonic hearing aid, cartilage conduction hearing aid, autocorrelation analysis

1. Introduction

When the ability to hear declines, people become uncomfortable during conversations and gradually begin to speak less and less. This worsening situation can lead to depression and an increased risk of dementia. In 2015, the Ministry of Health, Labour and Welfare in Japan published an initiative for preventing dementia (New Orange Plan), which states that hearing loss is a risk for declining cognitive function [1]. The first report to show the relationship between hearing impairment and dementia was published in 1989 [2], and several longitudinal studies that included auditory and nonauditory cognitive testing have shown that people with hearing loss have a 30–40% rate of accelerated cognitive decline [3] and an increased risk of incident all-cause dementia [4, 5]. The implications are that auditory stimulation that reaches the brain can delay aging of the brain and allow communication with family and society to continue. Thus, the earlier that people can receive audiological treatment and hearing aid prescriptions, the better.

2. The history of hearing aids

When we cannot hear what someone nearby is saying, we cup our hand behind our ears. This is actually a type of hand reflector, which can aid hearing by emphasizing in the middle and high frequency range (>500 Hz) between 5 and 10 dB and by blocking unnecessary noise from extraneous directions. The first documented evidence of a hearing aid dates back to the sixteenth century [6] and describes wooden panels that imitated animal auricles and were meant to be worn behind the ear. **Figure 1** shows a 1673 sketch depicting a hearing device called the *"Ellipsis Otica."* This is one of the oldest illustrations of a hearing aid and was published in *Phonurgia nova*, the first known book to deal with the nature of sound, acoustics, and music in 1673 [7]. Horn-shaped hearing aids called *"Ear Trumpets"* (**Figure 2**) became a common remedy for hearing loss for the next 300 years [8] until the development of electric hearing devices. Before the twentieth century, hearing aids were always thought of as sound collectors. The narrow end of the ear trumpet was inserted in the user's ear, and the broad end faced toward the speaker. Thus, like a cupped hand, the ear trumpet was used between two people standing at close range.

Early on, ear trumpets were made from animal horn, but over time people began making them from wood and metal. The preferred color was black because it blended in with the dark clothes that were often worn by European people of that time. This was perhaps an effort to avoid drawing attention to the horn for fear that one's hearing loss would be exposed. In the eighteenth and nineteenth centuries, hearing aids were designed to be hidden from public view, as can be seen in **Figure 3**. For females, the hearing aid body was placed into a hair band (**Figure 3a**, *Aurolese Phones*) or a handy fan (**Figure 3b**, air conduction fan), which they used in daily life. For men, the hearing aid body was covered by their own beard (**Figure 3c**). The

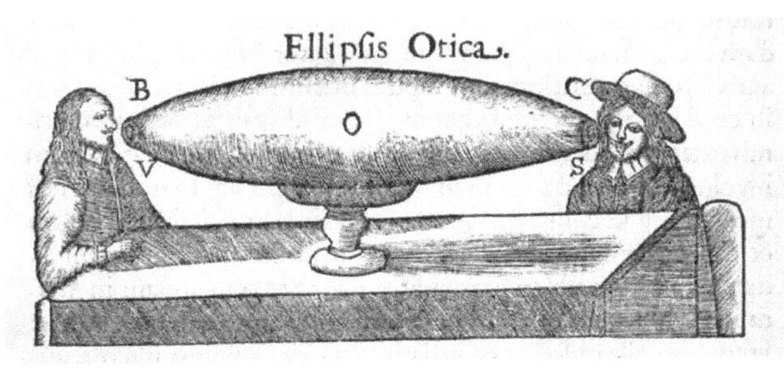

Figure 1. Speaking tubes (*Ellipsis Otica*) from *Phonurgia nova* (1673) [7].

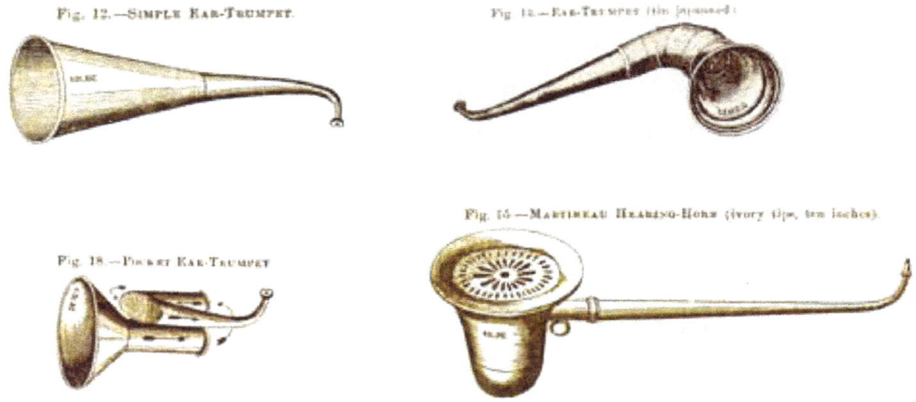

Figure 2. Illustrations of *Ear Trumpets* in *A clinical manual of the diseases of the ear* (1887) [8].

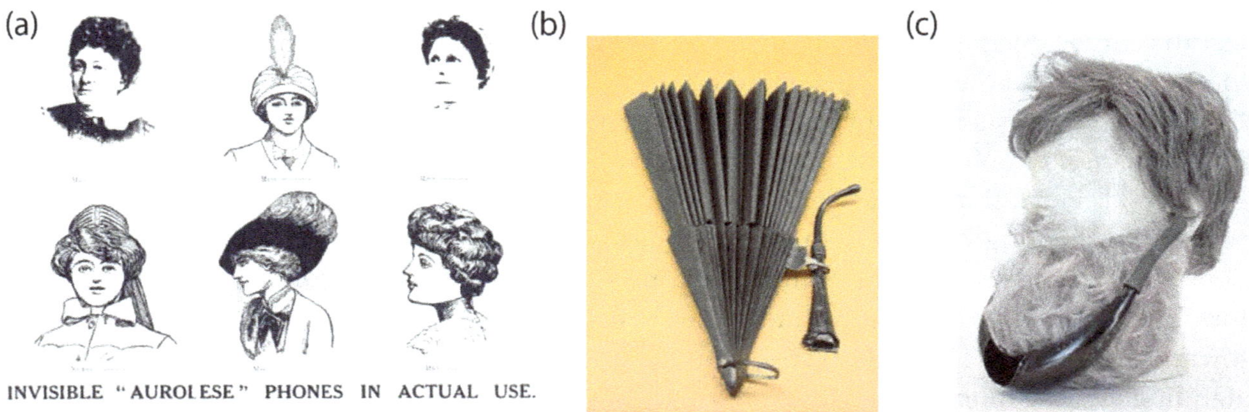

Figure 3. (a) *Aurolese Phones* simulated in hair bands (F. C. Rein co.) from the 1810s. (b) Acoustic fan with ear trumpet from the 1850s. (c) Beard receptacle (Hawksley co.) from the 1830s.

desire to hide hearing aids has not changed with new technology, as evidenced by the current popularity of small, skin-colored hearing aids.

In contrast to the wearable hearing aids described earlier, larger types of hearing aids were placed or mounted on furniture. **Figures 4a** and **b** show a flower-vase-type hearing aid that was placed in the center of a table to collect sound from a number of people conversing during a meal, while the user put the end of tube on his ear. **Figure 4c** shows a chair that was designed to function as a hearing aid. The mouths of the lions carved at the front of the wooden armrests gathered sound, and hollow cavities running through the armrests transmitted the amplified sound to the end of the tube that the user inserted into his ear. Because wearable hearing aids required the speakers to be at very close proximity, those in high positions or peerage used these types of acoustic thrones to keep a suitable distance from unknown speakers that might make them uncomfortable.

In the latter part of the nineteenth century, the invention of the telephone and microphone had a tremendous impact on hearing aid design. Once sound signals (longitudinal wave in air) could be converted into electric signals, hearing aids changed from classical sound collectors

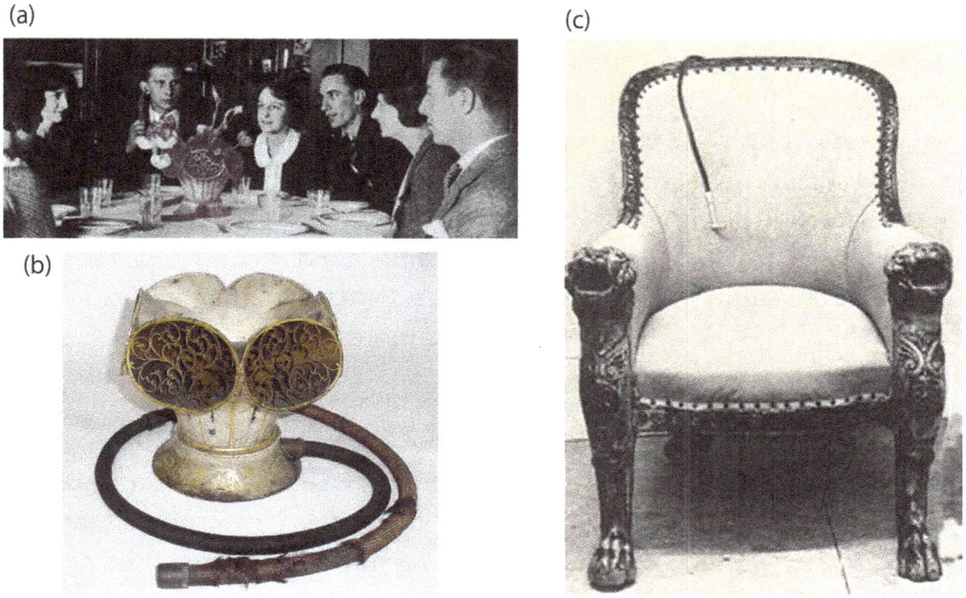

Figure 4. (a) and (b) Flower-vase-type hearing aid for gathering multiple speakers' voices (F. C. Rein Co.) in 1810. (c) Acoustic throne for European royalty in 1819.

to devices that could amplify sound through an electric circuit. The history of the electronic hearing aid is thus very similar to that of the technological evolution of the microphone, amplifier, and battery cell. Between 1989 and 1900, the Akouphone Company produced the first electronic hearing aids called "*Akoulallion*" and "*Akouphone,*" introducing a carbon microphone technique. The carbon transmitter was able to use an electric current to amplify weak signals by 20–30 dB [9]. The *Akoulallion* was large and was used on a table, while the *Akouphone* was portable. Miler Reese Hutchison—one of the company's founding presidents—established the Hutchison Acoustic Company in 1903 and produced "*Acousticon,*" an improved electric hearing aid that was further miniaturized (**Figure 5a**). Users wore the microphone and main body, put the battery in a bag, and held the earphone in their hands. The Danish company *Oticon* and the German company *Siemens* are two current makers of hearing aids that begun operations during this period.

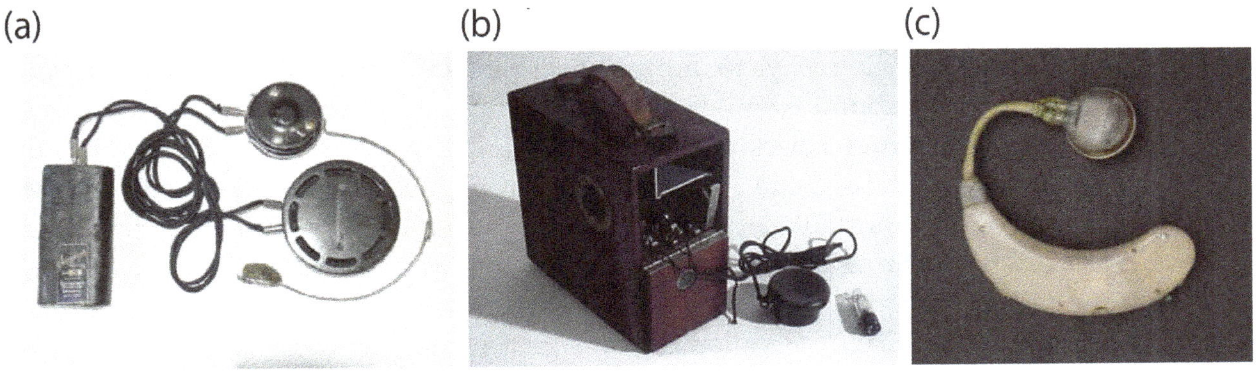

Figure 5. (a) Early electronic hearing aid with carbon components: *Acousticon* model A (Hutchison Acoustic Company, 1905). (b) Early vacuum tube hearing aid: *Vactuphone* (Globe Ear-phone Company, 1921). (c) Behind-the-ear hearing aid-embedded transistor amplifier (Zenith Diplomat Company, 1956).

In 1920, a new type of hearing aid was developed using vacuum tubes to amplify sound by 70–130 dB. The vacuum tube aid contains a filament (heated electron-emitting cathode) and a plate (the anode), and the amount of applied voltage can control the current traveling from cathode to anode. Although the vacuum tube hearing aid was able to have a high gain and accurate frequency response, it was quite large because two batteries were needed for heating the filament and controlling the electric circuit, and batteries at that time were not small. **Figure 5b** shows the earliest vacuum tube hearing aid, called the "*Vactuphone*" (1921). Because the body was about the same size as the box camera of its day, the "*Vactuphone*" included an unnecessary lens that helped disguise it as a box camera.

Over time, advances in vacuum tube and battery technology allowed hearing aids to be made much smaller, until eventually the vacuum tube hearing aid was small enough to be worn. However, the invention of the transistor 1952 put an end to the vacuum tube era. The transistor is a semiconductor device used to amplify or switch electronic signals and electrical power. The transistor was much smaller than the vacuum tube, consumed much less power, and thus allowed for much smaller battery sizes. A predecessor of a current behind-the-ear (BTE) hearing aid appeared in this period (**Figure 5c**). By wearing it on the head, noise from moving clothes was avoided, the direction of sound could be partially perceived, and the cord could be as short as possible. As technology advanced further with the integrated circuit (IC) and button-sized zinc-air battery (1960s–1970s), miniaturization and technical performance were further improved. The end of the twentieth century saw a steady progression of innovation from in-the-ear (ITE) hearing aids that fit into the concha (1980s) to in-the-canal (ITC) and completely-in-the-canal (CIC) hearing aids (1990s). ITC and CIC hearing aids allowed maximized sound collection from the auricle and sound insulation from environmental noises, as well as cut out wind noise. With these inventions, sound could be amplified by more than 100 dB and people with hearing loss could completely hide their problem with an invisible hearing aid.

3. Digital hearing aid

After achieving this level of hearing aid output gain and miniaturization, scientists and engineers began looking for further ways to improve hearing-aid convenience. For example, analog hearing aids amplify sound from all frequency ranges, which means that both speech and unnecessary background noises are amplified equally. Another problem was that the small size of the devices caused the speaker and microphone to be too close, and acoustic feedback generated uncomfortable levels of amplified sound. In 1996, these problems began to be addressed when hearing aids entered the age of digital sound. The digital hearing aid converts sound into a binary digital signal, which can then be modified by computer software. This type of signal modification is called digital signal processing (DSP) and is the biggest advantage of the digital hearing aid.

Figure 6 shows a computer interface through which the DSP installed in a hearing aid can be controlled after connecting the hearing aid to the computer. The most beneficial aspect

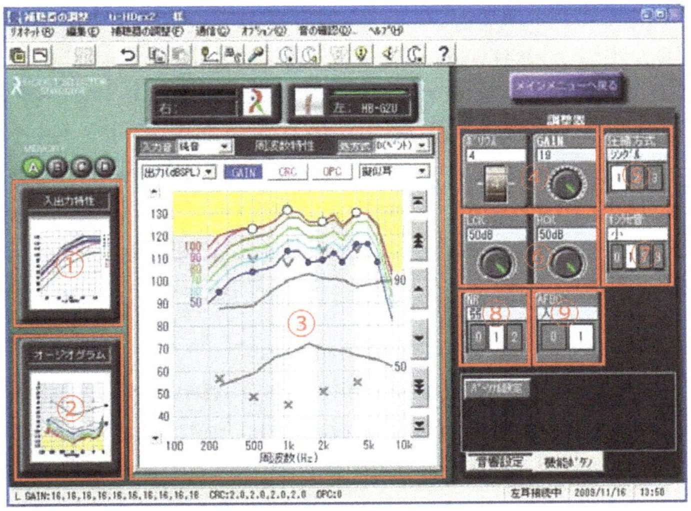

① Balance of output and input level
② Audiogram of user
③ Gain controller in each frequency band
④ Total volume controller
⑤ Selector of compression systems
⑥ Selector of compression ratio
⑦ Alarm sound volume
⑧ Slector of noise reduction system
⑨ Slector of acoustic feedback canceler

Figure 6. Example of software used to adjust a hearing aid's digital signal processing.

of the DSP is the ability to adjust the output gain in each one or one-third octave frequency band. The computer program designs the shape of a digital filter and modifies the signal passing through the filter (multichannel analysis). Because sound energy in human voice is distributed in a frequency range of 200 Hz to 4 kHz, unwanted noise can be weakened by amplifying only the desired frequency range. Audiograms of people with hearing loss differ according to individual sensitivity to each frequency band (e.g., high tone deafness, horizontal deafness, convex deafness, or concave deafness). The multichannel output can thus limit compensation to the frequency bands for which a person has difficulty in hearing.

The multichannel output is also useful for suppressing acoustic feedback. Acoustic feedback occurs when the following happens simultaneously: (1) attenuation of the speaker's voice by the time it reaches the microphone is less than the amount of sound gain and (2) the phases of the original and feedback signals are mostly overlapped. ITC and CIC hearing aids have a vent to reduce the uncomfortable feeling that can occur in the occluded ear, and the output sound transmitted through the vent can cause acoustic feedback. The solution is a feedback canceller in the hearing aid that identifies the offending frequency-repeating amplification and reduces the sound gain in the corresponding band.

The other important role of DSP is to create a compression system for the output sound. If a hearing aid amplifies sound linearly, it makes already loud sounds excessively loud. Patients with sensorineural hearing loss hear sounds above a certain sound level louder than normal listeners (recruitment hearing). Thus, the sound of a closing door or a cry from a child can annoy hearing aid users. The compression system suppresses the amplification of sounds above a certain sound level and instead fits them within the restricted dynamic range of the user. This system can therefore avoid unpleasant sounds, normalizes the perceived loudness, and improves speech intelligibility.

Another advantage of digital hearing aids is their ability to work wirelessly. In their times, the BTE hearing aid only had a short cord, and the ITC and CIC hearing aids did not require any cords or cables. However, in modern society, wireless function is increasingly useful for connecting hearing aids to other electronic devices. For example, because holding a smartphone near one's ear is difficult when wearing a hearing aid, the wireless hearing aid can receive speech signals directly from the smartphone using Bluetooth technology. In the near future, users will be able to control the DSP from a smartphone app. Wireless hearing aids can also help when watching television. By wirelessly connecting to the TV, users can hear clear sound from a TV program without the sound needing to travel through the air. Thus, environmental noise can be minimized and reverberations in a room can be ignored.

Digital hearing aids will likely continue to evolve and add new features and functions. For example, a hearing aid with Global Positioning System will make it easier to be found if it gets lost or misplaced. Like other wearable electronics, if hearing aids incorporate functions for measuring heart rate, step counts, and burned calories, they will become a type of wearable device that supports lifelong health.

4. User subjective assessment of hearing aids

Against a background of various technological advances, the hearing aid has continued to respond to user expectations. Are users today satisfied with the current hearing aid? Countries in Europe and Japan have conducted large-scale market research surveys called *EuroTrak* and *JapanTrak* since 2009 [10]. According to JapanTrak 2015, 1306 people with hearing loss filled out their marketing surveys. Along with a corresponding survey in the US (*MarkeTrak IX* in 2014), we can discuss how satisfied hearing-aid users are in countries whose citizens have access to the latest technology.

Figure 7 shows basic demographic information. The percentage of people with hearing loss is higher for countries with aging populations (i.e., Germany, Italy, and Japan). However, the percentage of people with hearing loss who own hearing aids is lower in these countries than

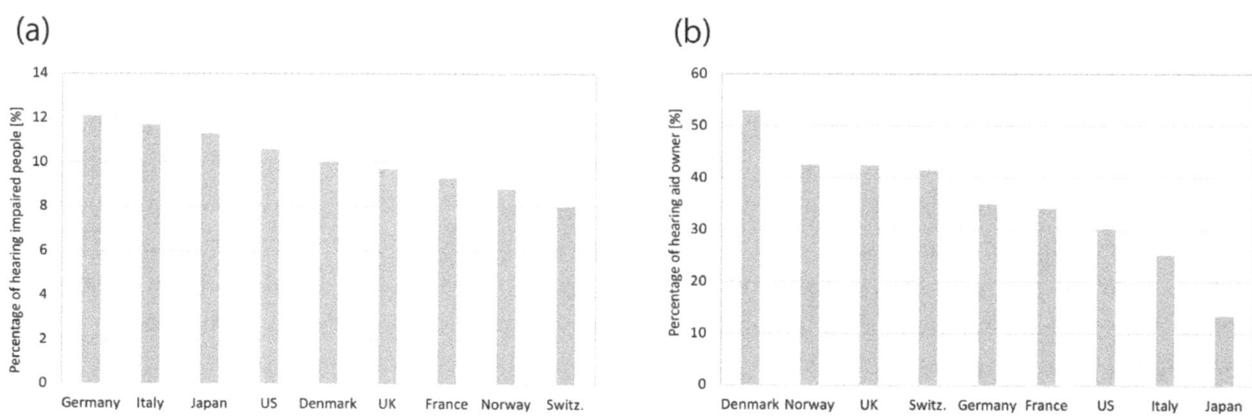

Figure 7. (a) Percentage of people with hearing loss in several high-tech countries. (b) Percentage of people using hearing aids to the number of people with hearing loss in each country.

Country	Amount granted
Denmark, Norway, UK	All expenses paid
Germany	840 Euro
Switzerland	840 CHF (about 740 Euro)
Italy	600 Euro
France	120 Euro
US	Almost none
Japan	Almost none

Table 1. Amount of money granted by governments for hearing aids.

in other countries. This trend is easy to understand after considering how much support people receive to mitigate the cost of hearings aids. **Table 1** shows public financial support for the purchase of hearing aids for each country listed in **Figure 7**. Not surprisingly, the countries showing the highest percentages of people with hearing aids are Denmark, Norway, and the UK, all of which prescribe hearing aids at no cost when a patient is diagnosed with hearing loss. We can thus say that government aid is needed to increase hearing aid distribution or the cost for these hearings aids is too high.

Figure 8 shows the percentage of people in each country who are satisfied with their hearing aids. It is interesting that people in different countries have different views about the performance of their hearing aids, even though the specification criteria are almost the same in all these countries. The countries with established social security systems are ranked in the bottom half, while more than 80% of the people with hearing loss in France, the US, and

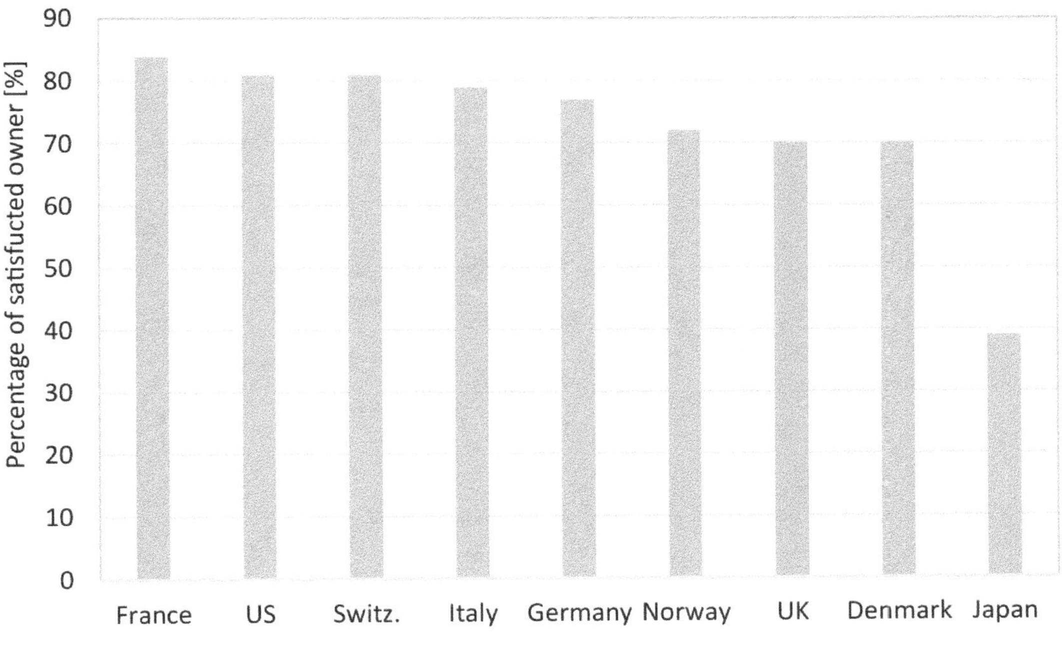

Figure 8. Percentage of people in each country who are satisfied with their hearing aids.

Switzerland (whose out-of-pocket expenses are higher) were satisfied with their hearing aids. This result seems to support the idea that the user's own expense adds value to the hearing aid. However, users in Japan who receive no public assistance feel the most dissatisfied among the surveyed countries and have one of the lowest percentages of people with hearing aids (**Figure 7b**). Aside from Japan, other countries believe that rehabilitation for hearing loss is a medical practice, and only a state-certified technician can permit a hearing aid to be sold or adjusted. In Japan, however, a private association (The Association for Technical Aids) certifies hearing aid technicians, who can then recommend people to buy hearing aids or to have their hearing aids adjusted. These data imply that a government guarantee earns the trust of hearing aid owners and is related to satisfaction. In terms of hearing aids, the role of government is not to disburse tax money but to make people with hearing loss feel secure. Thus, the current digital hearing aid has already reached the technical ceiling, and satisfaction will depend only on the user's feelings.

5. Implanted hearing devices

Although wearable hearing aids come close to the goal desired by people with hearing loss, implanted hearing devices allow room for further improvements. Several types of implanted hearing devices exist, with one being the bone-anchored hearing aid (BAHA), shown in **Figure 9a**. People have known for centuries that we can perceive sound when our skull bones vibrate, and bone conduction hearing was first described in the sixteenth century [11]. Currently, some commercially available hearing aids utilize bone conduction, and the user fixes a vibrator over the mastoid bone using a hair band. However, vibrating the skull through skin and fat tissue effectively is difficult. Therefore, the BAHA implants a titanium anchor on the temporal bone (behind the ear) to work as a bridge for vibration transmission [12, 13]. The other end of the anchor appears on the skin, and the user attaches the vibrator and receiver to the edge. Compared with previous bone

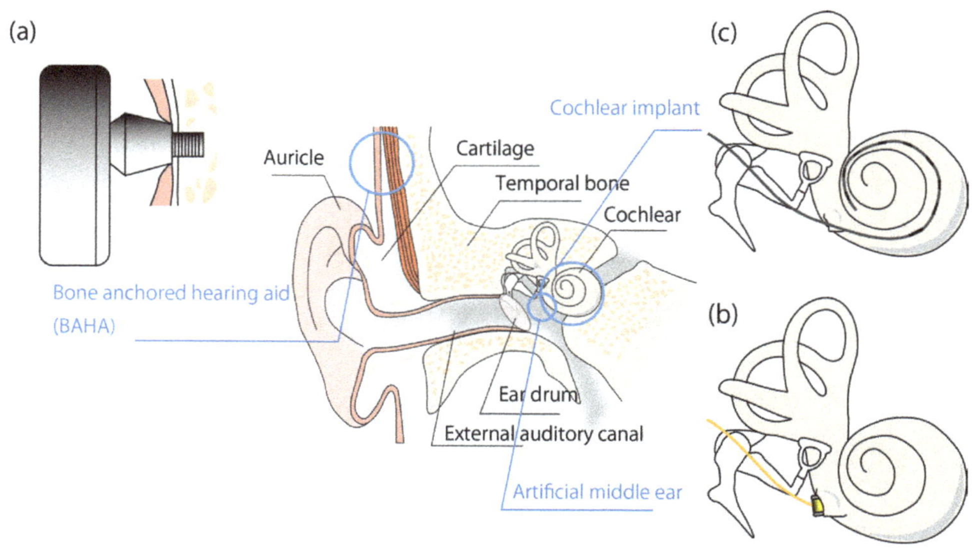

Figure 9. Implanted hearing devices: (a) bone-anchored hearing aid, (b) artificial middle ear and (c) cochlear implant.

conduction hearing aids, this technique has better amplification of higher frequency ranges, which improves speech intelligibility [14, 15].

Another implanted device is the artificial middle ear, which is used when vibration from the ear drum does not smoothly travel through the ear ossicles even after tympanoplasty operations (**Figure 9b**). A sound receiver with a built-in transmitting coil is magnetically attached behind the ear to an implanted receiving coil on the temporal bone, and the signal is transmitted through the skin by the reciprocation of the two coils. The receiving coil activates a transducer that touches the round window of the cochlea, which directly stimulates the basilar membrane. The artificial middle ear was originally developed by a Japanese hearing aid maker (RION Co., LTD.) in 1983, and other makers are currently developing a new stimulation approach using artificial ear ossicles [16].

A third device is the cochlear implant, which converts sound into an electrical current and directly stimulates hair cells in the cochlea using an implanted electrode (**Figure 9c**). The first prototype cochlear implant was conducted by William House and John Doyle in 1961 [17], making the history of this method older than either the BAHA or the artificial middle ear. Subsequently, Clark developed a multichannel electrode cochlear implant in 1977 and produced the first commercialized multielectrode device in 1978 [18]. The cochlear implant is adaptive for profound deafness (hearing level > 90 dB) in Japan. The cochlear implant is reported to be especially useful for children who have not acquired language skills for the linguistic development in the future.

Unlike implanted hearing devices, another future option could utilize stem cells, as inner ear stem cells were found in 1999 [19], and studies in regenerative medicine have developed even further since that time. This means that surgical approaches might become mainstream hearing-loss treatments. One irony is that in Japan, medical expenses for implanted hearing devices are more economic for the individual than the cost of hearing aids because they are considered within the scope of the health-care system.

6. Future of hearing aids

Although implanted hearing devices are a rapidly evolving research field and market, noninvasive hearing aids remain the first approach for treating hearing loss. Although these hearing aids have approximately achieved their aim, three severe problems are yet to be resolved.

The first is the adaptation for profound hearing loss (hearing level > 90 dB). Hearing aids are recommended when hearing level is higher than 40 dB but do not have much effect for profound hearing loss. The exception is the cochlear implant, which can work in some instances.

The second problem concerns how the hearing aids are worn. In the long history of hearing aids, some part is always inserted in the ear. The earplug occludes the external auditory canal, and the annoyance this causes is always a high-ranking reason for discontinuing use. Although the vent in CIC hearing aids as well as open-fitting hearing aids seems to reduce this feeling and the accentuation of the user's voice, they lead to acoustic feedback. Additionally, earplugs are not possible for patients with atresia of the external auditory canal or microtia, who do not have enough space to insert it.

The third problem deals with the adaptation for sensorineural hearing loss. Unlike conductive hearing loss that affects sound waves conduction anywhere along the route through the outer ear, tympanic membrane, and middle ear, the root cause of sensorineural hearing loss lies in the inner ear or between the auditory nerves and audio cortex in the brain. Some types of hearing loss, like presbycusis, have mixed causes. Patients with conductive hearing loss are able to achieve nearly 100% accuracy on speech intelligibility tests when the speech is presented at a sufficiently loud volume. However, patients with sensorineural hearing loss including presbycusis can only achieve the maximum peak accuracy between 40 and 80%, even when the speech is presented at an optimal volume. In this condition, patients can hear but cannot identify the syllables. Because the main function of a hearing aid is to amplify sound, it may offer limited benefits for sensorineural and mixed hearing loss when used during conversation.

The following subsections describe the solutions or potential clues for solving these three problems and introduce the next-generation hearing aids.

6.1. Bone-conducted ultrasonic hearing aid

Ultrasonic sound waves are those with frequencies greater than 20 kHz, which is the audible limit of human hearing. Although airborne ultrasound cannot be perceived, we can hear ultrasound delivered to the mastoid bone of the skull via a transducer [20]. Importantly, bone-conducted ultrasound can even be perceived by people with profound hearing impairment. One study has reported that these individuals are able to identify ultrasound amplitude-modulated speech signals as speech [21]. Additionally, Hosoi used magnetoencephalography and positron-emission tomography to show that bone-conducted ultrasound can activate auditory cortex of people with profound hearing loss [22]. Although the mechanisms underlying this phenomenon are still only hypotheses, the best guess at the moment is that bone-conducted ultrasound stimulates residual inner hair cells in the base of basilar membrane [23, 24].

An accumulation of research has led to the development of several different bone-conducted ultrasonic hearing aids (**Figure 10**). The HD-GU was a test model developed by Nara Medical University in Japan. Connected to a computer, parameters from various digital signal processors (e.g., noise reduction and nonlinear gain) were controlled on a monitor via software. AIST-BCUHA-003 and AIST-BCUHA-005 were developed by the National Institute of Advanced Industrial Science and Technology (AIST) in Japan [25]. AIST-BCUHA-003 was able to control amplitude and carrier frequency (i.e., ultrasound), while the AIST-BCUHA-005 contained digital signal processors and could control the degree of modulation. Another device was HiSonic, a commercial product that controlled sound amplitude for hearing aids and as therapy for suppressing tinnitus [26, 27]. Using these models, Shimokura was able to see vast improvement in speech intelligibility in a woman with profound hearing loss who he advised to try bone-conducted ultrasonic hearing aids. [28]. The results demonstrated significant improvement from the outset of therapy, and her perceived-speech intelligibility reached 60%, as measured by correctly answered questions in a closed-set test of word intelligibility

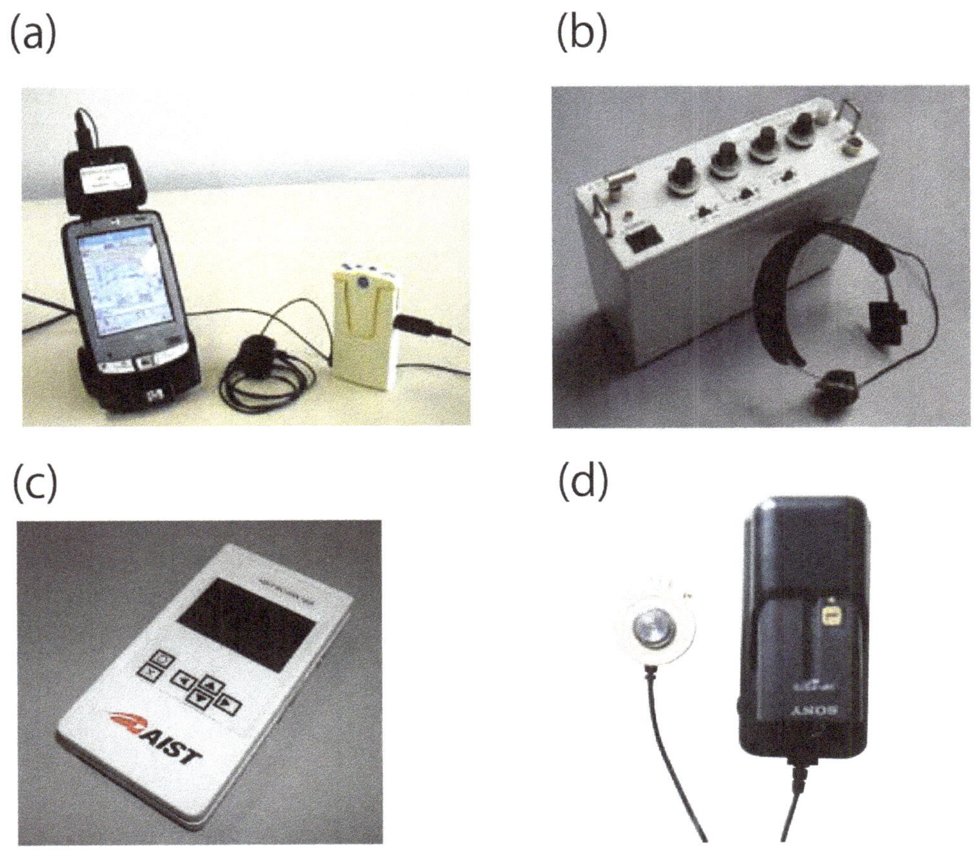

Figure 10. Bone-conducted hearing aids: (a) HD-GU, (b) AIST-BCUHA-003, (c) AIST-BCHA-005, and (d) HiSonic.

with three options. For patients with profound hearing loss, the bone-conducted ultrasonic hearing aid might be a good option before risking cochlear implant surgery.

6.2. Cartilage conduction hearing aid

The uncomfortable feeling that results from an occluded ear is a major hurdle for hearing aid users, and this feeling is always a top reason for discontinuing hearing-aid use. One study tried using active noise control to reduce this feeling [29]. Unlike this digital approach, a cartilage conduction hearing aid reduces the "full ear" feeling with an analog procedure. In 2004, Hosoi found that a specific type of transducer could be used to create clear audible sound when gently placed on aural cartilage [30, 31]. Aural cartilage comprises the outer ear and is distributed around the exterior half of the external auditory canal. Transducer-induced cartilage vibration generates sound directly in the external auditory canal as shown in **Figure 11b** [32–35]. In this case, the cartilage and transducer play the roles of a diaphragm and a loudspeaker voice coil, respectively. When the transducer is ring shaped, it can amplify the sound without occluding the ears (**Figure 11a**). Sound pressure levels in the canal show that the ring-shaped transducer produces an average gain of 35 dB for frequencies below 1 kHz [32]. Although the cartilage conduction hearing aid does not work for those with profound hearing loss, it can help those with moderate loss of hearing. One advantage of cartilage-conducted sound is its unique property of remaining in the canal regardless of the amount of ventilation, and the less sound leakage reduces the risk of acoustical feedback [36].

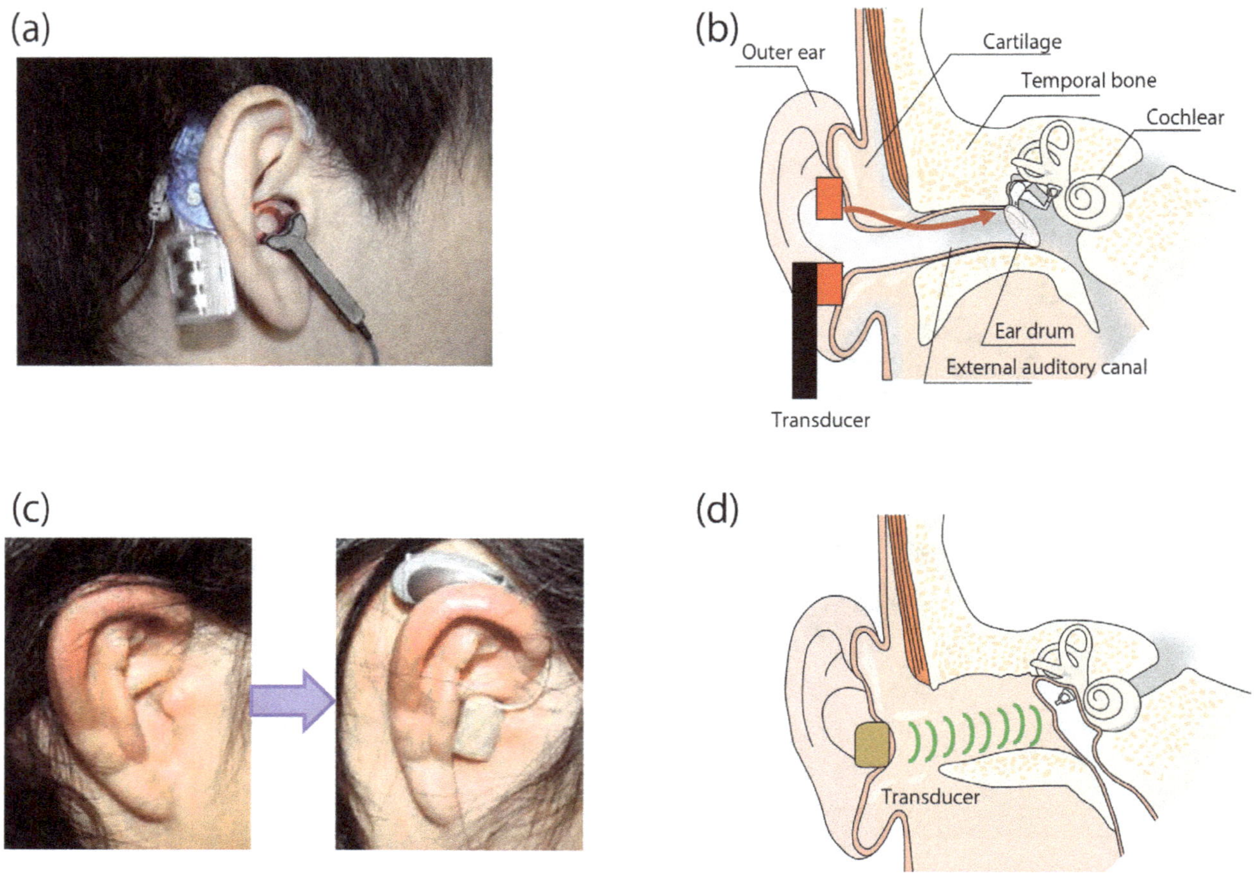

Figure 11. (a) Cartilage conduction hearing aid with a ring-shaped transducer. (b) Sound-transmission pathway in the ear. (c) Cartilage conduction hearing aid with a small transducer. (d) Sound-transmission pathway for people with atresia of the external auditory canal.

The cartilage conduction hearing aid can be used by patients with atresia of the external auditory canal [37, 38]. Because patients whose canal is occluded by fibrotic tissue cannot use a conventional hearing aid because they lack a sound pathway (**Figure 11c** and **d**), they are usually advised to use a bone conduction hearing aid or a BAHA. However, the bone conduction transducer must be pushed tightly against the head insufferably when using it for a long period of time, and the BAHA needs surgery. In contrast, the cartilage conduction transducer only needs to be softly put on the end of the canal because the excitation force required for light cartilage is much smaller than that for heavy skull bone. Despite this, hearing levels for bone and cartilage conduction are almost equivalent at frequencies below 2 kHz [38].

6.3. Autocorrelation analysis of speech signals

The third problem is the speech intelligibility for people with sensorineural hearing loss. As mentioned earlier, patients with sensorineural hearing loss can perceive sound but cannot recognize speech. For example, all Japanese medical institutions use the same list of monosyllable signals for an intelligibility test, which are delivered by a professional female speaker, and studies investigating speech intelligibility in patients with sensorineural hearing loss have identified the less discernible consonants within Japanese monosyllables [39–41]. According to [41], 90% of patients identified monosyllable /i/ correctly, while only 10% could identify /de/.

To explain the difference, studies have investigated several physical parameters. For example, voice onset time (VOT) is the length of time in milliseconds that passes between the release of a stop consonant and the onset of voicing [42]. Another example is the speech intelligibility index (SII), which is a measure of the proportion of a speech sound that is discernible under different listening conditions, such as filtering related to hearing decline or reverberation [43]. Loudness level [phon] can be calculated based on the averaged spectra of a signal, but the masking effects of neighboring auditory filters may be included [44].

All these parameters are related to mechanisms of peripheral perception in the auditory pathway. However, the causes of sensorineural hearing loss are in the inner ear or the auditory nerve. Therefore, subsequent processing after peripheral functions is complete and has to be considered when trying to explain speech intelligibility. A major candidate for imitating subsequent processing is autocorrelation function (ACF). ACF is an established method for temporally analyzing auditory nerve processes [45]. Neural representations that resemble the ACF of an acoustic stimulus have been detected in distributions of all-order interspike intervals in the auditory nerve [46, 47]. Mathematically, the normalized ACF and ACF can be represented by

$$\varnothing(\tau) = \frac{\Phi(\tau)}{\Phi(0)} \qquad (1)$$

where $\Phi(\tau) = \frac{1}{2T}\int_{-T}^{T} p'(t)\,p'(t+\tau)\,dt$ and where 2 T is the integral interval, τ is the time delay, and $p'(t)$ is the signal after it is passed through an A-weighting filter. **Figure 12** shows an example of the calculated monosyllable /sa/. In this case, the ACF was calculated for the integral interval (2 T = 80 ms) that moves with the duration of the monosyllable (running ACF). In the fricative consonant part of the sound (before 0.3 s), the normalized ACF decays suddenly to 0, while in the extended vowel portion of the sound (after 0.3 s), it gradually decays as a function of the delay time. To evaluate the slope of the decay, an effective duration (τ_e) has been proposed [48] that is defined by the delay such that the envelope of the normalized ACF becomes smaller than 0.1. When the consonant component-containing noise element (e.g., /s/ and /d/) occupies the monosyllable, τ_e becomes shorter because it expresses the amount of noise (i.e., $\tau_e = 0$ for white noise and $\tau_e = \infty$ for a pure tone). Indeed, τ_e represents the SN ratio (S: speech and N: noise or reverberation) of a monosyllable itself.

Figure 13 shows the relationships between the physical parameters and the percent of monosyllables articulation presented to patients with sensorineural hearing loss at an optimal volume [49]. Each symbol is the average for a consonant, and $(\tau_e)_{med}$ indicates the median of the time-varied τ_e of the running ACF. Among the four physical measures examined, only τ_e was correlated with speech intelligibility. Effective duration is a measure of temporal pattern persistence, that is, the duration over which a waveform maintains a stable pattern. These data have led to the hypothesis that poor speech recognition is related to the degraded perception of temporal fluctuation patterns. DSPs that prolong the effective duration (e.g., shorten the consonant length or smoothen the voicing frequency) may therefore improve speech intelligibility for those with sensorineural hearing loss.

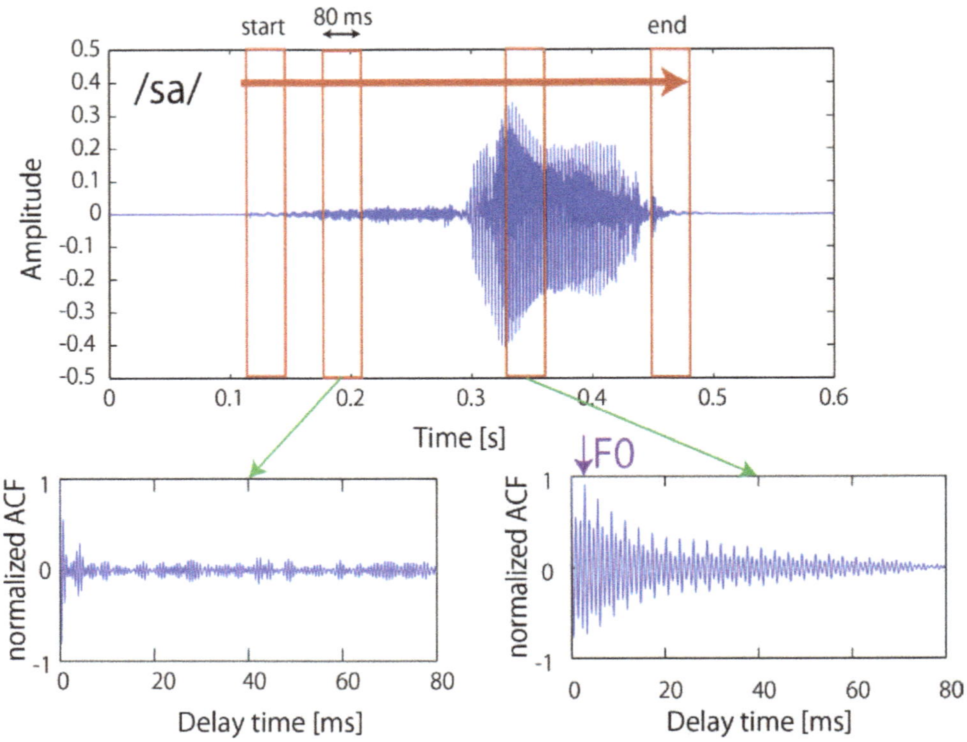

Figure 12. Example of an autocorrelation function calculated for the Japanese monosyllable /sa/ (F0: Fundamental frequency of voice).

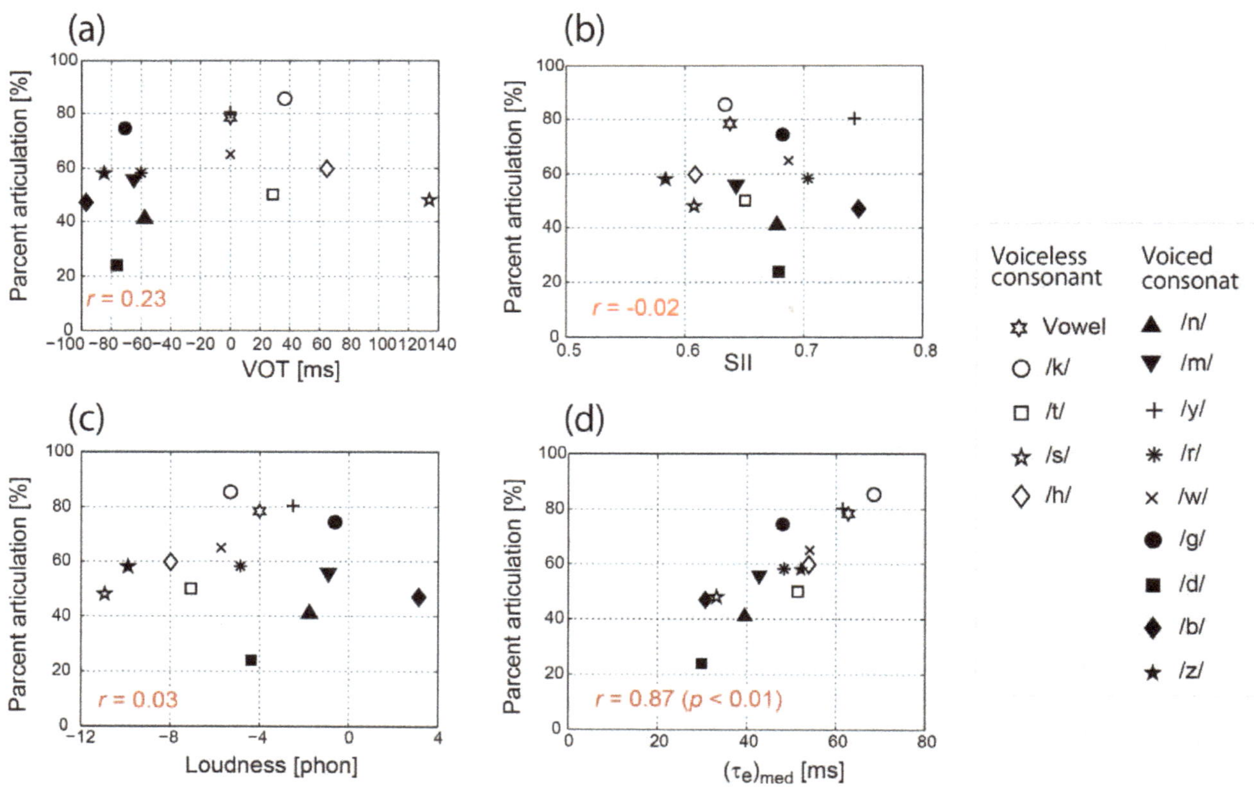

Figure 13. Relationship between the percent of articulation and four physical parameters: (a) VOT, (b) SII, (c) loudness, and (d) $(\tau_e)_{med}$ (R: Correlation coefficient). The different symbols indicate different consonants. Reproduced from (**Figure 5**) in [49].

7. Concluding comments

To avoid advanced hearing loss and instances of hearing loss-related dementia, it is important to recognize hearing loss at an early stage and provide treatment that prevents the loss of hair-cell or auditory-nerve stimulation. In particular, for those who wear hearing aids in only one ear, speech intelligibility is known to degrade more in the other ear [50, 51]. However, currently popular implanted hearing devices are a fairly large burden for people soon after they become aware of their hearing loss. For this reason, we tend to stick to wearable hearing aids that are easy to be put on and take off. Researches are therefore using the scientific method to remove technical barriers for hearing aids. Further, governments should try to remove other barriers by providing services such as financial support or public qualification for handling hearing aids, and companies that make hearing aids should charge less money. This will help slow down hearing loss and lead to a healthier society.

Index of technical terms

Active noise control, p11	Active noise control is a technique for minimizing undesired sound by acoustic interference with a secondary sound source.
Audiogram, p5	Audiogram represents hearing thresholds for standardized frequencies in a dB-scale.
Aural cartilage, p11	Aural cartilage is flexible fibrous tissue shaping an auricle and a part of external auditory canal.
Autocorrelation function (ACF), p12	Autocorrelation function is correlation of a signal with decayed copy of itself as a function of decay.
A-weighting filter, p12	A-weighting filter is designed by a loudness curve (IEC 61672:2003) around 40 phone, and the filtered sound pressure level can quantify the loudness partly.
Bone conducted ultrasonic hearing aid, p10	Bone conducted ultrasonic hearing aid has an ultrasonic transducer which is attached to a mastoid to transmit vibration in ultrasonic range modulated by speech waveform.
Bone-anchored hearing aid (BAHA), p8, p11	Bone-anchored hearing aid is a hearing device which transmit vibration to skull bone through the intermediary of an implanted titanium projection.

Cartilage conduction hearing aid, p11	Cartilage conduction hearing aid transmits sound information by vibrating aural cartilage.
Cochlear implant, p8	Cochlear implant bypasses the normal hearing process and stimulates hair cells in the cochlea using an implanted electrode directly.
Conductive hearing loss, p9	Conductive hearing loss occurs when there is a problem conducting sound waves anywhere along the route through the outer ear, tympanic membrane (eardrum), or middle ear (ossicles).
Effective duration (τ_e), p12	Effective duration is defined by the delay time at which the envelope along the early decay of the normalized autocorrelation becomes below 0.1, and signifies the degree of periodicity contained in a signal.
Fricative consonant, p12	Fricative consonant is produced by forcing air through a narrow channel made by placing two articulators close together.
Full ear, p11	Full ear is uncomfortable feeling when ears are occluded by something, and it emphasize excessively own voice and sound of mastication during a meal.
Loudness level, p12	Loudness level [phon] quantifies the subjective perception of sound pressure and is calculated by spectral energy applied to the equal loudness chart for each 1/3-octave band (ISO 532).
Magnetoencephalography, p10	Magnetoencephalography (MEG) is a non-invasive technique for measuring neuromagnetic signals generated by the brain.
Open-fitting hearing aid, p9	Open-fitting hearing aid has an earplug with a significant leak venting for the purpose of reducing the full ear.
Positron-emission tomography, p10	Positron-emission tomography is non-invasive technique for measuring a positron (positive electron) emitted by a nucleus after blood flow, metabolism, neurotransmitters, and radiolabelled drugs.
Profound hearing loss, p9	Profound hearing loss is an inability to hear sound even in 90 dB in silent condition.

Recruitment hearing, p6	Recruitment hearing is an auditory disorder to exaggerate loudness for sound over a certain amount of sound pressure.
Sensorineural hearing loss, p6, p9, p12	Sensorineural hearing loss is a type of hearing loss, in which the root cause lies in the inner ear or sensory organ (cochlea and associated structures) or the vestibulocochlear nerve (cranial nerve VIII) or neural part.
SN ratio, p13	Signal-to-noise (SN) ratio compares the level of a desired signal to the level of background noise.
Speech intelligibility index (SII), p12	Speech intelligibility index (SII) is a measure of the proportion of a speech sound that is discernible under different listening conditions, and is calculated according to the signal (i.e., speech) to noise (i.e., environmental noise) ratio and the hearing threshold (i.e., audiogram) of each 1/3-octave band.
Voice onset time (VOT), p12	Voice onset time (VOT) is the length of time in milliseconds that passes between the release of a stop consonant and the onset of voicing.

Author details

Ryota Shimokura

Address all correspondence to: rshimo@riko.shimane-u.ac.jp

Architecture and Production Design Engineering, Interdisciplinary Graduate School of Science and Engineering, Shimane University, Shimane, Japan

References

[1] Comprehensive Strategy to Accelerate Dementia Measures (in Japanese). Japan: Ministry of Health, Labour and Welfare. Available from: http://www.mhlw.go.jp/stf/seisakunitsuite/bunya/0000064084.html; 2015 [Accessed: 2017-9-29]

[2] Uhlmann RF, Larson EB, Rees TS, Koepsell TD, Duckert LG. Relationship of hearing impairment to dementia and cognitive dysfunction in older adults. Journal of the American Medical Association. 1989;**261**:1916-1919

[3] Lin FR, Ferrucci L, An Y, Goh JO, Doshi J, Metter EJ, Resnick SM. Association of hearing impairment with brain volume changes in older adults. NeuroImage. 2014;**90**:84-92

[4] Lin FR, Niparko JK, Ferrucci L. Hearing loss prevalence in the United States. Archives Internal Medicine. 2011;**171**:1851-1852

[5] Groshcel M, Gotze R, Ernst A, Basta D. Differential impact of temporary and permanent noise-induced hearing loss on neural cell density in the mouse central auditory pathway. Journal of Nuerotrauma. 2010;**27**:1499-1507

[6] Giambattista della Porta. Magia Naturalis; 1558

[7] Kircher A. Phonurgia Nova Sive Conjugium Mechanic-Physicum Artis & Naturae Paranymta Phonosophia Concinnatum. Rudolpho Dreherr: Kempten; 1673

[8] Turnbull L. A Clinical Manual of the Diseases of the Ear. 2nd edition, revised ed. Philadelphia: J.B. Lippincott Company; 1887

[9] Mills M. Hearing aids and the history of electronics miniaturization. IEEE Annals of the History of Computing. 2011;**33**:24-44

[10] Documents of EuroTrak, JapanTrak, and MarkeTrak (European Hearing Instrument Manufacturers Association). Avairable from: http://www.ehima.com/documents/ [Accessed: 2017-9-28]

[11] Girolama Cardano. De Subtilitate. 1550

[12] Håkansson B, Tjellström A, Rosenhall U. Hearing thresholds with direct bone conduction versus conventional bone conduction. Scandinavian Audiology. 1984;**13**:3-13

[13] Håkansson B, Tjellström A, Rosenhall U. Acceleration levels at hearing threshold with direct bone conduction versus conventional bone conduction. Acta Oto-Laryngologica. 1985;**100**:240-252

[14] Stenfelt S, Wild T, Hato N, Goode RL. Factors contributing to bone conduction: The outer ear. Journal of the Acoustical Society of America. 2003;**113**:902-913

[15] Stenfelt S, Hato N, Goode RL. Round window membrane motion with air conduction and bone conduction stimulation. Hearing Research. 2004;**198**:10-24

[16] Canale A, Dagna F, Cassandro C, Giordano P, Caranzano F, Lacilla M, Albera R. Oval and round window vibroplasty: A comparison of hearing results, risks and failures. European Archives of Oto-Rhino-Laryngology. 2014;**271**:90-94

[17] House LR. Cochlear implants. The Laryngoscope. 1987;**97**:996-997

[18] Clark GM, Tong YC, Black R, Forster IC, Patrick JF, Dewhurst DJ. A multiple electrode cochlear implant. Journal of Laryngology & Otology. 1977;**91**:935-945

[19] Bermingham NA, Hassan BA, Price SD, Vollrath MA, Ben-Arie N, Eatock RA, Bellen HJ, Lysakowski A, Zoghbi HY. Math1: An essential gene for the generation of inner ear hair cells. Science. 1999;**284**:1837-1841

[20] Gavreau V. Audibillite de sons de frequence elevee. Compte Rendu. 1948;**226**:2053-2054

[21] Lenhardt ML, Skellett R, Wang P, Clarke AM. Human ultrasonic speech perception. Science. 1991;**253**:82-85

[22] Hosoi H, Imaizumi S, Sakaguchi T, Tonoike M, Murata K. Activation of the auditory cortex by ultrasound. Lancet. 1998;**351**:496-497

[23] Nishimura T, Nakagawa S, Sakaguchi T, Hosoi H. Ultrasonic masker clarifies ultrasonic perception in man. Hearing Research. 2003;**175**:171-177

[24] Nishimura T, Okayasu T, Uratani Y, Fukuda F, Saito O, Hosoi H. Peripheral perception mechanism of ultrasonic hearing. Hearing Research. 2011;**277**:176-183

[25] Nakagawa S, Okamoto Y, Fujisaka Y. Development of bone-conducted ultrasonic hearing aid for the profoundly deaf. Transactions of Japanese Society for Medical and Biological Engineering. 2006;**44**:184-189

[26] Goldstein BA, Shulman A, Lenhardt ML. Ultra-high-frequency ultrasonic external acoustic stimulation for tinnitus relief: A method for patient selection. International Tinnitus Journal. 2005;**11**:111-114

[27] Lenhardt ML, Shulman A, Goldstein BA. Bone-conduction propagation in human body: Implications for high-frequency therapy. International Tinnitus Journal. 2007;**13**:81-86

[28] Shimokura R, Fukuda F, Hosoi H. A case study of auditory rehabilitation in a profoundly deaf participant using a bone-conducted ultrasonic hearing aid. Behavioral Science Research. 2012;**50**:1-12

[29] Sunohara M, Watanuki K, Tateno M. An occlusion reduction method for hearing aids using adaptive filter. IEICE Technical Report. 2013;**113**:91-96 (in Japanese)

[30] Hosoi H. Receiver. Japanese Patent Application Number 166644 (June 4, 2004)

[31] Hosoi H. Approach in the use of cartilage conduction speaker. Japanese Patent Number 4541111 (November 17, 2004)

[32] Shimokura R, Hosoi H, Nishimura T, Yamanaka T, Levitt H. Cartilage conduction hearing. Journal of the Acoustical Society of America. 2014;**135**:1959-1966

[33] Nishimura T, Hosoi H, Saito O, Miyamae R, Shimokura R, Matsui T, Yamanaka T, Levitt H. Is cartilage conduction classified into air or bone conduction? The Laryngoscope. 2014;**124**:1214-1219

[34] Nishimura T, Hosoi H, Saito O, Miyamae R, Shimokura R, Matsui T, Yamanaka T, Kitahara T, Levitt H. Cartilage conduction efficiently generates airborne sound in the ear canal. Auris, Nasus, Larynx. 2015;**42**:15-19

[35] Nishimura T, Hosoi H, Saito O, Miyamae R, Shimokura R, Yamanaka T, Kitahara T, Levitt H. Cartilage conduction is charcterized by vibrations of the cartilaginous portion of the ear canal. PLoS One. 2015;**10**:1-11

[36] Shimokura R, Hosoi H, Iwakura T, Nishimura T, Matsui T. Development of monaural and binaural behind-the-ear cartilage conduction hearing aids. Applied Acoustics. 2013;**74**:1234-1240

[37] Nishimura T, Hosoi H, Saito O, Miyamae R, Shimokura R, Matsui T, Iwakura T. Benefit of a new hearing device utilizing cartilage conduction. Auris, Nasus, Larynx. 2013;**40**:440-446

[38] Morimoto C, Nishimura T, Hosoi H, Saito O, Fukuda F, Shimokura R, Yamanaka T. Sound transmission of cartilage conduction in the ear with fibrotic aural atresia. Journal of Rehabilitation Research and Development. 2014;**51**:325-332

[39] Kodera K, Akai S, Demizu M, Hirota E, Miura M, Yabe S. Classifications of sensorineural hearing loss by consonant confusion. Audiology Japan. 1992;**35**:582-587 (in Japanese)

[40] Kodera K, Akai S, Hirota E, Miura M, Yabe S. Study on consonant confusion in Japanese patients with sensorineural hearing loss. Journal of Oto-rhino-Laryngological Society of Japan. 1993;**96**:1404-1409 (in Japanese)

[41] Akasaka S, Nishimura T, Okayasu T, Hosoi H. Percentage of correct answers to 57-S individual Japanese monosyllabic words in the hearing impaired. Audiology Japan. 2010;**53**:69-75 (in Japanese)

[42] Lisker L, Abramson A. Some effects of context on voice onset time in English stops. Language and Speech. 1967;**10**:1-28

[43] ANSI S3.5-1997. American National Standard Methods for the Calculation of the Speech Intelligibility Index. New York: American National Standards Institute; 1997

[44] ISO-532. Acoustics—Method for Calculating Loudness Level. Basel, Switzerland: International Standards Organization; 1975

[45] Licklider JCR. A duplex theory of pitch perception. Experientia. 1951;**7**:128-133

[46] Cariani PA, Delgutte B. Neural correlates of the pitch of complex tones. I. Pitch and pitch salience. Journal of Neurophysiology. 1996;**76**:1698-1716

[47] Cariani PA. Temporal coding of periodicity pitch in the auditory system: An overview. Neural Plasticity. 1999;**6**:147-172

[48] Ando Y. Subjective preference in relation to objective parameters of music sound fields with a single echo. Journal of the Acoustical Society of America. 1977;**62**:1436-1441

[49] Shimokura R, Akasaka S, Nishimura T, Hosoi H, Matsui T. Autocorrelation factors and intelligibility of Japanese monosyllables in individuals with sensorineural hearing loss. Journal of the Acoustical Society of America. 2017;**141**:1065-1073

[50] Silman S, Gelfand SA, Silverman CA. Late-onset auditory deprivation: Effects of monaural versus binaural hearing aids. Journal of the Acoustical Society of America. 1984;**76**:1357-1362

[51] Hattori H. Ear dominance for nonsense-syllable recognition ability in sensorineural hearing-impaired children: Monaural versus binaural amplification. Journal of the American Academy of Audiology. 1993;**4**:319-340

10

Electrophysiology in Ménière's Disease

Pauliana Lamounier

Abstract

Ménière's disease (MD) is a progressive inner ear disorder that affects at least 0.2% of the population in EUA. The symptoms triad of fluctuating hearing loss, tinnitus, and vertigo was described by Prosper Ménière for more than a century and its pathophysiology is still unknown. MD has a fluctuating course and in many cases, difficult clinical management. Progressive hearing loss and intense dizzying seizures becomes more frequent as the disease progresses. All of this increases the challenges of accurate identification and has probably led to the trial of several tests for identifying MD. The tests are useful tools to assist the otolaryngologist both in diagnosis and prognosis of MD. These tests includes audiometry, otoacustic emission (OAE), electrocochleography (EcochG), vestibular evoked myogenic potentials (VEMP), cochlear hydrops analysis masking procedure (CHAMP) and video head impulse test (vHIT).

Keywords: Meniere's disease, endolymphatic hydrops, electrocochleography, VEMP, CHAMP, vHIT

1. Introduction

Ménière's disease (MD) is a progressive inner ear disorder that affects at least 0.2% of the population in EUA [1]. The symptoms triad of fluctuating hearing loss, tinnitus, and vertigo was described by Prosper Ménière for more than a century and its pathophysiology is still unknown.

For a long time, it was believed that endolymphatic hydrops would be the histopathological substrate of the disease. The cause of hydrops is still unknown and most of the theories are based on altered endolymph production or reabsorption. The hydrops occurs more often in the cochlea and saccule, followed by the utricle and semicircular channels [2]. Recent studies have indicated that hydrops is a finding of the MD, together with the symptoms, since it alone does not explain all the clinical features, including the progression of hearing loss and the frequency of vertigo attacks [3].

According to the criteria of the Bárány Society, MD is classified as definite or probable. In definite MD, the patient should have had two or more spontaneous episodes of vertigo, each lasting from 20 min to 12 h, documented mild to moderate sensorineural hearing loss, aural symptoms (hearing, tinnitus, and fullness) in the affected ear, and exclusion of other vestibular disorders that explain the symptoms. In probable MD, the patient should have had two or more episodes of vertigo or loss of balance, each lasting from 20 min to 24 h, floating aural symptoms (hearing, tinnitus, or fullness) in that ear, and exclusion of other vestibular disorders that explain the symptoms [4].

MD has a fluctuating course and in many cases difficult in clinical management. Progressive hearing loss becomes more frequent and intense dizzying seizures as the disease progresses. All of this increases the challenges of accurate identification, and has probably led to the trial of several tests for identifying MD. The tests are useful tools to assist the otolaryngologist both in diagnosis and prognosis of MD. Identify the site of hydrops, even in cases of severe hearing loss and possible involvement of the asymptomatic ear are useful information on disease management.

These tests includes tonal and speech audiometry /impedance, otoacustic emissions (OAE), electrocochleography (EcochG), vestibular evoked myogenic potentials (VEMP), cochlear hydrops analysis masking procedure (CHAMP) and video head impulse test (vHIT).

2. Electrophysiology

2.1. Tonal and speech audiometry/Impedance

Audiometry is helpful to confirm the diagnosis and it is a part of the criteria of the Bárány Society. In the early stages of the disease, there is a low frequency sensorineural hearing loss that fluctuates in time. In some cases, it also affects high frequency, setting the pattern of inverted U. In later stages, the hearing loss would increase and the audiogram would become more and more flat. Sometimes, a decreased speech discrimination is also mentioned as a common symptom of MD [5]. Hearing loss initially resolves after attacks, but with the disease progression, patients may experience loss of auditory nerve fibers. The impedance is helpful to exclude middle ear pathology.

2.2. Otoacoustic emission (OAE)

Otoacoustic emissions are subliminal sounds detected in the external auditory canal and generated by the outer hair cells. They are useful in the diagnosis of many cochleopathies, including MD.

Authors believe that hydrops causes changes in the hydrodynamic and cochlear biomechanical micromechanism, due to changes in the interciliary bridges caused by the distension of membranes and cells within the cochlear duct. These changes could affect the transmission of the stimulus by outer hair cells, but not necessarily loss of them. The selective atrophy of the short and medium stereocilia at the cochlea's apex is correlated with the hearing loss in low frequencies that occur in the early phase of MD. The OEA can reveal early lesions due to alterations of the cochlear micromechanism not correlated with the auditory thresholds detected in tone audiometry [6].

The distortion product otoacoustic emission (DPOAE) was considered more appropriate than transient otoacoustic emission (TEOAE) for monitoring during glycerol test because of its high sensitivity in the detection of changes in cochlear function. DPOAE is a complementary test to pure tone audiometry during the glycerol test. It is very useful and will improve the diagnosis of endolymphatic hydrops [7].

2.3. Electrocochleography (EcochG)

Electrocochleography records the three mechanoelectrical potentials of the cochlea. The cochlear microphonic is considered the first step to the neural impulse. It reflects the sum of the intracellular potentials generated in the hair cells of the basal portion of the cochlea during depolarization [8]. Hall in 2007, Durrant, Ding and Salvi in 1998, affirm that the inner hair cells play a central role in the generation of SP, while other authors, such as Burkand et al. believe that it is generated by both internal and external hair cell [8–10]. Action potential (AP) is the sum of the synchrony of individual neural APs of the cochlear nerve.

Electrocochleography is the test capable of measuring endolymphatic hydrops in the cochlea. The test is usually performed with a transthympanic or extrathympanic electrode (**Figure 1**). Hydrops changes the mechanical properties of the cochlea, leading to asymmetric movements of the basilar membrane, which may exacerbate the SP, and consequently, increases the ratio between the amplitudes of SP and AP. The increase in SP amplitude will change according to the existing pressure and volume of the intralabirintic fluid [10, 11] (**Figure 2**).

The SP/AP ratio thresholds are variable in the literature. Pappas et al. believe that any result above 0.5 in an extratympanic EcochG is suggestive of endolymphatic hydrops [12], while Iseli and Gibson established a value of 0.33 in a transtympanic EcoghG [13].

Lamounier et al. in a systematic review reported that in 25–54% of patients with MD, the electrocochleography presented normal results, with the sensitive of the test ranging from 57 to 71% and a specificity ranging from 92 to 96%. In most studies selected, the transtympanic electrode is the most widely used. EcochG in MD presents a variable sensitivity, as in cases of hearing loss due to disease progression, patients may experience a reduction in the amplitude of AP due to loss of auditory nerve fibers [14–17].

On comparing the results of the transtympanic and extratympanic electrocochleography in 20 patients with Ménière's disease and 20 control patients, Ghosh et al. reported a significant difference between the SP/AP ratios of the cases and control groups. For an SP/AP ratio of 0.29, they found 100% sensitivity, 90% specificity to transtympanic, and 90% and 80% to the extratympanic EcochG, respectively, and concluded that extratympanic EcochG is a non-invasive method, effective and easier to carry out in clinical practice than transtympanic EcochG [15].

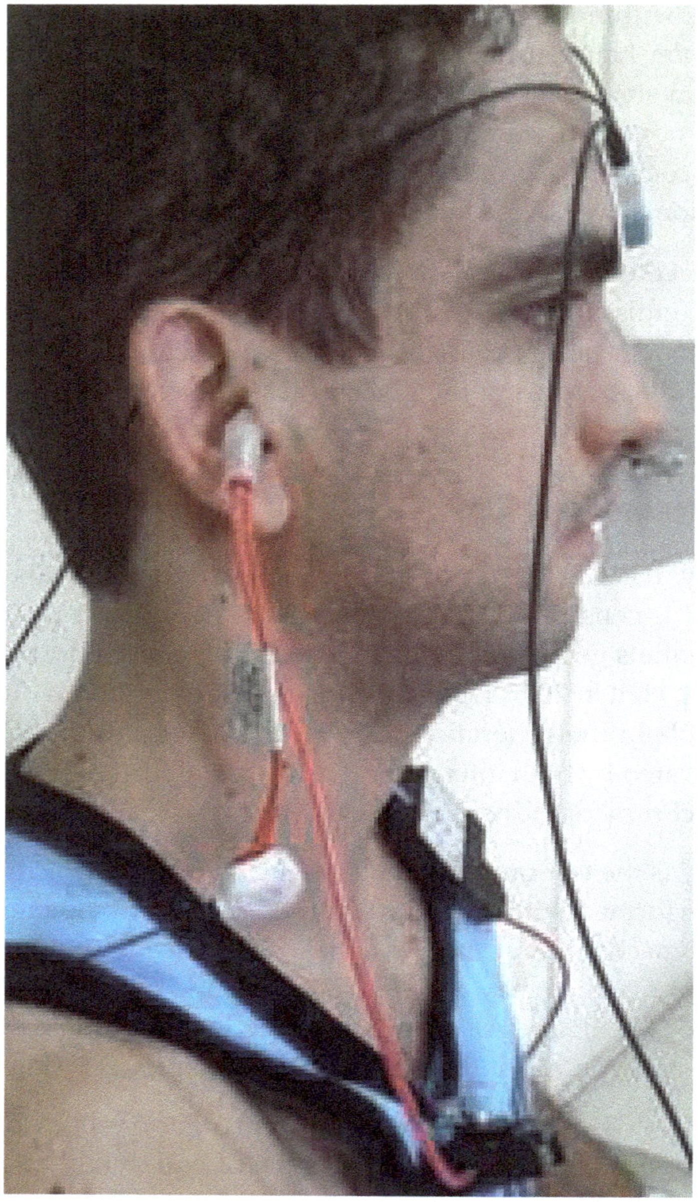

Figure 1. Position of EcochG´s electrodes.

Lamounier et al. also found in the systematic review that the analysis of the SP/AP ratio curve of the transtympanic electrocochleography did not necessarily increase sensitivity in the diagnosis of hydrops when compared with the SP/AP amplitude [14, 16–18].

Gibson et al. compared EcochG results in ears with Ménière's disease and healthy ears with similar hearing loss and concluded that click SP/AP measurements are not helpful in making this differentiation but that tone burst SP amplitude measurements were significantly different between these populations [19].

Colon and Gibson showed that the sensitivity of transtympanic electrocochleography increased to 85% when 1 kHz of tone burst was used to measure SP. They reported that the majority of

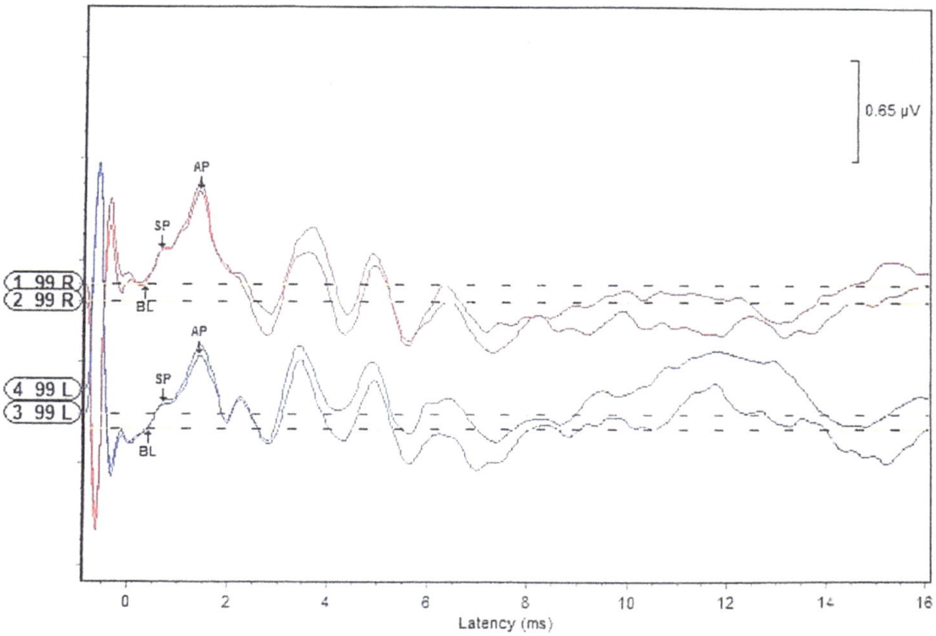

Figure 2. EcochG.

specialists or 58.6%, use click stimuli as opposed to 17.2%, who use tone burst, and 24.3% who use both stimuli [20]. Lopes et al. evaluated the sensitivity and specificity of the SP/AP ratio and graphic angular measurement in electrocochleographies of 71 ears of 41 MD patients and 14 normal-hearing control patients. They concluded that the graphic angular measurement is not sensitive or specific enough to diagnose MD. The association of the SP/AP ratio and graphic angular measurement in conjunction improved the sensitivity to the detriment of the specificity of the test [21].

Electrocochleography is a valuable tool in the diagnosis of cochlear hydrops, as it is noninvasive, easy to handle, and offers new techniques to increase the sensitivity of the test.

2.4. Vestibular evoked myogenic potentials (VEMP)

Vestibular evoked myogenic potentials (VEMP) emerged as a recent and complementary way of vestibular system assessment with the specific analysis of the saccular function and inferior vestibular nerve.

In 1992, Colebatch and Halmagyi proposed that the saccular macula was the peripheral receptor of the vestibular-spinal reflex and in 1994 reported surface potential in the sternocleidomastoid (SCM) muscle in response to clicks through high-intensity air conduction (100 dB), accessing the Sacculo-collic reflex [22].

VEMP is, therefore, a short latency myogenic response, generated after a sound stimulus, originating in the sacculo and conducted by the inferior division of the inferior vestibular nerve to the central nervous system, generating inhibitory electrical responses captured by surface electrodes on the muscles, during muscular contraction. This neural response is a reflex arc of three neurons that surround the inner ear, the brainstem, and the vestibular-spinal pathway [22–24] (**Figure 3**).

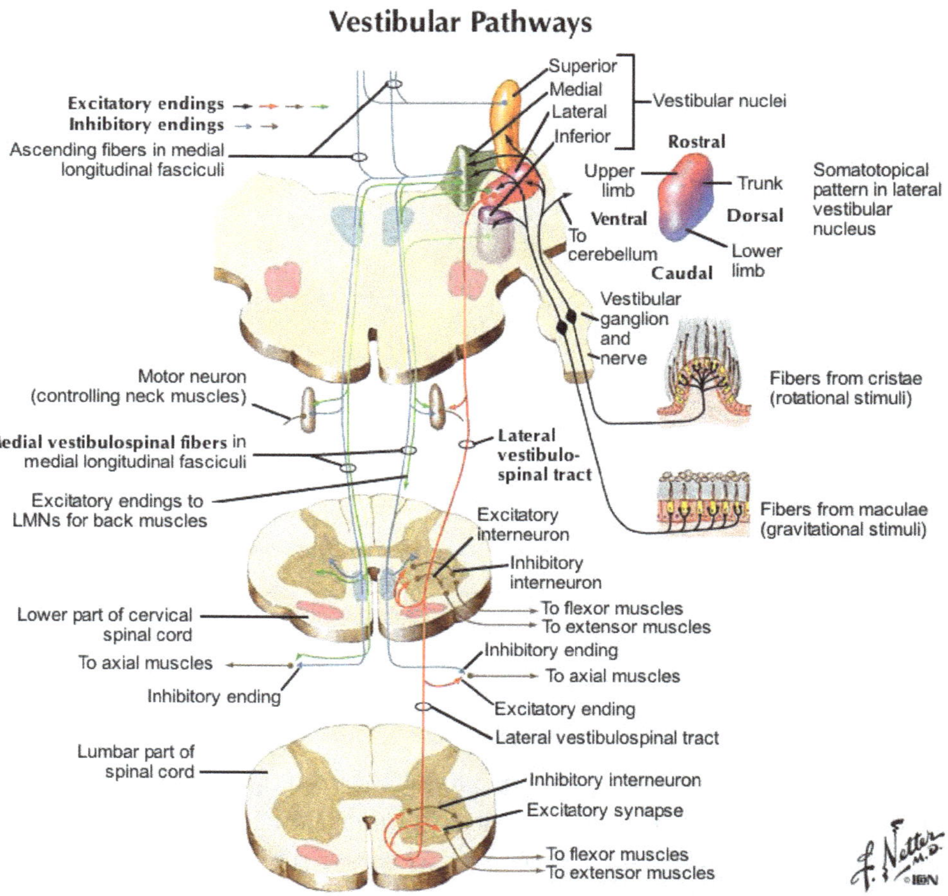

Figure 3. Neural pathway of VEMP.

Similar myogenic responses have been captured in other muscle groups. The responses captured in SCM are called cervical VEMP (cVEMP) and those collected in the extraocular musculature are called ocular VEMP (oVEMP). VEMP can be obtained by air and bone conduction and galvanic stimulation, using tone burst or clicks stimulus [23–25] (**Figure 4**).

The electrical responses of these potentials consist of two biphasic waves, the first negative wave, with latency around 13 ms, known as p13. This is followed by another wave, this time positive, with latency around 23 ms, known as n23. There is also a second biphasic complex known as n34-p44, but due to the lack of replicability of this second complex, only the first complex is considered. The electromyographic potential recording waves are usually defined by: latency, wave morphology, peak-to-peak amplitude, or the difference in values between the most positive point of one wave and the most negative point of another wave [26] (**Figure 5**).

The large variation in the amplitude of the responses, due to the different degrees of muscular contracture obtained for each individual, justifies the analysis of the VEMP responses through the interaural asymmetry index. The literature review showed that VEMP is considered altered by the absence of reproducible waves and or asymmetry index of interaural responses greater than 34% [26].

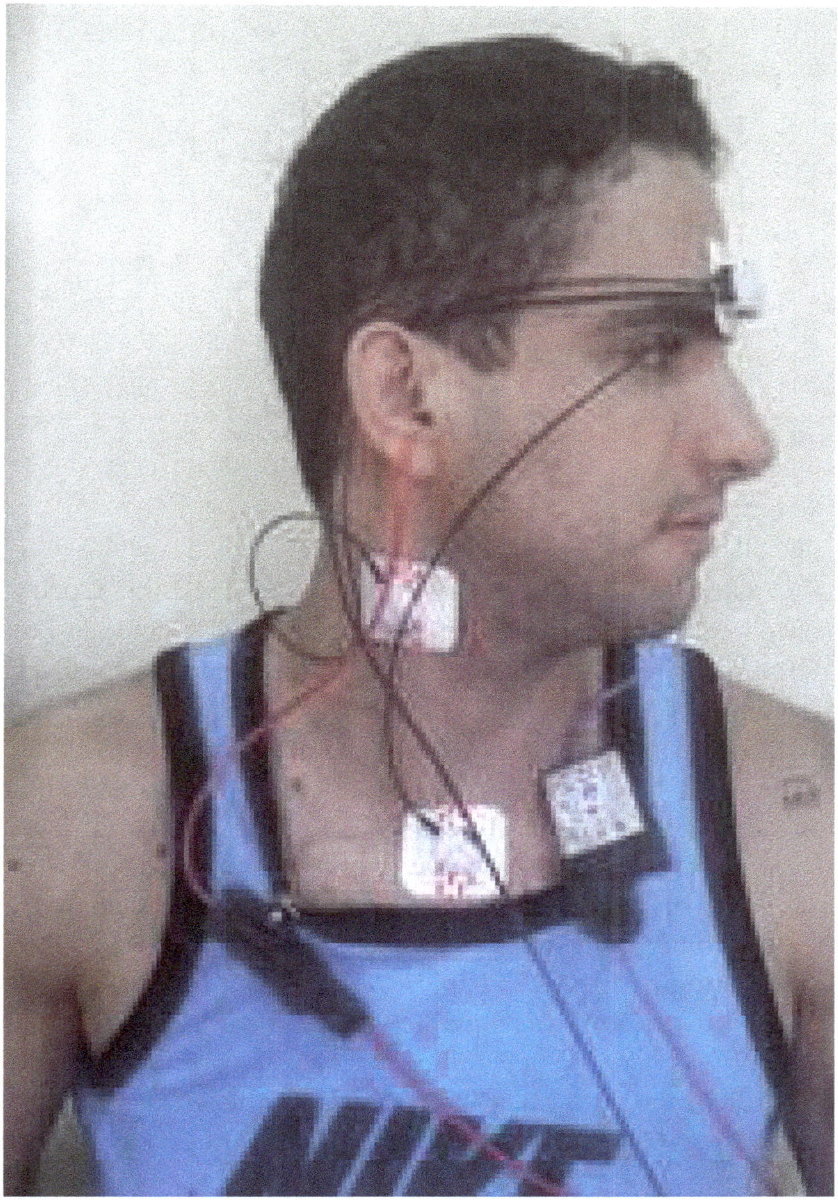

Figure 4. Position of cervical VEMP's electrodes.

The cVEMP is more sensitive for deep bass. Stimuli with frequencies near 500 Hz have higher response amplitudes. Air conducted (AC) sound is the most commonly used stimulus for eliciting cVEMPs. Tone bursts are preferable above clicks because the latter have less reliable results and need higher absolute intensities to evoke a response [26].

The cVEMP is absent or decreased by 30–54% in patients with MD [22, 23]. It may be increased in the early stages of MD, perhaps by the pressure of saccular hydrops against the stapes footplate, increasing sensitivity sacular to intense sound. Its measurement may be floating, with a tendency to disappear with the progression of the disease, as well as 24 h post-crisis, which may reappear after 48 h or with the use of drugs to reduce endolymphatic hydrops [25–27].

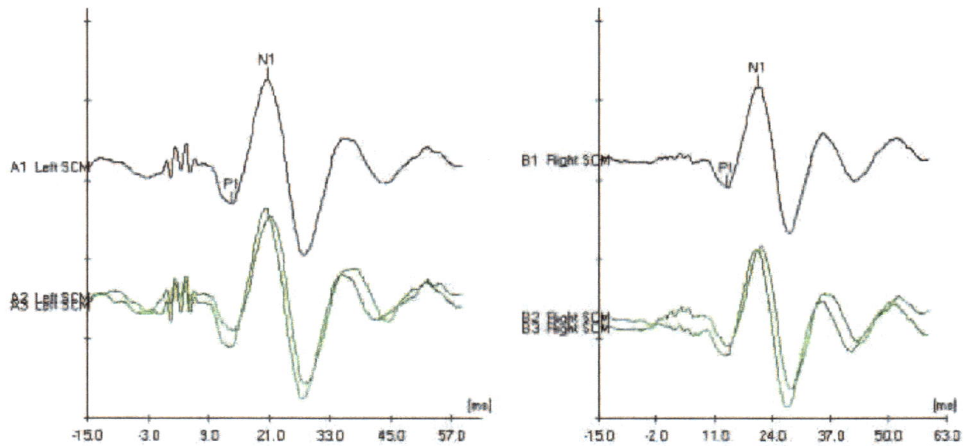

Figure 5. VEMP ´s waves.

Lamounier et al. evaluated the sensitivity and specificity of VEMP and EcochG in the diagnosis of definite MD compared with the clinical diagnosis. The study includes 12 patients (24 ears) diagnosed with definite MD defined according to the clinical criteria proposed by the American Academy of Otolaryngology Head and Neck Surgery (AAO-HNS) in 1995, as well as 12 healthy volunteers allocated to the control group (24 ears). A clinical diagnosis by the AAO-HNS criteria was considered as the gold standard. All patients underwent an otoneurological examination, including pure tone and speech audiometry, cVEMP and extratympanic EcochG. The sensitivity and specificity to detect the presence or absence of disease were calculated. In both tests and in both ears, the ability to diagnose healthy cases was high, with specificity ranging from 84.6 to 100%. Moreover, the ability of the tests to diagnose the disease varied from low to moderate sensitivity, with values ranging from 37.5 to 63.6%. The agreement of both tests in the right ear, measured by the kappa coefficient, was equal to 0.54 indicating a moderate agreement. In the left ear, that agreement was equal to 0.07 indicating a weak correlation between the tests. The sensitivity of the VEMP for the right ear was 63.6% and for the left ear, 62.5%. The sensitivity of EcochG for the right ear was 63.6% and 37.5% for the left ear. They concluded that the specificity of both tests was high, and the sensitivity of VEMP was higher than that of EcochG [3].

Similar to cVEMPs, oVEMPs can also be augmented in MD [28].

The ocular VEMP (oVEMP) is a more recently described reflex, which is thought to reflect predominantly utricular otolith function and can be understood as part of the vestibulo-ocular reflex (VOR). Patients with MD have higher rates of attenuated or absent oVEMPs than normal subjects, increasing with advancing disease [28–30].

Wen et al. recruited unilateral MD patients with either augmented or reduced oVEMPs (asymmetry >40 and <100%) in response to bone-conducted vibration and found that augmented oVEMPs were seen more frequently in patients with early stage MD. Augmented responses might also be more likely when recorded during an attack [31].

Winters et al. examined air-conducted oVEMPs in MD patients and found lower response rates with smaller amplitudes and higher thresholds compared to normal subjects. Interestingly, this effect was observed not only in the affected, but to a lesser extent also in the clinically unaffected ears [32].

The VEMP is easy to perform, does not cause discomfort to patient and does not vary with hearing loss. The ability to predict the presence of abnormalities in an asymptomatic ear is one of the great features of VEMP [33].

2.5. Cochlear hydrops analysis masking procedure (CHAMP)

The cochlear hydrops analysis masking procedure (CHAMP) was introduced in 2005 as a new test to diagnose MD. Don et al. showed that endolymphatic hydrops in patients diagnosed with MD causes changes in the response properties of the basilar membrane that lead to impaired high-pass noise masking of auditory brainstem response (ABR) to clicks in staked ABR. The latency delay in normal-hearing ears, between wave V for the click alone response and the 0.5 kHz high-pass masking noise condition, is significantly longer than that in MD ears. This difference is known as the latency delay [34].

The increased velocity of the traveling wave would affect the properties of the basilar membrane but cannot affect the tonotopic organization along the basilar membrane. The increased velocity of the traveling wave is more likely to impact the low frequencies as they are represented toward the apical end on the basilar membrane. When ABR latencies are obtained by presenting clicks along with the high-pass masking noise in individuals with Méniére's disease, the altered motion mechanics of the basilar membrane limits the ability of low-frequency noise to mask the activity in high frequency [35, 36] (**Figure 6**).

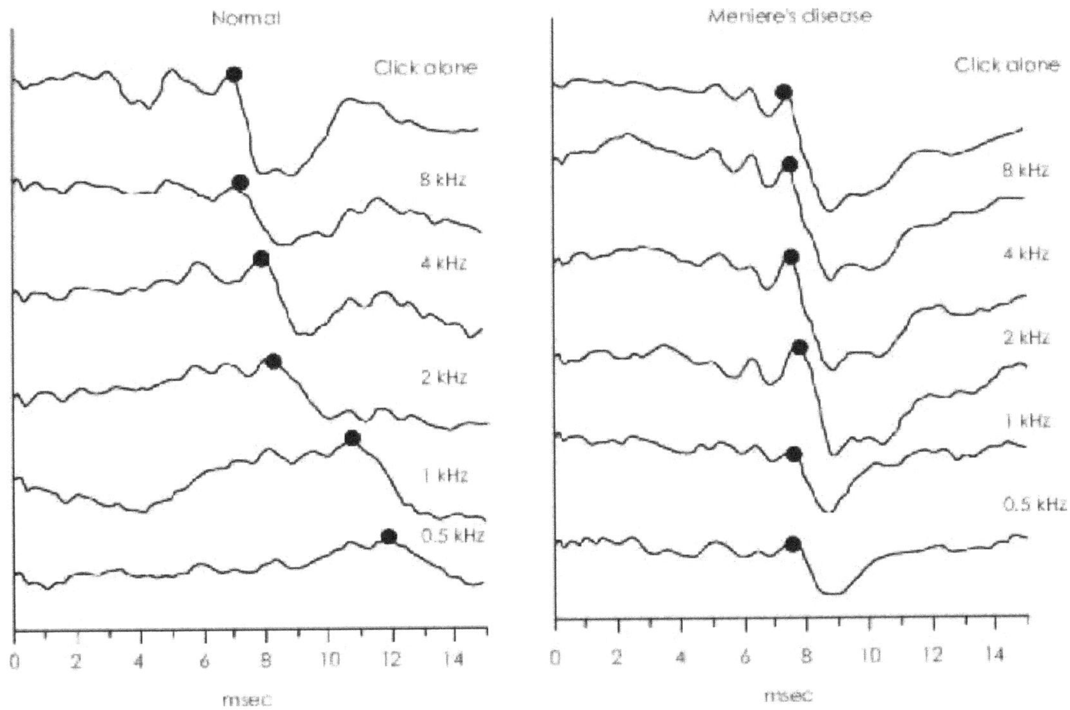

Figure 6. CHAMP.

In individuals with MD, we can observe the phenomenon of undermasking in high-pass responses, whereas the undermasking phenomenon is not seen in normal individuals. This would in turn result in lesser latency difference between click alone and click with 500 Hz high-pass masking noise condition in ears with MD than unaffected or normal ears [37].

Don et al. conducted the test in 23 definite MD patients and compared the results with 38 non-MD normal-hearing subjects. Their measures did not demonstrate an overlap between the Ménière's and nonMénière's groups, and therefore, the authors concluded that the test had an extremely high, even 100%, sensitivity and 100% specificity for diagnostic use in individual patients [34].

However, some studies have questioned these findings by reporting significantly lower sensitivity and specificity values. De Valck et al. evaluated CHAMP performance in Ménière patients and normal controls, and revealed no discriminative value in differentiating Ménière's from non-MD subjects with otovestibular symptoms [37].

Kingma investigated the usefulness of the cochlear hydrops analysis masking procedure (CHAMP) as an additional diagnostic test in patients with definite unilateral Ménière's disease. With less than 0.3 ms criterion and including the ears in which no delay could be measured, the sensitivity of the CHAMP is 32% and concluded that abnormal latency delays for CHAMP are delays shorter than 2 ms. Earlier results with CHAMP should be reconsidered using this criterion, instead of 0.3 ms [38].

Lee et al. suggest that the CHAMP seems to be more valuable in detection of definite MD than is extratympanic EcochG [39].

Furthermore, CHAMP can only be recorded for losses not exceeding moderate degree, which limits its use to identify Meniere's disease with lesser degree of hearing losses only.

The literature indicates a need for continued exploration of these tests in order to establish the usefulness or lack of it in the diagnosis for MD.

2.6. Video head impulse test (vHIT)

A new quantitative test of vestibular function known as the video head impulse test (vHIT) has recently emerged that now allows for discrete measurements of the vestibulo-ocular reflex (VOR) during evaluation of the extremely high-frequency head movements. Although the bithermal caloric test is useful for assessing low-frequency vestibular system function, the head impulse test (HIT), as described by Halmagyi and Curthoys, is a method for testing the function in a frequency region encountered in everyday life in the vestibular system [40, 41].

The primary differences between the vHIT and caloric tests are the mode of stimulus delivery (thermal gradient vs. natural head motion) as well as the temporal frequency of each examination (caloric stimulus represents a low-frequency stimulus and the vHIT a high-frequency stimulus). It is well known that the vHIT and caloric tests are sensitive to detection of a certain percentage of patients with MD [42, 43].

The test involves examiner-initiated high velocity, high-acceleration, and yet, small-amplitude head movements while the patient is instructed to stare at a stationary target located at center gaze. If the VOR is intact, the patient will be able to maintain foveal vision of the target during the head impulse. If the VOR is impaired, rotation of the head toward the ipsilesional semicircular canal will drive the eyes off the target, forcing the patient to generate a volitional catch-up saccade to bring eyes back to the target [40] (**Figures 7** and **8**).

The receptor of the angular VOR is the crista ampullaris. This structure consists of both type I and type II hair cells as well as regularly and irregularly discharging afferent neurons. Type I hair cells populate the central part of the crista ampullaris. Irregular afferents primarily connect to type I hair cells or a mixture of type I and type II. These hair cells encode high-frequency, high-acceleration head movements. Type II cells populate the periphery of the crista. Regular afferents carry the output of type II hair cells or a mixture of type I and type II and likely encode low-frequency, low acceleration movement [44, 45].

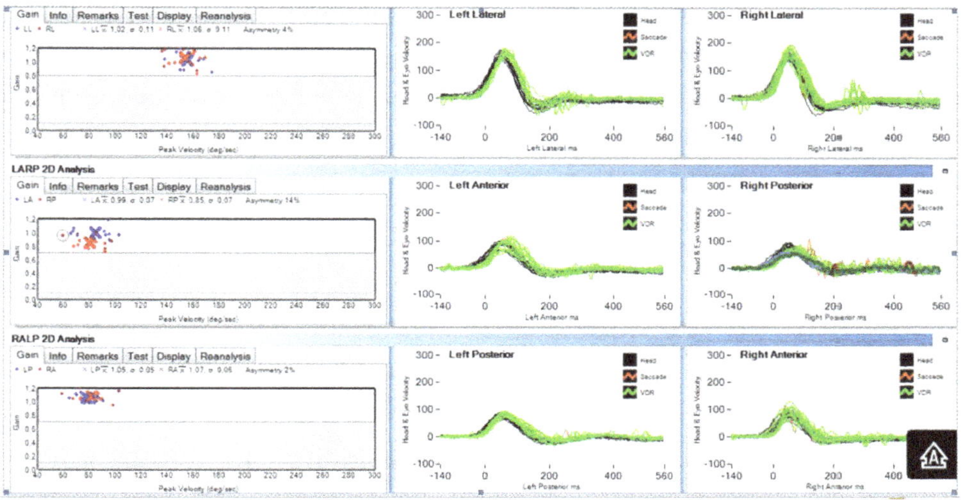

Figure 7. VHIT : Speed of the head in black = speed the eyes in green. There is no record of ccrrective saccades. (Figure provided by borgesdecarvalhootorrinos.com.br).

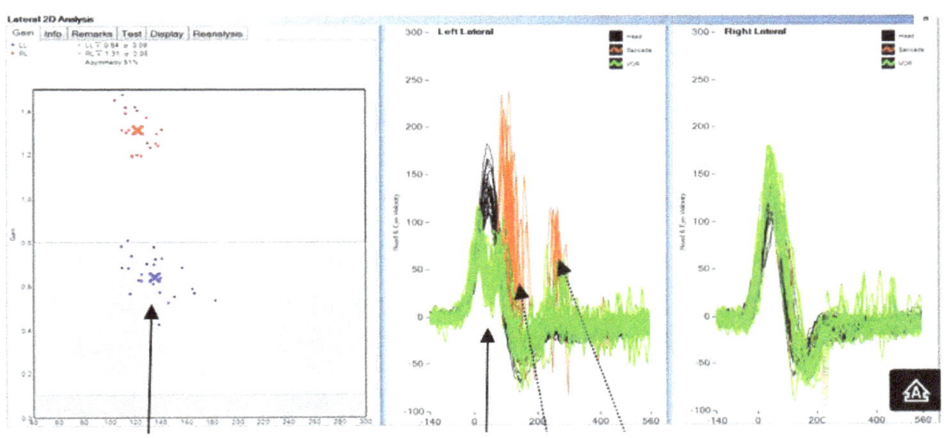

Figure 8. VHIT: Lower eye velocity than head. Presence of saccades. (Figure provided by borgesdecarvalhootorrinos.com.br).

Tsuji et al. reported that although MD affected the structure and function of type II hair cells, the density and number of type I hair cells appeared unchanged in patients with MD [46].

Maire and van Melle showed that, in early stages of MD, VOR gain was higher when the patient was rotated toward the affected ear, but this observed enhancement diminished as the disease progressed [47].

McCaslin et al. presented three cases of patients with Ménière's disease with asymptomatic vestibular dysfunction demonstrated with videonystagmography (VNG) testing, which provided a quantitative measure of VOR gain. The authors found a dissociation between the caloric test and VHIT results, and they explained these findings by understanding the different dynamic response properties of the two primary populations of neurons in the crista [40].

The assessment of cochlear function with audiometry, EcochG and CHAMP, of the saccule through cervical VEMP, of the utricle through ocular VEMP, of the lateral semicircular canal with the caloric tests, and all of the semicircular canals by the vHIT demonstrates the advancements of research in the vestibular diagnosis. New paths are open to the discovery of the pathophysiological mechanism of a disease that was first described over a century ago and still has no defined treatment protocol.

Author details

Pauliana Lamounier

Address all correspondence to: paulilamounier@yahoo.com.br

Centro de Reabilitação e Readaptação Dr Henrique Santillo—CRER, Goiânia, GO, Brazil

References

[1] Lacour M, van de Heyning PH, Novotny M, Brahim T. Betahistine in the treatment of Ménière's disease. Neuropsychiatric Disease and Treatment. 2007;**3**(4):429-440

[2] Okuno T, Sando I. Localization, frequency and severity of endolymphatic hydrops and the pathology of the labyrinthine membrane in Méniére's disease. The Annals of Otology, Rhinology, and Laryngology. 1987;**96**:438-445

[3] Lamounier P, de Souza TSA, Gobbo DA, Bahmad Jr. F. Evaluation of vestibular evoked myogenic potentials (VEMP) and electrocochleography for the diagnosis of Ménière's disease. Brazilian Journal of Otorhinolaryngology. 2016. DOI: 10.1016/j.bjorl.2016.04.021

[4] Escamez JAL, Carey J, Chung WH, Goebel JA, Magnusson M, Mandala M, et al. Diagnostic criteria for Menière's disease. Consensus document of the Bárány Society, The Japan Society for Equilibrium Research, the European Academy of Otology and Neurotology (EAONO), the American Academy of Otolaryngology-Head and Neck

Surgery (AAO-HNS) and theKorean Balance Society. Acta Otorrinolaringológica Española. 2016;**67**(1):1-7

[5] Mateijsen DJM, Van Hengel PWJ, Van Huffelen WM, Wit HP, Albers FWJ. Pure-tone and speech audiometry in patients with Meniere's disease. Clinical Otolaryngology. 2001;**26**:379-387

[6] Aquino AMCM, Massaro CAM, Tiradentes JB, Garzon JCV, Oliveira JAA. Otoacoustic emissions in early diagnosis of cochlear lesions in Méniére's disease. Revista Brasileira de Otorrinolaringologia. 2002;**68**(5):761-765

[7] Sakashita T, Kubo T, Kyunai K, Ueno K, Hikawa C, et al. Changes in otoacoustic emission during the glycerol test in the ears of patients with Ménière's disease. Nihon Jibiinkoka Gakkai Kaiho. 2001;**104**(6):682-693

[8] Burkard RF, Eggermont JJ, Don M. Auditory evoked potentials: Basic principles and clinical application. In: Electric and Magnetic Fields of Synchronous Neural Activity. Baltimore: Lippincott Williams & Wilkins; 2007. pp.2-21

[9] Hall JW, Antonelli PJ. Assessment of peripheral and central auditory function. In: Bailey BJ, Jackler RK, Pillsbury HC 3rd, Lambert PR, editors. Head and Neck Surgery-Otolaryngology. 3rd ed. Lippincott, Philadelphia: Williams and Wilkins; 2001. p. 1666

[10] Durrant J, Wang J, Ding D, Salvi R. Are inner or outer hair cells the source of summating potentials recorded from the round window? Journal of the Acoustical Society of America. 1998;**104**:370-377

[11] Nguyen LT, Harris JP, Nguyen QT. Clinical utility of electrocochleography in the diagnosis and management of Ménière's disease: AOS and ANS member ship survey data. Otology & Neurotology. 2010;**31**:455-459

[12] Pappas DGJ, Pappas DGS, Carmichael L, Hyatt DP, Toohey LM. Extratympanic electrocochleography: Diagnostic and predictive value. American Journal of Otolaryngology. 2000;**21**:81-87

[13] Iseli C, Gibson WA. Comparison of three methods of using transtympanic electrocochleography for the diagnosis of Ménière's disease: Click summating potential measurements, tone burst summating potential amplitude measurements, and biasing of the summating potential using a low frequency tone. Acta Oto-Laryngologica. 2010;**130**:95-101

[14] Lamounier P, Gobbo DA, de Souza TS, de Oliveira CA, Bahmad F Jr. Electrocochleography for Ménière's disease: Is it reliable? Brazilian Journal of Otorhinolaryngology. 2014; **80**:527-532

[15] Ghosh S, Gupta AK, Mann SS. Can electrocochleography in Meniere's disease be noninvasive? The Journal of Otolaryngology. 2002;**31**:371-375

[16] Baba A, Takasaki K, Tanaka F, Tsukasaki N, Kumagami H, Takahashi H. Amplitude and area ratios of summating potential/action potential (SP/AP) in Ménière's disease. Acta Oto-Laryngologica. 2009;**129**:25-29

[17] Chung WH, Cho DY, Choi JY, Hong SH. Clinical usefulness of extratympanic electrocochleography in the diagnosis of Ménière's disease. Otology & Neurotology. 2004;**25**: 144-149

[18] Devaiah AK, Dawson KL, Ferraro JA, Ator GA. Utility of area curve ratio electrocochleography in early Meniere disease. Archives of Otolaryngology–Head and Neck Surgery. 2003;**129**:547-551

[19] Gibson WP. A comparison of two methods of using transtympanic electrocochleography for the diagnosis of Meniere's disease: Click summating potential/action potential ratio measurements and toneburst summating potential measurements. Acta Oto-Laryngologica. 2009. Suppl;38-42

[20] Conlon BJ, Gibson WP. Electrocochleography in the diagnosis of Meniere's disease. Acta Oto-Laryngologica. 2000;**120**:480-483

[21] Lopes KC, Munhoz MSL, Santos MAR, Moraes MFD, Chaves AG. A medida angular gráfica como parâmetro de avaliação da eletrococleografia. Brazilian Journal of Otorhinolaryngology. 2011;**77**(2):214-220

[22] Rosengren SM, Welgampola MS, Colebatch JG. Vestibular evoked myogenic potentials: Past, present and future. Clinical Neurophysiology. 2010;**121**:636-651

[23] Egami N, Ushio M, Yamasoba T, Yamaguchi T, Murofushi T,Iwasaki S. The diagnostic value of vestibular evoked myogenic potentials in patients with Ménière's disease. Journal of Vestibular Research. 2013;**23**:249-257

[24] Ribeiro S, Almeida RR, Caovilla HH, Ganança MM. Dos potenciais evocados miogênicos vestibulares nas orelhas comprometida e assintomática na Doença de Ménière unilateral. Revista Brasileria Otorrinolaringologia. 2005;**71**:60-66

[25] Young YH, Huang TW, Cheng PW. Assessing the stage of Ménière's disease using vestibular evoked myogenic potentials. Archives of Otolaryngology–Head and Neck Surgery. 2003;**129**:815-818

[26] Duarte PLS. Avaliação dos Potenciais Evocados Miogênicos Vestibulares e Eletrococleografia no diagnóstico da Doença de Ménière. Brasília: Universidade de Brasília; 2015

[27] Kuo SW, Yang TH, Young YH. Changes in vestibular evoked myogenic potentials after Meniere attacks. The Annals of Otology, Rhinology, and Laryngology. 2005;**114**(9):717-721

[28] Weber KP, Rosengren SM. Clinical utility of ocular vestibular-evoked myogenic potentials (oVEMPs). Current Neurology and Neuroscience Reports. 2015;**15**:22

[29] Huang CH, Wang SJ, Young YH. Localization and prevalence of hydrops formation in Meniere's disease using a test battery. Audiology & Neuro-Otology. 2011;**16**(1):41-48

[30] Taylor RL, Wijewardene AA, Gibson WP, Black DA, Halmagyi GM, Welgampola MS. The vestibular evoked-potential profile of Meniere's disease. Clinical Neurophysiology: Official Journal of the International Federation of Clinical Neurophysiology. 2011;**122**(6): 1256-1263

[31] Wen MH, Cheng PW, Young YH. Augmentation of ocular vestibular-evoked myogenic potentials via bone-conducted vibration stimuli in Meniere disease. Otolaryngology–Head and Neck Surgery: Official Journal of American Academy of Otolaryngology–Head and Neck Surgery. 2012;**146**(5):797-803

[32] Winters SM, Campschroer T, Grolman W, Klis SF. Ocular vestibular evoked myogenic potentials in response to air-conducted sound in Meniere's disease. Otolaryngology–Head and Neck Surgery: Official Journal of American Academy of Otolaryngology–Head and Neck Surgery. 2011;**32**(8):1273-1280

[33] Adams ME, Heidenreich KD, Kileny PR. Audiovestibular testing in patients with Ménière's disease. Otolaryngologic Clinics of North America 2010;**43**:995-1009

[34] Don M, Kwong B, Tanaka C. A diagnostic test for Meniere's disease and cochlear hydrops: Impaired high-pass noise masking of auditory brainstem response. Otology & Neurotology. 2005;**26**(4):711-722

[35] Donaldson GS, Ruth RA. Derived-band auditory brainstem response estimates of traveling wave velocity in humans: II. Subjects with noise-induced hearing loss and Meniere's disease. Journal of Speech, Language, and Hearing Research. 1996;**39**(3):534-545

[36] Singh NK, Krishnamurthy R, Premkumar PK. Relative efficiency of cochlear hydrops analysis masking procedure and cervical vestibular evoked myogenic potential in identification of Meniere's disease. Advances in Otolaryngology. 2015. DOI: 10.1155/2015/978161

[37] De Valck CFJ, Claes GME, Wuyts FL, Van de Heyning PH. Lack of diagnostic value of high-pass noise masking of auditory brainstem responses in Ménière's disease. Otology & Neurotology. 2007;**28**:700-707

[38] Kingma CM, Wit HP. Cochlear hydrops analysis masking procedure results in patients with unilateral Ménière's disease. Otology & Neurotology. 2010;**31**(6):1004-1008

[39] Lee JB, et al. Diagnostic efficiency of the cochlear hydrops analysis masking procedure in Meniere's disease. Otology & Neurotology. 2011;**32**:1486-1491

[40] McCaslin DL, Rivas A, Jacobson GP, Bennett ML. The dissociation of video head impulse test (Vhit) and bithermal caloric test results provide topological localization of vestibular system impairment in patients with "Definite" Ménière's disease. American Journal of Audiology. 2015;**24**:1-10

[41] Halmagyi GM, Curthoys IS. A clinical sign of canal paresis. Archives of Neurology. 1988 Jul;**45**(7):737-739

[42] McCaslin DL, Jacobson GP. Current role of the videonystagmography examination in the context of the multidimensional balance function test battery. Seminars in Hearing. 2009;**30**(4):242-252

[43] McCaslin DL, Jacobson GP, Bennett ML, Gruenwald JM, Green AP. Predictive properties of the video head impulse test: Measures of caloric symmetry and self-report dizziness handicap. Ear and Hearing. 2014;**35**(5):185-191

[44] Hullar TE, Della Santina CC, Hirvonen T, Lasker DM, Carey JP, Minor LB. Responses of irregularly discharging chinchilla semicircular canal vestibular-nerve afferents during high-frequency head rotations. Journal of Neurophysiology. 2005;**93**(5):2777-2786

[45] Hullar TE, Minor LB. High-frequency dynamics of regularly discharging canal afferents provide a linear signal for angular vestibuloocular reflexes. Journal of Neurophysiology. 1999 Oct;**82**(4):2000-2005

[46] Tsuji K, Velázquez-Villaseñor L, Rauch SD, Glynn RJ, Wall C 3rd, Merchant SN. Temporal bone studies of the human peripheral vestibular system. Meniere's disease. The Annals of Otology, Rhinology, and Laryngology. Suppl. 2000 May;**181**:26-31

[47] Maire R, van Melle G. Vestibulo-ocular reflex characteristics in patients with unilateral Ménière's disease. Otology & Neurotology. 2008 Aug;**29**(5):693-698

11

Effects of Genetic Background on Susceptibility and the Acceleration of Hearing Loss in Mice

Shumpei P. Yasuda, Yuki Miyasaka and Yoshiaki Kikkawa

Abstract

Acquired hearing loss, which includes age-related hearing loss and noise-induced hearing loss, is a common hearing impairment and shows phenotypic variability. One reason for phenotypic variability is influence of genetic background. The modifiers underlying genetic background are modulated and advance the hearing phenotypes through gene-gene interactions with other etiological genetic factors. Moreover, the modifiers play a role in the susceptibility of environmental hearing risk factors, namely, the strength and weakness of environmental susceptibility often modulate and advance hearing phenotypes via gene-environment interactions. The complicated gene-gene and gene-environment interactions make genetic analysis of acquired hearing loss difficult. In particular, the effects of environmental factors cannot be completely excluded or controlled. Although genome-wide approaches to identify genetic modifiers have proven challenging in humans, the responsible genes and mutations are widely unknown. In this chapter, we suggest that mouse models are useful for studying genetic background effects for acquired hearing loss. The genetic analysis of mouse models identified the genetic modifiers. We review the genetic research in mouse models for acquired hearing loss to identify and confirm the modifiers by both forward and reverse genetics approaches.

Keywords: genetic background effects, mouse model, quantitative trait loci (QTL), genetic modifiers, genetic interaction, epistasis, genome editing

1. Introduction

Hearing loss is the most common sensory disorder, which affects approximately 0.1–0.2% of newborns [1]. A genetic etiology of congenital hearing loss accounts for an estimate of at least 50–60% of hearing loss cases, whereas the remaining 40–50% develops from a nongenetic etiology, such as effects of risk factors for neonates and birth conditions [1–3]. To date, many mutations responsible for hearing loss have been recently identified in approximately 100 human genes [3, 4]. However, most mutations are primarily associated with congenital and severe hearing loss developed at newborn and childhood stages caused by a single gene. The identification of the more common "acquired hearing loss," such as age-related hearing loss (ARHL) and noise-induced hearing loss (NIHL) is currently understudied.

Acquired common hearing loss is a complex multifactorial disease influenced by genetic backgrounds and environments. In ARHL, an accurate estimation of the genetic etiology has not been reported. However, it is estimated that ARHL develops through the effects of genetic modifier(s) because the onset time and severity of hearing loss vary greatly among individuals [5, 6]. Moreover, there is a significant heritability of hearing phenotypes [6]. The heritability ranges from low to high [6–10], suggesting that multiple genetic modifiers and environmental factors contribute to the onset and severity of hearing loss. The documented risk factors of ARHL and acquired hearing loss are noise, smoking, alcohol consumption, diet and reduced exercise, complication of other diseases, and uses of ototoxic drugs [6, 11]. It is known that one major risk factor is exposure to loud noise, accounting for approximately 16% of the population worldwide [12]. Genetic factors from a genetic background might also play an important role in the susceptibility of NIHL [13]. However, the identification of genetic background effects in ARHL and NIHL is difficult in humans because of lower heritability of this phenotype and the influence of environmental risk factors mentioned above. In addition, genetic differences among individuals disturb genetic analysis.

To investigate genetic background effects associated with hearing loss, we propose that mouse models have several advantages to overcome weaknesses in the genetic analysis of ARHL and NIHL in humans. Mice can be controlled to avoid environmental risk factors. The techniques for evaluation of hearing, such as measurements of the auditory brainstem response (ABR) and distortion product otoacoustic emission (DPOAE), have been established [14–18]. Based on the techniques, it is known that there is phenotypic heterogeneity of ARHL and NIHL caused by genetic background effects [3, 6, 11]; therefore, the genetic background effects can be analyzed using the quantitative trait loci (QTL) analysis and genome-wide association study (GWAS) of experimental populations produced by mating susceptible and resistant strains of ARHL and NIHL. This chapter applies the advantages of a genetic analysis by using mouse models to study the genetic background effects of hearing loss.

2. What is a genetic background effect?

First, we will explain the basic mechanisms of background effect in phenotypic modification to readers in a way that they will understand the importance of this chapter.

2.1. Gene-gene interaction

A complex disease is one that lacks a one-to-one correspondence of mutation and phenotype [19, 20], namely, the expression of phenotype is influenced by genetic modifier(s) underlying the genetic background. **Figure 1A** shows a simple model of the genetic background effect. In most cases, the genetic background effects are revealed by the expression of different phenotypes caused by the same genetic mutation in different genetic backgrounds. Let us assume that a gene associated with hearing loss was mutated by gene targeting in mice (strain R). We performed the hearing test of knock-out (KO) mice using measurements of ABR. The KO mouse exhibited latency peak responses for peaks I–V as well as the wild-type mouse; however, the amplitudes of all the peaks were weak and delayed. Next, we performed the gene targeting of the same gene in mice of different genetic backgrounds (strain S). The mouse had no discernable ABR waveform, indicating that the hearing loss of the mouse became more severe due to variation in the genetic background. These results suggest the presence of a genetic modifier, which affects the phenotype developed by the mutation of the causative gene, with respect to the genetic background of strain R. Moreover, it is assumed that the modifier interacts with the causative gene in the acceleration of hearing loss. The genetic interaction could be separated into nonadditive and additive effects to

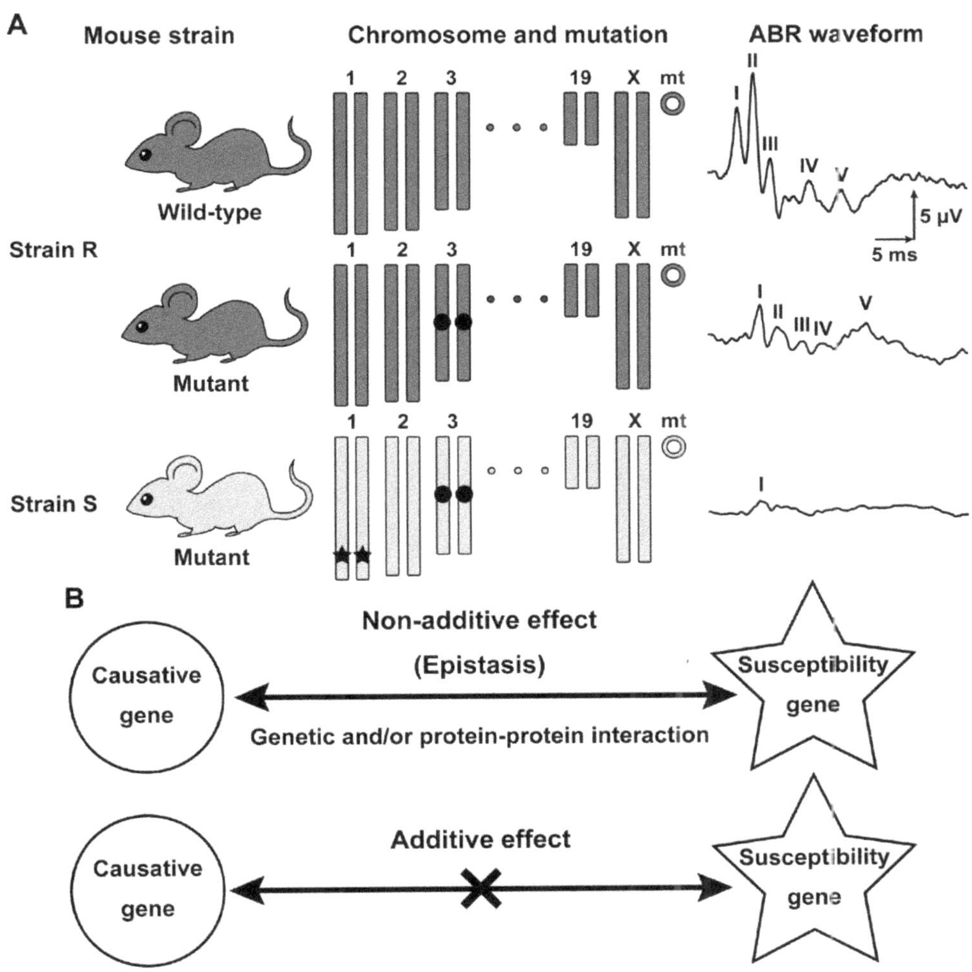

Figure 1. Simple models for genetic background effect in phenotypic modification. (A) Schematic representation of the genetic background effect in hearing of mice. Illustrations show the differences of auditory brainstem response (ABR) waveforms by the effects of the susceptible allele (black stars) in the hearing loss mutant. Black circles indicate mutation associated with hearing loss. The locations of ABR peaks I–V are indicated with ranges (µV) of the negative wave apex and latency (ms). (B) Definition of additive (top) and nonadditive (bottom) interaction in phenotypic modification.

evaluate whether the gene-gene, gene-protein, and protein-protein interaction are present in the regulatory pathway of the phenotype (**Figure 1B**). The nonadditive effect is called "epistasis" in technical terms of genetics, stating that there is a direct interaction between two or more genes [19, 20]. The additive effect states that phenotypic acceleration and modification occur by accumulation of mutations in genes of similar function in different molecular pathways (**Figure 1B**) [20].

2.2. Gene-environment interaction

In a complex disease, the expression of phenotype is also influenced by environmental factor(s), along with the interaction between the environment and genes in genetic background. A model is shown in **Figure 2A**. Let us assume that we performed an experiment of noise exposure to mice. We performed the experiment in strains R and S and then measured ABR. The ABR responses between the two strains were different. The peaks of the ABR

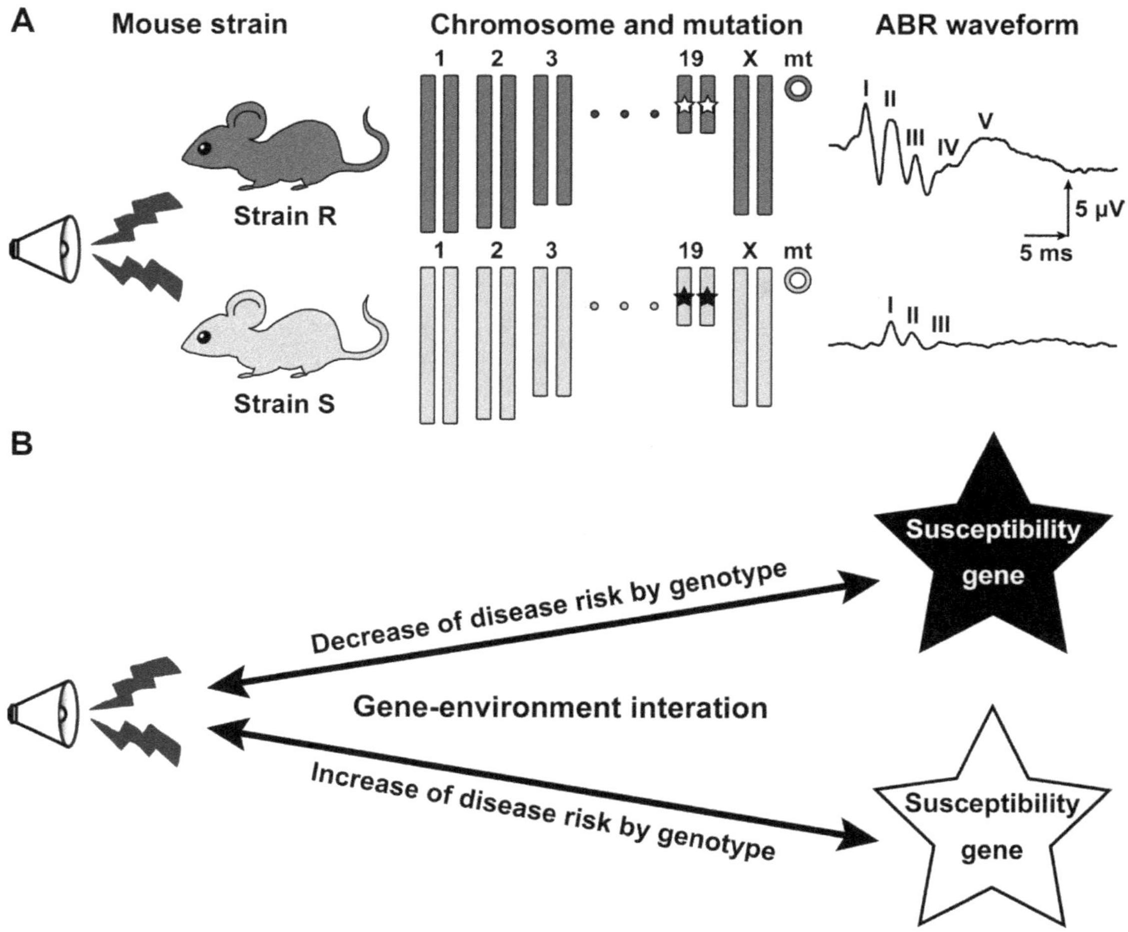

Figure 2. Simple models for genetic background effect in the susceptibility of environmental factors. (A) Schematic representation of the genetic background effect in noise-induced hearing loss of mice. Illustrations show the differences between strain R and S of ABR waveforms by the effects of the noise exposure and susceptible allele (black stars). The locations of ABR peaks I–V are indicated with ranges (μV) of the negative wave apex and latency (ms). (B) a model for genetic background effect in the susceptibility of environmental factors.

waveform in strain S were significantly lower than those in strain R. This result suggests that strain R is a noise-resistant strain, whereas strain S is a noise-susceptible strain. In addition, the genetic mechanism for noise sensitivity in both strains can be explained by the presence of resistance and susceptibility alleles in addition to the risk of noise exposure, namely, a gene-environment interaction contributes to the development of NIHL (**Figure 2B**) based on a genetic background effect. Thus, the genetic background effect is important in the study of the influence of environmental factors on complex diseases.

There is one thing to note. Although we explained the gene-environment interaction using a model that would be easy to understand, this model is admittedly simple because it only considers the effect of one gene and one environmental factor. In the case of human diseases, the gene-environment interactions are more complicated because the interactions involve multiple genes, multiple environmental factors, genetic heterogeneity, and heterogeneity of environmental exposure [20].

3. Phenotypic variations of hearing caused by genetic backgrounds in mouse inbred strains

Laboratory mice are one of the best experimental models to investigate the genetic background effect for ARHL as mentioned in Section 1. Moreover, the classical inbred strains have been established in large numbers and exhibit variable hearing ability and onset time of ARHL caused by genetic background [21, 22]. **Figure 3** shows the means of ABR thresholds to tone-pip stimuli at 4, 8, 16, and 32 kHz in mice from MSM/Ms, C3H/HeN, C57BL/6J, A/J, and DBA/2J at 4 months of age, as cited in our previous studies [23–25]. The hearing phenotypes of these strains can be classified into two groups: normal hearing and early onset ARHL. The MSM/Ms and C3H/HeN comprise the normal hearing group. The ABR thresholds are stable at all frequencies. The C57BL/6J mice also show normal ABR thresholds at 4, 8, and 16 kHz. However, the ABR threshold at 32 kHz of C57BL/6J mice is significantly higher than that of MSM/Ms and C3H/HeN mice, indicating that C57BL/6J developed high-frequency-specific ARHL. The A/J mice exhibit an ARHL that is more severe for high-frequency stimuli. In addition, the ABR thresholds of the A/J mice at other frequencies are clearly increased when compared with those of C57BL/6J mice. Moreover, the DBA/2J mice developed more severe hearing loss. The ABR thresholds of the DBA/2J mice exhibited levels of severe (71–90 dB SPL) and profound (<91 dB SPL) hearing loss in sound stimuli at 4/8 and 16/32 kHz, respectively, which were significantly higher than those of A/J mice at 4, 8, and 16 kHz.

The difference between the normal hearing and early onset ARHL groups can be explained by a mutation of the Cadherin 23 gene (*Cdh23*). The responsible $Cdh23^{c.753G>A}$ mutation was identified at one base before the splice-donor site, leading to partial skipping of a single exon [21, 24, 26] and age-related stereocilia degeneration in cochlear hair cells [23, 24, 27]. The A/J mice have another strain-specific mutation (p.His55Asn) in the citrate synthase gene (*Cs*) [28]. By identifying $Cs^{p.His55Asn}$ mutation, A/J mice were shown to have developed severe ARHL

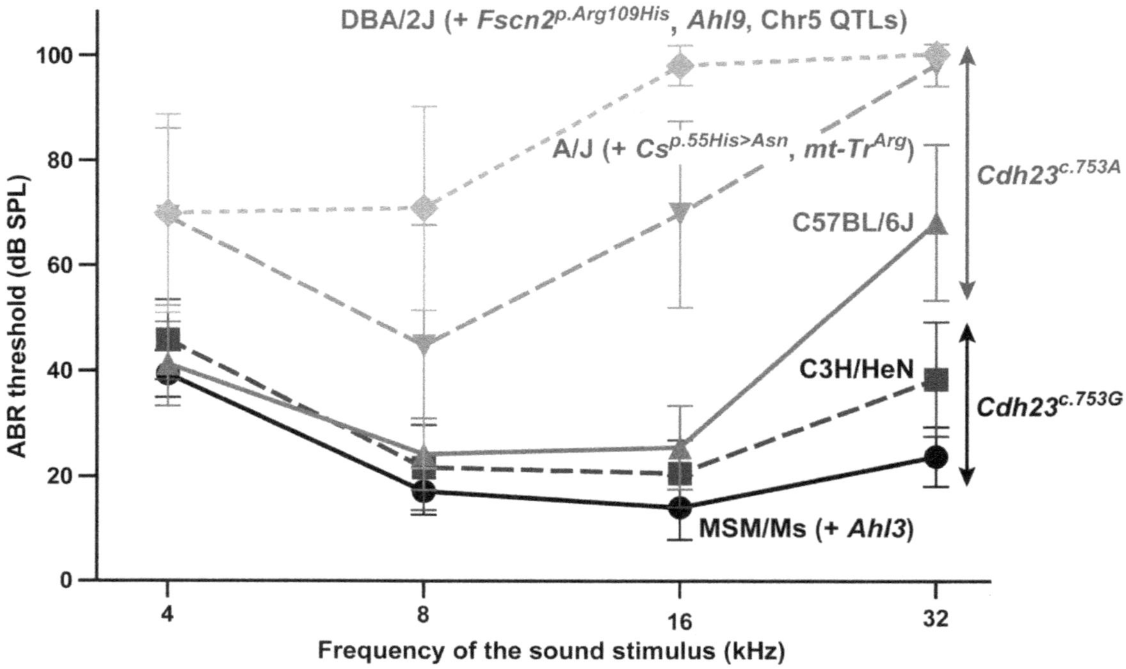

Figure 3. Comparison of hearing levels among the mouse inbred strains. The means (circles, squares, diamonds, and upper and lower triangles) and standard deviations (error bars) of ABR thresholds for 4, 8, 16, and 32 kHz sound stimuli are shown for MSM/Ms, C3H/HeN, DBA/2J, C57BL/6J, and A/J mice at 4 months of age. The graph was created by using data from our previous studies [23–25].

by interaction between $Cdh23^{c.753G>A}$ and $Cs^{p.His55Asn}$ mutations. The CDH23 is a member of the calcium-dependent cell-cell adhesion and tip link component [21, 29, 30]. In contrast, CS is the first enzyme of the tricarboxylic acid cycle, generating citrate and free coenzyme A [31]. Therefore, both proteins seem to contribute different functions in the inner ear for hearing, suggesting that A/J mice develop early onset hearing loss from additive effects of different functional mutations, as described in the previous section (**Figure 1B**). In addition, A/J mice carried a single adenine insertion in the mitochondrial tRNA-Arg gene ($mt\text{-}Tr^{Arg}$) [32]. CS is transported into the mitochondrial matrix and plays an important role in condensing mitochondrial acetyl-coenzyme A and oxaloacetate for transporting of acetyl-coenzyme A from the mitochondrial matrix to the cytosol [31], suggesting that mitochondrial dysfunction by epistasis (**Figure 1B**) between $Cs^{p.His55Asn}$ and $mt\text{-}Tr^{Arg}$ mutations is accelerated in ARHL of A/J mice. The DBA/2J mice also have a strain-specific mutation (p.Arg109His) in the fascin 2 gene (*Fscn2*) [33]. DBA/2J mice exhibit progressive shortening of the stereocilia, and this phenotype only develops with homozygosity of both the $Cdh23^{c.753G>A}$ and $Fscn2^{p.Arg109His}$ mutations [34]. FSCN2 is an actin crosslinking protein and localizes along the length of stereocilia at especially high concentration around the stereocilia tips [33, 34]. Although the pathological mechanisms in the genetic interaction between the $Cdh23^{c.753G>A}$ and $Fscn2^{p.Arg109His}$ mutations are widely unknown, the degeneration of stereocilia in DBA/2J mice may be explained by epistasis. Moreover, the other QTLs related to ARHL were detected in DBA/2J mice. The QTLs, *Ahl9* [35] and *Chr5* QTL [25, 36], are likely to contribute to frequency-specific ARHL. Although the causative genes and mutations are still unknown, these QTLs lead to severe hearing loss by additive or epistatic interaction with the *Cdh23*$^{c.753G>A}$ and *Fscn2*$^{p.Arg109His}$ mutations. Thus, the differences of hearing levels among the inbred strains are regulated by background effects through the epistatic and additive effects.

4. Identification of the genetic modifiers in mice

We have described in the previous section that several mouse inbred strains developed ARHL by genetic background effects. In this section, we introduce approaches to identify genetic modifiers and susceptibility loci of hearing loss underlying the genetic backgrounds.

4.1. Classical forward genetics approach

The forward genetics approach is phenotype-driven, with a foundation that associates the detection of chromosomal location with phenotype by linkage analysis. The start of the experiments included production of chromosomal recombinants, F_2 and N_2 mice, by crossing between the susceptible and resistant strains in phenotype (**Figure 4A**). The linkage analysis is based on meiotic recombination events that occur in sperm and egg precursor cells of F_1 hybrid, which have heterozygous chromosomes derived from both the susceptible and resistant strains. Accordingly, the F_2 and N_2 progenies were produced by intercrossing between F_1 mice and backcrossing of F_1 mice to one parental strain, respectively, and inherited chromosomes that underwent recombination events. The recombinant region on the chromosomes was detected by using a genetic marker, such as microsatellites and SNPs, which recognized genetic polymorphisms compared to parental strains. Finally, the phenotypes of F_2 and N_2 mice were investigated to determine whether there is linkage with the recombinant regions of F_2 and N_2 mice. This approach has been a powerful and productive method to identify QTL-associated ARHL. Johnson et al. [37] detected the first QTL *ahl* locus for ARHL that displayed a *Cdh23*$^{c.753G>A}$ mutation by using N_2 backcross mice between ARHL-susceptible C57BL/6J and -resistant CAST/Ei.

As mentioned earlier, there are many modifiers in the genome of inbred strains. To evaluate the effect of a single QTL identified in the mapping by avoiding the effects from other modifiers, congenic mice have become a powerful tool. Congenic mice are defined as having part of the mutation or a chromosomal segment from one inbred genetic background (donor) to another (host) [38] (**Figure 4B**). The creation of congenic mice is based on backcrossing the system for at least seven times. Although this process is long, the resolution of the phenotype greatly improves when compared with F_2 and N_2 mice. The most successful example of this strategy is the study of *moth1* locus [39, 40]. The *tubby* mice, which are a mutant of tubby bipartite transcription factor gene (*Tub*), exhibit severe hearing loss caused by cochlear degeneration in C57BL/6J background [39]. However, some F_2 mice produced by intercrossing with AKR/J and CAST/Ei showed normal hearing. Ikeda et al. [39] mapped the modifier, *moth1*, via linkage analysis using both F_2 mice and confirmed the locus by creating congenic mice. This study led to the successful identification of the association of the modification of hearing loss with a strain-specific mutation in microtubule-associated protein 1 gene (*Map1a*), which was the first elucidated causative gene caused by the background effect in hearing [40].

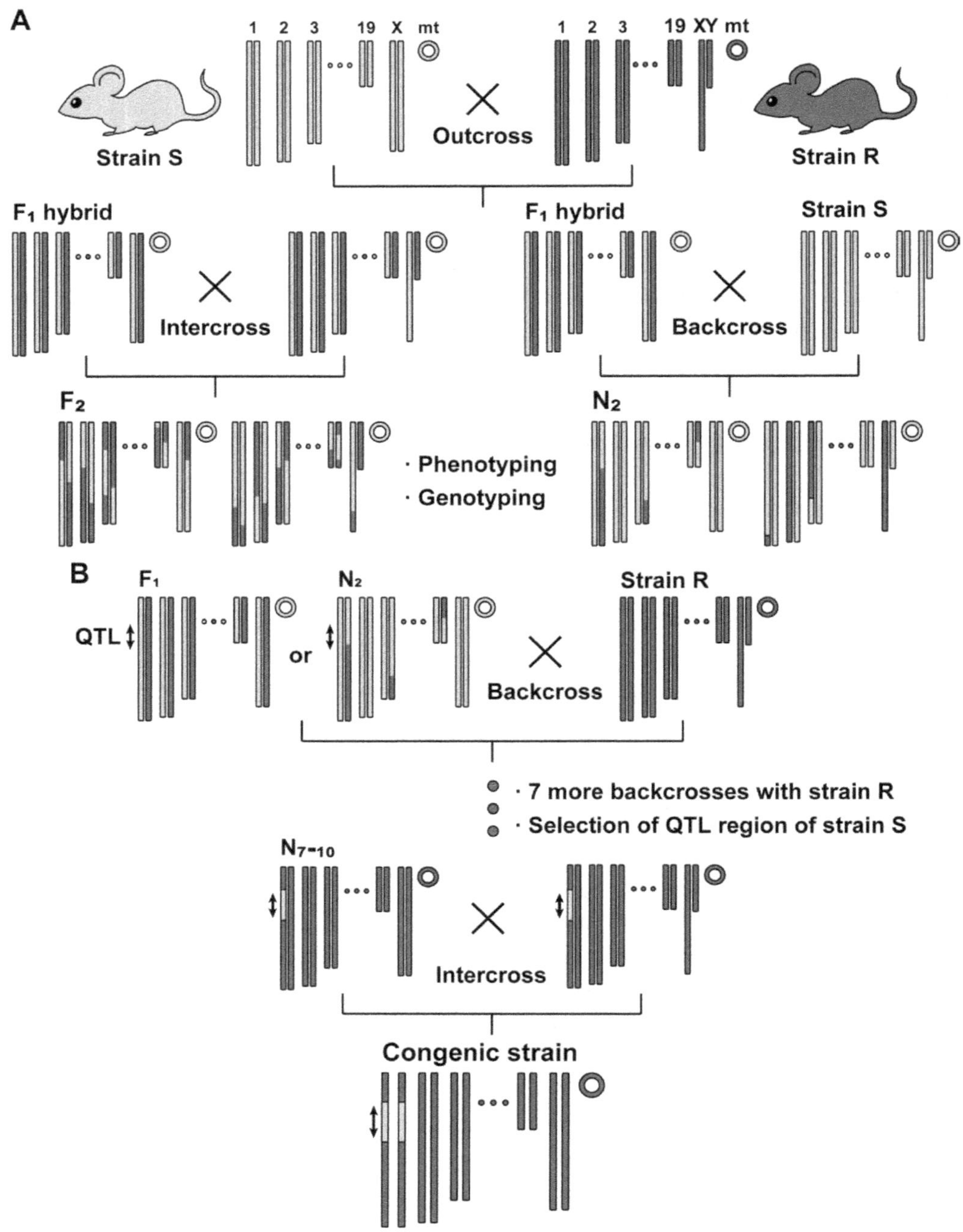

Figure 4. Schematic representation of the virtual genomic structures of experimental cross (F_2 and N_2) (A) for genetic mapping and congenic mouse (B). The rectangles and circles represent chromosome and mitochondrial DNA, respectively. The different strain-derived chromosomal regions are distinguished by light and dark gray colors. Bidirectional arrows indicate quantitative trait locus (QTL) regions.

4.2. Forward genetics approaches using genetic reference populations of mice

Currently, we believe that a classical forward genetics approach using F_2, N_2, and congenic mice is useful to identify the modifiers from genetic background in mice. However, productions of the F_2, N_2, and congenic mice consume great amount of time and costs for breeding. Large numbers of mice are required to increase mapping resolution. Moreover, the F_2 and N_2 mice must be used for genome-wide genotyping because their genome architectures are uniquely mixed between parental chromosomes. Therefore, the genotyping cost is enormous. Here, we introduce the public genetic reference populations of mice. These populations have several advantages owing to established QTL mapping.

4.2.1. Recombinant inbred strain (RIS)

Recombinant inbred strain (RIS) panel is a genetic reference population of mice and can serve as a powerful tool for QTL mapping. It is produced by mating sibling F_2 mice until the resulting progeny, at least 20 generations later, is fully inbred and displays a mosaic of parental genomes (**Figure 5A**) [41, 42]. RIS panel has several advantages for QTL mapping; if the genotyping is performed once, it does not require genotyping in each individual and is available in public databases; individual, environmental, and measurement variability can be reduced; it has greater mapping resolution because the breakpoints in the genome are denser than those that occur in any one meiosis, such as F_2 and N_2 mice [41].

RIS panels have been successfully applied to several QTL mappings for ARHL. The strategy includes only evaluating the hearing abilities of each individual RIS panel performed by

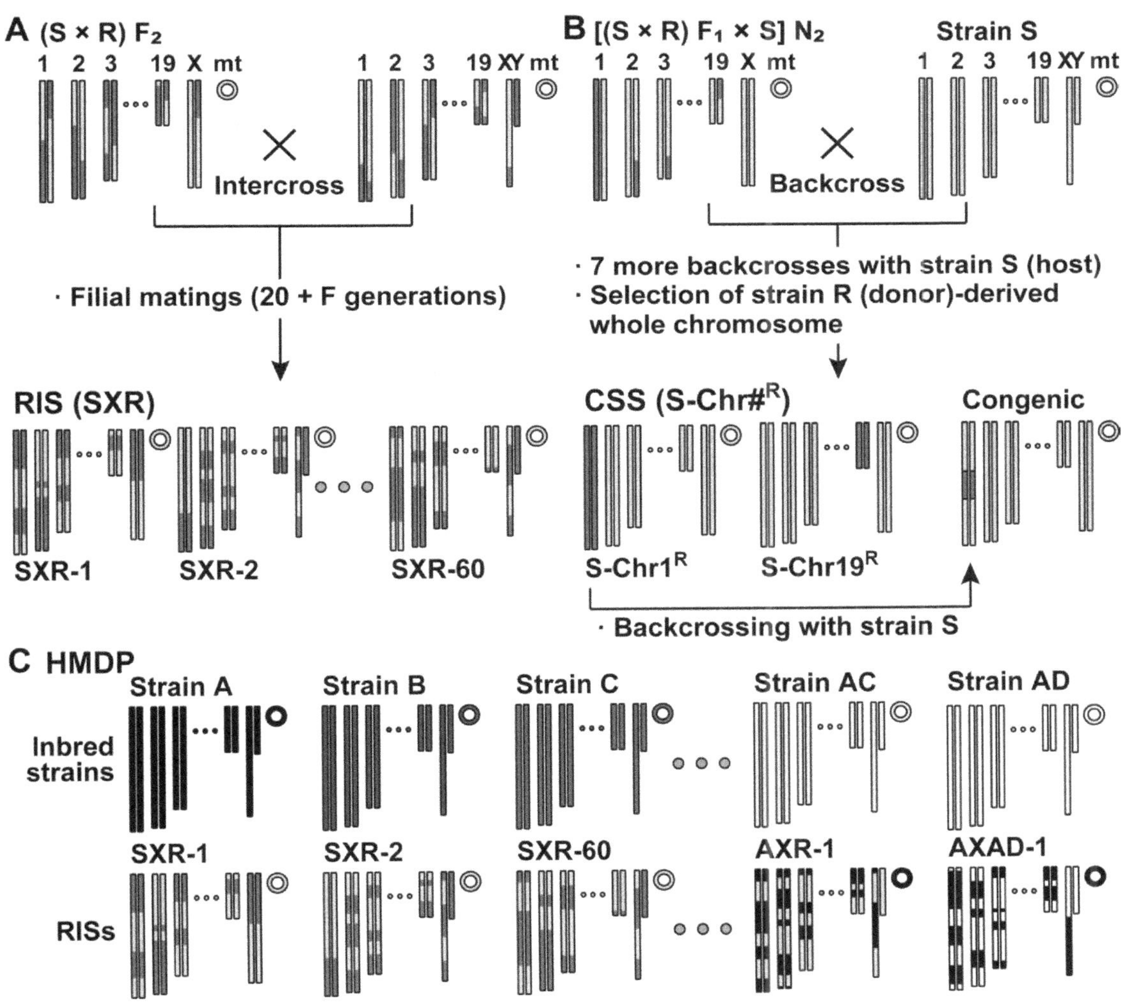

Figure 5. Schematic representation of the virtual genomic structures of the recombinant inbred strains (RIS) (A), consomic strain (CSS) (B), and hybrid mouse diversity panel (HMDP) (C) for QTL analysis and genome-wide association study (GWAS). The rectangles and circles represent chromosomes and mitochondrial DNA, respectively. Each strain-derived chromosomal region is distinguished by a different color.

measurements of ABR thresholds and then performing QTL linkage analysis using WebQTL [43], which collects genotypes of microsatellite and SNPs in each RIS panel. By this strategy, the QTLs *ahl4* (*Cs*$^{p.His55Asn}$) [44], *ahl8* (*Fscn2*$^{p.Arg109His}$) [45], *Ahl9* [35], and *Snhl* [18] were mapped using the AXB/BXA [46], BXD [47], BXD and LXS [48], and RIS panels, respectively (**Table 1**). The other RIS panels, such as CXB [49], BXH [50], and SMXA [51], have been established by sibling mating between several inbred strains and will become useful resources to identify new loci associated with ARHL and NIHL.

4.2.2. Consomic strains (CSS)

Consomic strains (CSS), also called chromosome substitution strains, are combined genomes of two founder inbred strains that have a substitution of one whole chromosome pair from the donor strain into the genetic background of the host strain (**Figure 5B**) [52, 53]. The productive strategy is the same with congenic mice. Usually, a full set of CSSs will consist of 22 strains, which includes 19 pairs of autosomal chromosomes, X and Y sex chromosomes, and a mitochondrial genome, although the introgression into the host background of a whole chromosome from the donor is difficult in some cases [53]. The main advantage of CSS is mapping of the phenotype to single chromosomes. The *Ahl3* [54] and *ahl4* [44] loci have

Population	Panel	Origin	QTL or QTN	Gene
Recombinant inbred strain (RIS)	AXB [46]	(A/J × C57BL/6J) F_1	*ahl4* [44]	*Cs* [28]
	BXA [46]	(C57BL/6J × A/J) F_1		
	BXD [47]	(C57BL/6J × DBA/2J) F_1	*ahl8* [45]	*Fscn2* [34]
			Ahl9 [35]	Unknown
	LXS [48]	* (ILS × ISS) F_1	*Snhl* [18]	Unknown
Consomic strain (CSS)	C57BL/6J-Chr#$^{A/J}$ [52]	Host: C57BL/6J, donor: A/J	*ahl4* [44]	*Cs* [28]
	C57BL/6J-Chr#$^{MSM/Ms}$ [53]	Host: C57BL/6J, donor: MSM/Ms	*Ahl3* [54]	Unknown
			*mjs*** [24]	*Cdh23* [24]
Inbred strain population	Hybrid mouse diversity panel (HMDP) [56]	30 classic inbred strains and 70 recombinant inbred strains	rs33652818 [17]	*Nox3* [17]
			rs37517079 [60]	Unknown
Outbred stock (OS)	Black Swiss [62]	NIH Swiss, C57BL/6J	*Ahl5* [63]	*Gipc3* [14]
			Ahl6 [63]	Unknown
	NIH Swiss [64]	NIH GP colony	*Hfhl1* [15]	Unknown
			Hfhl2 [15]	Unknown
			Hfhl3 [16]	Unknown

*Inbred long sleep (ILS) and inbred short sleep (ISS) mouse strains, which were derived from a multi-generation cross of eight inbred strains.

**Modifier of *js* (tentative symbol).

Table 1. Genetic reference population contributed for identification of the loci and SNPs associated with hearing loss underlying in genetic background of mice by QTL analysis and GWAS.

been mapped to a single chromosome by ABR measurements in CSSs of partial and full sets (**Table 1**). Moreover, congenic mice for QTL mapping can be easily and quickly produced by intercrossing (CSS × host strain) F_1 and backcrossing (CSS × host strain) F_1 × host strain (**Figure 5B**). The genotyping is only required in one chromosome for progeny. By this strategy, we have previously mapped the *Ahl3* [54] and a modifier [24] responsible for the acceleration of ARHL of heterozygotes of Jackson shaker mice (*Ush1g^{js}*) (**Table 1**).

In addition, CSS may be used to study epistasis in detail. An example is *Ahl3* [54], which was mapped to chromosome 17 using C57BL/6J-Chr17$^{MSM/Ms}$ CSS. The donor strain, MSM/Ms, is an inbred derived from the Japanese wild mouse, *Mus musculus molossinus*. By introgression of the genomic segment including *Ahl3*, the ARHL of C57BL/6J was dramatically suppressed despite having the homozygous *Cdh23$^{c.753A}$* allele in the genome. Although we predicted that *Ahl3* is the resistance allele for ARHL in MSM/Ms mice, the resistant effects of *Ahl3* were not detected in the other mapping system of the C57BL/6J and MSM/Ms strain [24]. The genetic divergence between C57BL/6J and MSM/Ms is extremely high [55]; therefore, the resistant effect of *Ahl3* was caused by incompatibility by chromosomal substitution. We detected a similar situation in CSSs of another chromosome [54] (Yasuda et al. unpublished data). There is some possibility that the incompatibility is caused by a *cis/trans* change via chromosomal substitution; therefore, the analysis of CSS may allow for the study of cross talk between genes on different chromosomes, namely, *cis-* and *trans*-regulation of the variation of gene expression in hearing research.

4.2.3. Hybrid mouse diversity panel (HMDP)

Although the classical genetic crosses, RIS and CSS, are powerful tools to identify modifiers in genetic backgrounds, the phenotypic and genetic variations are low because of the inclusion of only two parental strains. Moreover, the low genetic variation is not suitable for GWAS. The hybrid mouse diversity panel (HMDP) was developed to increase the statistical power and resolution of the classical QTL mapping [56]. The HMDP consists of 30 classical inbred strains and four set of RISs (AXB/BXA, BXD, BXH, and CXB) (**Figure 5C** and **Table 1**), which are genotyped with 140,000 SNPs [57]. By using the HMDP, a high statistical power and high resolution of QTL mapping were provided from the RISs and classical inbred strains, respectively.

HMDP contributed to the identification of the gene and locus associated with NIHL. Lavinsky et al. [17] investigated the noise susceptibility in five-week female mice in 64 strains selected from HMDP. The noise susceptibilities of strains varied widely, and GWAS analysis picked up five quantitative trait nucleotides (QTNs) with statistically significant p values ($p < 4.1E{-}06$) [17]. Consequently, candidate genes were screened by expression QTL (eQTL) analysis after which NADPH oxidase-3 gene (*Nox3*) was selected as a candidate (**Table 1**). Moreover, the study identified that the *Nox3* KO mice showed noise sensitivity [17]. This is the first study to have reported the NIHL-related gene. Till date, noise sensitivity of 100 stock strains from HMDP has been reported [58], and phenotype data have also been collected continuously [59]. Additionally, a QTN at chromosome 6 associated with noise susceptibility was detected (**Table 1**) [60].

4.2.4. Outbred stock (OS)

QTL analysis using inbred strains is limited to the phenotypes and alleles associated with ARHL and NIHL. Although the genotyping is required, outbred stock (OS) is a colony with maintained phenotypic and genetic diversity kept in laboratory settings and thus exhibits a high degree of both genetic and phenotypic diversity, allowing high-resolution genetic mapping for a wide variety of traits by crossing with another population [42, 61].

In a study of ARHL, Black Swiss [62], which is derived from NIH Swiss outbred stock and C57BL/6J, was first used in OS for QTL linkage mapping. Drayton and Noben-Trauth [62] performed QTL linkage mapping using [(Black Swiss × CAST/Ei) F_1 × Black Swiss] N_2 backcross mice and mapped two QTLs: *Ahl5* and *Ahl6*. Subsequently, the responsible mutation for *Ahl5* was detected in the GIPC PDZ domain containing family member 3 gene (*Gipc3*), which is associated with audiogenic seizures and sensorineural hearing loss in mice and humans [14]. The *Gipc3*$^{p.Gly115Arg}$ mutation was absent in inbred strain, indicating that OS is a powerful tool to identify new ARHL-related genes. Moreover, NIH Swiss mice [63] also contributed to the detection of three loci (*Hfhl1–3*) associated with high-frequency hearing loss (HFHL) (**Table 1**) [15, 16].

Heterogeneous stock (HS) and diversity outcross stock (DO) could be considered variants of OS and display a similar advantage with OS for QTL mapping [42, 61]. These populations are available and probably will contribute to the identification of QTL and genes responsible for ARHL and NIHL.

4.3. Elucidation of genetic background effects by using reverse genetics approaches

When the candidate gene and mutation are detected by forward genetics approach, the next step is elucidation of the real causative gene and mutation. The reverse genetics technique is immensely helpful with this elucidation. An approach is production and phenotypic analysis of KO mice of candidate gene *Nox3* as mentioned earlier [17]. However, rescue of phenotype is required for full proof.

Transgenic expression of bacterial artificial chromosome (BAC) clones in mice is commonly used for *in vivo* complementation tests. The test BAC contains wild-type allele and is simple since BAC contains the wild-type allele to be injected into the susceptible strain with the candidate mutation. The *Fscn2*$^{p.Arg109His}$ mutation of DBA/2J is confirmed by this complementation test [33]. The disadvantage of BAC transgenesis is that genes of large sizes exceeding the BAC clone (average size between 120 and 250 kb) cannot be rescued. Moreover, the rescue of the phenotype caused by dominant-negative and gain-of-function mutations is difficult. In addition, the strains of available BAC libraries are limited [64, 65].

An advanced approach is rescue by the knock-in (KI) method mediated by the CRISPR/Cas9 genome editing system. This system can efficiently and quickly repair the candidate mutation of the KI donor oligonucleotide containing the wild-type allele via a homology-directed repair (HDR) [66]. We previously reported utility of this method [24]. C57BL/6J-*Ush1g*$^{js/+}$ heterozygous mice exhibit severe early onset ARHL caused by progressive degeneration in the stereocilia of outer hair cells. We mapped a locus associated with early onset ARHL of *Ush1g*$^{js/+}$ mice in an interval of chromosome 10 that harbors the *Cdh23*$^{c.753G>A}$ mutation, which is also responsible for ARHL of C57BL/6J mice as mentioned above. We injected Cas9 mRNA, single guide RNA (sgRNA) and a donor oligonucleotide that contained *Cdh23*$^{c.753G}$ (**Figure 6A**) to produce KI mice. In KI mice, early onset ARHL and stereocilia degeneration were completely rescued (**Figure 6B**). This is the first report that confirms the phenotypic effect of modifiers at the mutation level in hearing research.

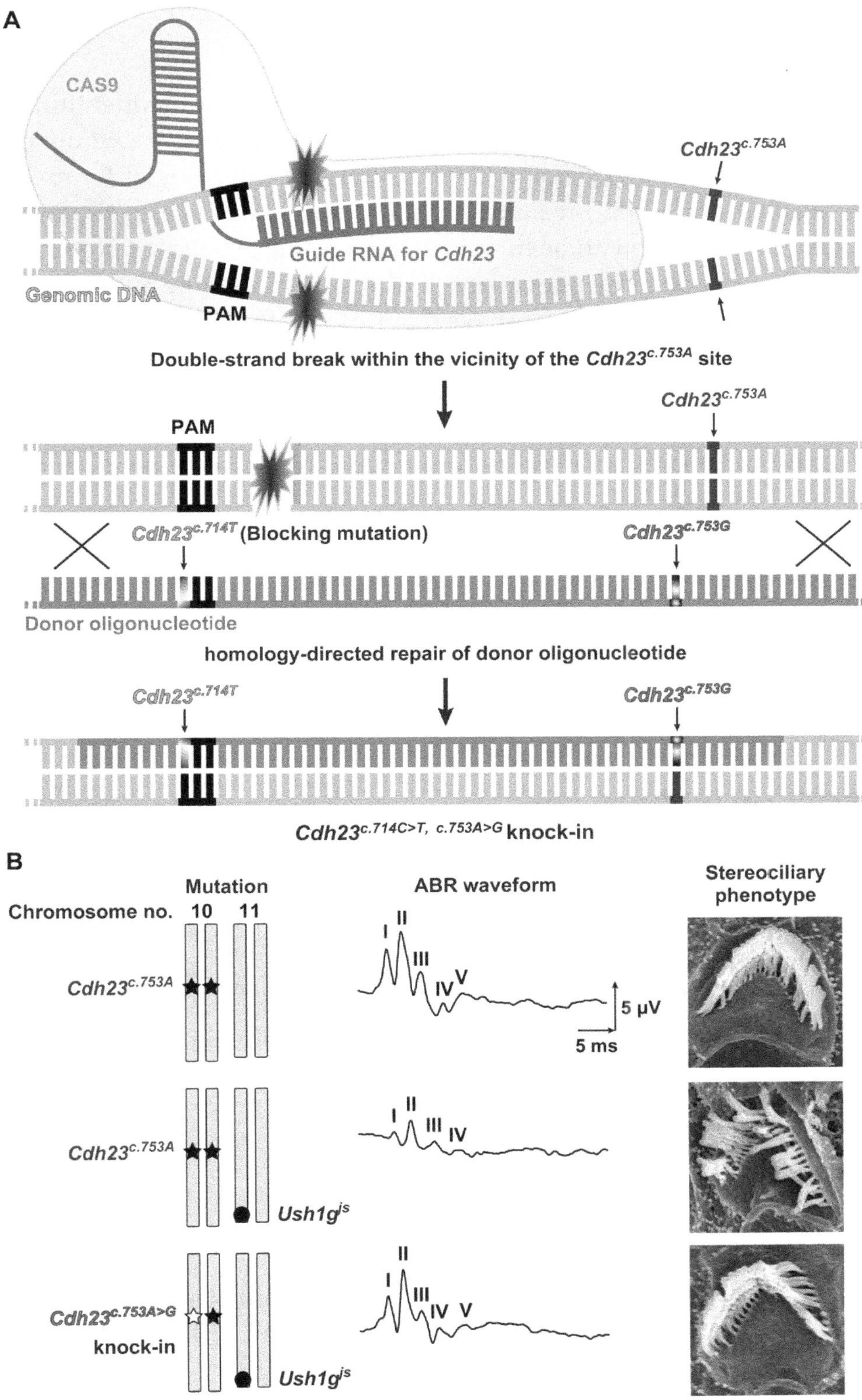

Figure 6. Phenotypic rescue of hearing loss in mice caused by genetic background effect using the CRISPR/Cas9-mediated KI method. (A) Schematic representation of the *Cdh23*$^{c.753A>G}$ KI using double-strand break within the vicinity of the *Cdh23*$^{c.753A}$ site of C57BL/6J mice by CRISPR/Cas9 and homology-directed repair of single-stranded donor oligonucleotide. The donor oligonucleotide was designed to include c.753A>G with a synonymous blocking of the c.714C>T mutation to avoid cleavage by Cas9 [24]. (B) Comparison of the hearing phenotypes among the C57BL/6J (top), C57BL/6J-*Ush1g*$^{js/+}$ (middle) and -*Ush1g*$^{js/+}$ *Cdh23*$^{c.753A/G}$ (bottom) mice. Illustrations of left panels represent combination of the *Cdh23*$^{c.753A>G}$ (★>☆) on chromosome 10 and *Ush1g*^{js} (●) on chromosome 11. Middle and right panels show ABR waveforms and stereocilia phenotypes, respectively, in each mouse.

5. Conclusions

In this chapter, we attempt to highlight several issues regarding the identification of background effects in mice. To identify the modifiers underlying genetic background effects, several strains were established for QTL and GWAS. Thus, the technologies for forward genetics in mice have enabled important breakthroughs and will contribute to the identification of new loci and genes associated with hearing loss. The reverse genetics approach has also been developed based on technological innovations, that is, genome editing and will be increasingly applied. An increasing number of studies have reported that the hearing loss phenotype resulting from a single gene mutation in humans is modulated by the genetic background in which the mutation is maintained (e.g., see [67].). Using genome editing, mutations discovered in the genetic background of patients with hearing loss can be conveniently manipulated in mice, and the effects of the candidate mutation can be confirmed *in vivo* by phenotypic analyses of mice.

Acknowledgements

We thank Emiko Wakatsuki for the drawing the illustrations. This review was supported by JSPS KAKENHI (Grant Number JP15H04291).

Index of technical terms

μV: microvolts

ABR: auditory brainstem response

ahl, *Ahl3*, *ahl4*, *Ahl5*, *Ahl6*, *ahl8* and *Ahl9*: loci for age-related hearing loss in mice

A/J, C3H/HeN, C57BL/6J, CAST/Ei, DBA/2J and MSM/Ms: mice inbred strains

ARHL: age-related hearing loss

AXB, BXA, BXD, BXH, CXB, LXS and SMXA: mice recombinant inbred strains

BAC: bacterial artificial chromosome

Black Swiss and NIH Swiss: mice outbred strains

C57BL/6J-Chr17$^{MSM/Ms}$: a consomic (chromosome substitution) strain, which contain MSM/Ms-derived chromosome 17 in the genetic background of the C57BL/6J strain

Cas9: CRISPR associated protein 9

Cdh23: cadherin 23 gene

Cdh23$^{c.753G>A}$: a guanine-to-adenine substitution at nucleotide position 753 of cadherin 23 gene

Chr5 QTL: QTL on chromosome 5

CRISPR: clustered regularly interspaced short palindromic repeat

Cs: citrate synthase gene

Cs$^{p.His55Asn}$: a histidine-to-asparagine substitution at amino acid position 55 of citrate synthase (CS) protein

CSS: consomic (chromosome substitution) strains

dB SPL: decibel sound pressure level

DPOAE: distortion product otoacoustic emission

DO: diversity outcross stock

eQTL: expression QTL

Fscn2: fascin 2 gene

Fscn2$^{p.Arg109His}$: an arginine-to-histidine substitution at amino acid position 109 amino acid of fascin 2 (FSCN2) protein

Gipc3: GIPC PDZ domain containing family member 3

GWAS: genome-wide association study

HDR: homology-directed repair

HFHL: high-frequency hearing loss

Hfhl1, 2 and *3*: loci for high-frequency hearing loss in mice

HMDP: hybrid mouse diversity panel

HS: heterogeneous stock

kHz: kilohertz

KI: knock-in

KO: knock-out

Map1a: microtubule-associated protein 1

moth1: modifier of tubby hearing

ms: milliseconds

mt-Tr^{Arg}: mitochondrial tRNA-Arg

NIHL: noise-induced hearing loss

Nox3: NADPH oxidase-3

OS: outbred stock

QTL: quantitative trait loci

QTN: quantitative trait nucleotides

RIS: recombinant inbred strain

sgRNA: single guide RNA

Snhl: a locus for sensorineural hearing loss in mice

SNP: single nucleotide polymorphism

Tub: tubby bipartite transcription factor gene

Ush1g: USH1 protein network component sans gene

Ush1g^{js}: Jackson shaker mouse

Author details

Shumpei P. Yasuda[1], Yuki Miyasaka[1,2] and Yoshiaki Kikkawa[1]*

*Address all correspondence to: kikkawa-ys@igakuken.or.jp

1 Mammalian Genetics Project, Tokyo Metropolitan Institute of Medical Science, Tokyo, Japan

2 Division of Experimental Animals, Center for Promotion of Medical Research and Education, Graduate School of Medicine, Nagoya University, Nagoya, Aichi, Japan

References

[1] Morton CC, Nance WE. Newborn hearing screening—A silent revolution. The New England Journal of Medicine. 2006;**354**(20):2151-2164. DOI: 10.1056/NEJMra050700

[2] Roizen NJ. Nongenetic causes of hearing loss. Mental Retardation and Developmental Disabilities Research Reviews. 2003;**9**(2):120-127. DOI: 10.1002/mrdd.10068

[3] Vona B, Hofrichter MAH, Chioza BA, Crosby AH, Nanda I, Haaf T. Genetic elucidation of nonsyndromic hearing loss in the high-throughput sequencing era. In: Vona B, Haaf T, editors. Genetics of Deafness. Monographs in Human Genetics. Vol. 20. Basel: Karger; 2016. pp. 56-72. DOI: 10.1159/000444599

[4] Camp GV, Smith R. Hereditary Hearing Loss Homepage [Internet]. [Updated: 2017-03-13]. Available from: http://hereditaryhearingloss.org/ [Accessed: 2017-09-13]

[5] Cruickshanks KJ, Wiley TL, Tweed TS, Klein BE, Klein R, Mares-Perlman JA, Nondahl DM. Prevalence of hearing loss in older adults in beaver dam, Wisconsin. The epidemiology of hearing loss study. American Journal of Epidemiology. 1998;**148**(9):879-886. DOI: 10.1093/oxfordjournals.aje.a009713

[6] Dawes P, Payton A. Genetics of age-related hearing loss. In: Vona B, Haaf T, editors. Genetics of Deafness. Monographs in Human Genetics. Vol. 20. Basel: Karger; 2016. pp. 84-96. DOI: 10.1159/000444565

[7] Christensen K, Frederiksen H, Hoffman HJ. Genetic and environmental influences on self-reported reduced hearing in the old and oldest old. Journal of the American Geriatrics Society. 2001;**49**(11):1512-1517. DOI: 10.1046/j.1532-5415.2001.4911245.x

[8] Gates GA, Couropmitree NN, Myers RH. Genetic associations in age-related hearing thresholds. Archives of Otolaryngology – Head & Neck Surgery. 1999;**125**(6):654-659. DOI: 10.1001/archotol.125.6.654

[9] Karlsson KK, Harris JR, Svartengren M. Description and primary results from an audiometric study of male twins. Ear and Hearing. 1997;**18**(2):114-120

[10] Viljanen A, Era P, Kaprio J, Pyykkö I, Koskenvuo M, Rantanen T. Genetic and environmental influences on hearing in older women. The Journals of Gerontology. Series A, Biological Sciences and Medical Sciences. 2007;**62**(4):447-452. DOI: 10.1093/gerona/62.4.447

[11] McMahon CM. Hearing loss in older age and its effect on the individuals, their families and the community. In: Vona B, Haaf T, editors. Genetics of Deafness. Monographs in Human Genetics. Vol. 20. Basel: Karger; 2016. pp. 9-18. DOI: 10.1159/000444561

[12] Nelson DI, Nelson RY, Concha-Barrientos M, Fingerhut M. The global burden of occupational noise-induced hearing loss. American Journal of Industrial Medicine. 2005;**48**(6):446-458. DOI: 10.1002/ajim.20223

[13] Sliwinska-Kowalska M, Pawelczyk M. Contribution of genetic factors to noise-induced hearing loss: A human studies review. Mutation Research. 2013;**252**(1):61-65. DOI: 10.1016/j.mrrev.2012.11.001

[14] Charizopoulou N, Lelli A, Schraders M, Ray K, Hildebrand MS, Ramesh A, Srisailapathy CR, Oostrik J, Admiraal RJ, Neely HR, Latoche JR, Smith RJ, Northup JK, Kremer H, Holt JR, Noben-Trauth K. *Gipc3* mutations associated with audiogenic seizures and sensorineural hearing loss in mouse and human. Nature Communications. 2011;**2**:201. DOI: 1038/ncomms1200

[15] Keller JM, Neely HR, Latoche JR, Noben-Trauth K. High-frequency sensorineural hearing loss and its underlying genetics (*Hfhl1* and *Hfhl2*) in NIH Swiss mice. Journal of the Association for Research in Otolaryngology. 2011;**12**(5):617-631. DOI: 10.1007/s10162-011-0270-7

[16] Keller JM, Noben-Trauth K. Genome-wide linkage analyses identify *Hfhl1* and *Hfhl3* with frequency-specific effects on the hearing spectrum of NIH Swiss mice. BMC Genetics. 2012;**13**:32. DOI: 10.1186/1471-2156-13-32

[17] Lavinsky J, Crow AL, Pan C, Wang J, Aaron KA, Ho MK, Li Q, Salehide P, Myint A, Monges-Hernadez M, Eskin E, Allayee H, Lusis AJ, Friedman RA. Genome-wide association study identifies *Nox3* as a critical gene for susceptibility to noise-induced hearing loss. PLoS Genetics. 2015;**11**(4):e1005094. DOI: 10.1371/journal.pgen.1005094

[18] Noben-Trauth K, Latoche JR, Neely HR, Bennett B. Phenotype and genetics of progressive sensorineural hearing loss (*Snhl1*) in the LXS set of recombinant inbred strains of mice. PLoS One. 2010;**5**(7):e11459. DOI: 10.1371/journal.pone.0011459

[19] Cordell HJ. Epistasis: What it means, what it doesn't mean, and statistical methods to detect it in humans. Human Molecular Genetics. 2002;**11**(20):2463-2468. DOI: 10.1093/hmg/11.20.2463

[20] Scott WK, Schildkraut JM. Complex genetic interactions. In: Haines JL, Pericak-Vance M, editors. Genetic Analysis of Complex Disease. 2nd ed. Hoboken: Wiley; 2006. pp. 397-421. DOI: 10.1002/0471781142

[21] Kikkawa Y, Miyasaka Y. Genetic modifiers of hearing loss in mice: The case of phenotypic modification in homozygous *Cdh23*^{ahl} age-related hearing loss. In: Vona B, Haaf T, editors. Genetics of Deafness. Monographs in Human Genetics. Vol. 20. Basel: Karger; 2016. pp. 97-109. DOI: 10.1159/000444568

[22] Zheng QY, Johnson KR, Erway LC. Assessment of hearing in 80 inbred strains of mice by ABR threshold analyses. Hearing Research. 1999;**130**(1-2):94-107. DOI: 10.1016/S0378-5955(99)00003-9

[23] Miyasaka Y, Suzuki S, Ohshiba Y, Watanabe K, Sagara Y, Yasuda SP, Matsuoka K, Shitara H, Yonekawa H, Kominami R, Kikkawa Y. Compound heterozygosity of the functionally null *Cdh23*$^{v-ngt}$ and hypomorphic *Cdh23*^{ahl} alleles leads to early-onset progressive hearing loss in mice. Experimental Animals. 2013;**62**(4):333-346. DOI: 10.1538/expanim.62.333

[24] Miyasaka Y, Shitara H, Suzuki S, Yoshimoto S, Seki Y, Ohshiba Y, Okumura K, Taya C, Tokano H, Kitamura K, Takada T, Hibino H, Shiroishi T, Kominami R, Yonekawa H, Kikkawa Y. Heterozygous mutation of *Ush1g/Sans* in mice causes early-onset progressive hearing loss, which is recovered by reconstituting the strain-specific mutation in *Cdh23*. Human Molecular Genetics. 2016;**25**(10):2045-2059. DOI: 10.1093/hmg/ddw078

[25] Suzuki S, Ishikawa M, Ueda T, Ohshiba Y, Miyasaka Y, Okumura K, Yokohama M, Taya C, Matsuoka K, Kikkawa Y. Quantitative trait loci on chromosome 5 for susceptibility to frequency-specific effects on hearing in DBA/2J mice. Experimental Animals. 2015;**64**(3):241-251. DOI: 10.1538/expanim.14-0110

[26] Noben-Trauth K, Zheng QY, Johnson KR. Association of cadherin 23 with polygenic inheritance and genetic modification of sensorineural hearing loss. Nature Genetics. 2003;**35**(1):21-23. DOI: 10.1038/ng1226

[27] Mianné J, Chessum L, Kumar S, Aguilar C, Codner G, Hutchison M, Parker A, Mallon AM, Wells S, Simon MM, Teboul L, Brown SD, Bowl MR. Correction of the auditory phenotype in C57BL/6N mice via CRISPR/Cas9-mediated homology directed repair. Genome Medicine. 2016;**8**(1):16. DOI: 10.1186/s13073-016-0273-4

[28] Johnson KR, Gagnon LH, Longo-Guess C, Kane KL. Association of a citrate synthase missense mutation with age-related hearing loss in A/J mice. Neurobiology of Aging. 2012;**33**(8):1720-1729. DOI: 10.1016/j.neurobiolaging.2011.05.009

[29] Kazmierczak P, Sakaguchi H, Tokita J, Wilson-Kubalek EM, Milligan RA, Müller U, Kachar B. Cadherin 23 and protocadherin 15 interact to form tip-link filaments in sensory hair cells. Nature. 2007;**449**(7158):87-91. DOI: 10.1038/nature06091

[30] Sotomayor M, Weihofen WA, Gaudet R, Corey DP. Structure of a force-conveying cadherin bond essential for inner-ear mechanotransduction. Nature. 2012;**492**(7427):128-132. DOI: 10.1038/nature11590

[31] Pietrocola F, Galluzzi L, Bravo-San Pedro JM, Madeo F, Kroemer G. Acetyl coenzyme a: A central metabolite and second messenger. Cell Metabolism. 2015;**21**(6):805-821. DOI: 10.1016/j.cmet.2015.05.014

[32] Johnson KR, Zheng QY, Bykhovskaya Y, Spirina O, Fischel-Ghodsian N. A nuclear-mitochondrial DNA interaction affecting hearing impairment in mice. Nature Genetics. 2001;**27**(2):191-194. DOI: 10.1038/84831

[33] Shin JB, Longo-Guess CM, Gagnon LH, Saylor KW, Dumont RA, Spinelli KJ, Pagana JM, Wilmarth PA, David LL, Gillespie PG, Johnson K. The R109H variant of fascin-2, a developmentally regulated actin crosslinker in hair-cell stereocilia, underlies early-onset hearing loss of DBA/2J mice. The Journal of Neuroscience. 2010;**30**(29):9683-9694. DOI: 10.1523/JNEUROSCI.1541-10.2010

[34] Perrin BJ, Strandjord DM, Narayanan P, Henderson DM, Johnson KR, Ervasti JM. β-actin and fascin-2 cooperate to maintain stereocilia length. The Journal of Neuroscience. 2013; **33**(19):8114-8121. DOI: 10.1523/JNEUROSCI.0238-13.2013

[35] Nagtegaal AP, Spijker S, Crins TT, Neuro-Bsik Mouse Phenomics Consortium, Borst JG. A novel QTL underlying early-onset, low-frequency hearing loss in BXD recombinant inbred strains. Genes, Brain, and Behavior. 2012;**11**(8):911-920. DOI: 10.1111/j.1601-183X.2012.00845.x

[36] Johnson KR, Longo-Guess CM, Gagnon LH. A QTL on Chr 5 modifies hearing loss associated with the fascin-2 variant of DBA/2J mice. Mammalian Genome. 2015;**26**(7-8):338-347. DOI: 10.1007/s00335-015-9574-y

[37] Johnson KR, Erway LC, Cook SA, Willott JF, Zheng QY. A major gene affecting age-related hearing loss in C57BL/6J mice. Hearing Research. 1997;**114**(1-2):83-92. DOI: 10.1016/S0378-5955(97)00155-X

[38] Montagutelli X. Effect of the genetic background on the phenotype of mouse mutations. Journal of the American Society of Nephrology. 2000;**11**(Suppl 2):S101-S105

[39] Ikeda A, Zheng QY, Rosenstiel P, Maddatu T, Zuberi AR, Roopenian DC, North MA, Naggert JK, Johnson KR, Nishina PM. Genetic modification of hearing in tubby mice: Evidence for the existence of a major gene (*moth1*) which protects tubby mice from hearing loss. Human Molecular Genetics. 1999;**8**(9):1761-1767. DOI: 10.1093/hmg/8.9.1761

[40] Ikeda A, Zheng QY, Zuberi AR, Johnson KR, Naggert JK, Nishina PM. Microtubule-associated protein 1A is a modifier of tubby hearing (*moth1*). Nature Genetics. 2002;**30**(4):401-405. DOI: 10.1038/ng838

[41] Broman KW. The genomes of recombinant inbred lines. Genetics. 2005;**169**(2):1133-1146. DOI: 10.1534/genetics.104.035212

[42] Flint J, Eskin E. Genome-wide association studies in mice. Nature Reviews. Genetics. 2012;**13**(11):807-817. DOI: 10.1038/nrg3335

[43] Williams R, Yan L, Prins P, Sloan Z, Centeno A. The GeneNetwork [Internet]. 1994. [Updated: 2001-06-15]. Available from: http://www.genenetwork.org/webqtl/main.py [Accessed: 2017-09-13]

[44] Zheng QY, Ding D, Yu H, Salvi RJ, Johnson KR. A locus on distal chromosome 10 (*ahl4*) affecting age-related hearing loss in A/J mice. Neurobiology of Aging. 2009;**30**(10):1693-1705. DOI: 10.1016/j.neurobiolaging.2007.12.011

[45] Johnson KR, Longo-Guess C, Gagnon LH, Yu H, Zheng QY. A locus on distal chromosome 11 (*ahl8*) and its interaction with *Cdh23*^{ahl} underlie the early onset, age-related hearing loss of DBA/2J mice. Genomics. 2008;**92**(4):219-225. DOI: 10.1016/j.ygeno.2008.06.007

[46] Nesbitt MN, Skamene E. Recombinant inbred mouse strains derived from A/J and C57BL/6J: A tool for the study of genetic mechanisms in host resistance to infection and malignancy. Journal of Leukocyte Biology. 1984;**36**(3):357-364

[47] Seyfried TN, RK Y, Glaser GH. Genetic analysis of audiogenic seizure susceptibility in C57BL/6J × DBA/2J recombinant inbred strains of mice. Genetics. 1980;**94**(3):701-718

[48] DeFries JC, Wilson JR, Erwin VG, Petersen DR. LS × SS recombinant inbred strains of mice: Initial characterization. Alcoholism, Clinical and Experimental Research. 1989;**13**(2): 196-200

[49] Bailey DW. Recombinant-inbred strains. An aid to finding identity, linkage, and function of histocompatibility and other genes. Transplantation. 1971;**11**(3):325-327

[50] Watson J, Riblet R, Taylor BA. The response of recombinant inbred strains of mice to bacterial lipopolysaccharides. Journal of Immunology. 1977;**118**(6):2088-2093

[51] Nishimura M, Hirayama N, Serikawa T, Kanehira K, Matsushima Y, Katoh H, Wakana S, Kojima A, Hiai H. The SMXA: A new set of recombinant inbred strain of mice consisting of 26 substrains and their genetic profile. Mammalian Genome. 1995;**6**(12):850-857. DOI: 10.1007/BF00292434

[52] Singer JB, Hill AE, Burrage LC, Olszens KR, Song J, Justice M, O'Brien WE, Conti DV, Witte JS, Lander ES, Nadeau JH. Genetic dissection of complex traits with chromosome substitution strains of mice. Science. 2004;**304**(5669):445-458. DOI: 10.1126/science.1093139

[53] Takada T, Mita A, Maeno A, Sakai T, Shitara H, Kikkawa Y, Moriwaki K, Yonekawa H, Shiroishi T. Mouse inter-subspecific consomic strains for genetic dissection of quantitative complex traits. Genome Research. 2008;**18**(3):500-508. DOI: 10.1101/gr.7175308

[54] Nemoto M, Morita Y, Mishima Y, Takahashi S, Nomura T, Ushiki T, Shiroishi T, Kikkawa Y, Yonekawa H, Kominami R. *Ahl3*, a third locus on mouse chromosome 17 affecting age-related hearing loss. Biochemical and Biophysical Research Communications. 2004;**324**(4):1283-1288. DOI: 10.1016/j.bbrc.2004.09.186

[55] Takada T, Ebata T, Noguchi H, Keane TM, Adams DJ, Narita T, Shin I-T, Fujisawa H, Toyoda A, Abe K, Obata Y, Sakaki Y, Moriwaki K, Fujiyama A, Kohara Y, Shiroishi T. The ancestor of extant Japanese fancy mice contributed to the mosaic genomes of classical inbred strains. Genome Research. 2013;**23**(8):1329-1338. DOI: 10.1101/gr.156497.113

[56] Bennett BJ, Farber CR, Orozco L, Kang HM, Ghazalpour A, Siemers N, Neubauer M, Neuhaus I, Yordanova R, Guan B, Truong A, Yang WP, He A, Kayne P, Gargalovic P, Kirchgessner T, Pan C, Castellani LW, Kostem E, Furlotte N, Drake TA, Eskin E, Lusis AJ. A high-resolution association mapping panel for the dissection of complex traits in mice. Genome Research. 2010;**20**(2):281-290. DOI: 10.1101/gr.099234.109

[57] Ghazalpour A, Rau CD, Farber CR, Bennett BJ, Orozco LD, van Nas A, Pan C, Allayee H, Beaven SW, Civelek M, Davis RC, Drake TA, Friedman RA, Furlotte N, Hui ST, Jentsch JD, Kostem E, Kang HM, Kang EY, Joo JW, Korshunov VA, Laughlin RE, Martin LJ, Ohmen JD, Parks BW, Pellegrini M, Reue K, Smith DJ, Tetradis S, Wang J, Wang Y, Weiss JN, Kirchgessner T, Gargalovic PS, Eskin E, Lusis AJ, LeBoeuf RC. Hybrid mouse diversity panel: A panel of inbred mouse strains suitable for analysis of complex genetic traits. Mammalian Genome. 2012;**23**(9-10):680-692. DOI: 10.1007/s00335-012-9411-5

[58] Myint A, White CH, Ohmen JD, Li X, Wang J, Lavinsky J, Salehi P, Crow AL, Ohyama T, Friedman RA. Large-scale phenotyping of noise-induced hearing loss in 100 strains of mice. Hearing Research. 2016;**332**:113-120. DOI: 10.1016/j.heares.2015.12.006

[59] Grubb SC, Bult CJ, Bogue MA. Mouse phenome database. Nucleic Acids Research. 2014;**42**(D1):D825-D834. DOI: 10.1093/nar/gkt1159

[60] Lavinsky J, Ge M, Crow AL, Pan C, Wang J, Salehi P, Myint A, Eskin E, Allayee H, Lusis AJ, Friedman RA. The genetic architecture of noise-induced hearing loss: Evidence for a gene-by-environment interaction. G3 (Bethesda). 2016;**6**(10):3219-3228. DOI: 10.1534/g3.116.032516

[61] Williams RW, Williams EG. Resources for systems genetics. In: Schughart K, Williams RW, editors. Systems Genetics: Methods and Protocols, Methods in Molecular Biology. Vol. 1488. New York: Springer Science+Business Media; 2017. pp. 3-29. DOI: 10.1007/978-1-4939-6427-7_1

[62] Drayton M, Noben-Trauth K. Mapping quantitative trait loci for hearing loss in black Swiss mice. Hearing Research. 2006;**212**(1-2):128-139. DOI: 10.1016/j.heares.2005.11.006

[63] Chia R, Achilli F, Festing MF, Fisher EM. The origins and uses of mouse outbred stocks. Nature Genetics. 2005;**37**(11):1181-1186. DOI: 10.1038/ng1665

[64] Children's Hospital Oakland Research Institute. BACPAC Resources Center (BPRC) [Internet]. [Updated: 2017-01-09]. Available from: https://bacpacresources.org/home.htm [Accessed: 2017-09-13]

[65] RIKEN BRC Gene Engineering Division. MSM/Ms mouse BAC clone [Internet]. [Updated: 2017]. Available from: http://dna.brc.riken.jp/en/msm_bac_en [Accessed: 2017-09-13]

[66] Kan Y, Ruis B, Takasugi T, Hendrickson EA. Mechanisms of precise genome editing using oligonucleotide donors. Genome Research. 2017;**27**(7):1099-1111. DOI: 10.1101/gr.214775.116

[67] Vona B, Müller T, Nanda I, Neuner C, Hofrichter MA, Schröder J, Bartsch O, Läßig A, Keilmann A, Schraven S, Kraus F, Shehata-Dieler W, Haaf T. Targeted next-generation sequencing of deafness genes in hearing-impaired individuals uncovers informative mutations. Genetics in Medicine. 2014;**16**(12):945-953. DOI: 10.1038/gim.2014.65, 10.1038/gim.2014.65

12

Cochlear Implants: An Excursus into the Technologies and Clinical Applications

Mohammad Hossein Khosravi, Ali Kouhi,
Sasan Dabiri, Pedram Borghei and
Masoumeh Saeedi

Abstract

Hearing loss causes severe alterations in social function and daily communications. Cochlear device implantation (CDI) is the only beneficiary method for auditory rehabilitation in patients with severe to profound sensorineural hearing loss (SNHL). Regarding a report in 2014, over 300,000 people had received cochlear implants throughout the world since December 2012 among which about 60,000 were adults and 40,000 were children in the United States. In this chapter, we discuss the history, origin, mechanism of action, and type of cochlear implants, as well as method of surgery and complications.

Keywords: cochlear implantation, hearing loss, complications, clinical applications, surgical technique, epidemiology

1. History and introduction

Most of the patients with significant social dysfunction due to hearing loss can be treated by nonsurgical interventions. Many ways such as selective seating closer or with the better ear near important sound sources or using hearing aids can be utilized for these situations [1].

Cochlear device implantation (CDI) is the only beneficiary method for auditory rehabilitation in patients with severe to profound sensorineural hearing loss (SNHL). Regarding a report in 2014, over 300,000 people had received cochlear implants throughout the world since December 2012, among which about 60,000 were adults and 40,000 were children in the United States [2].

A 60-year-old history protects cochlear implantation technology, which has experienced multiple changes in devices and speech processing strategies. It was about 200 years ago when Alessandro Volta described the early auditory percepts induced by applying a large voltage between his own ears in 1790 [3–6]. Further investigations by Weaver and Bray were focused and resulted in this concept that it might be possible to generate electrical signals mimicking auditory input stimulus [7].

In 1957, an electrode with receiver coil was successfully implanted for a patient with resected cochlear nerve due to cholesteatoma, which was able to stimulate the apparatus for months, and shockingly, the patient had sound awareness and simple word recognition [8–10]. Following Djourno and Eyries, House started his work in the early 1960s who implanted simple wires, wires with ball electrodes, and even simple arrays into the scala tympani, which finally led into production of implantable device in 1972; this was a beginning point for clinical trials [3, 11].

At the beginning, there was a resistance from scientific community especially neurophysiologists and otologists against CI; however, the national institute of health (NIH) approved the use of electrical stimulation of auditory nerves as a rehabilitation method in 1977, while evaluating the outcome in patients with single channel implants [3, 4, 12, 13].

Multichannel CIs were produced in greater numbers due to the food and drug administration (FDA) approval because of their ability of open-set word recognition and better frequency spectrum percepts [3, 6, 14]. Another remarkable progress was occurred in 1991, while continuous interleaved sampling (CIS) strategy was introduced, which developed improved open-set word recognition in comparison with previous analogue methods, so that all currently available strategies are based on CIS [15].

2. Structure and mechanism of action

Sensory hair cells within the cochlea have the responsibility for transforming sound vibration to neural signal in healthy individuals; then, the signal continues its way to auditory cortex through cochlear nerve. Cochlear implants take the place of these cells using electrodes which stimulate the nerve fiber electrically. **Figure 1** illustrates a cochlear implant device. Common cochlear implants have two parts: external component as a hearing aid and internal component which is surgically inserted in mastoid [16].

The external part is consisted of three parts: a microphone for gathering sounds, a speech processor analyzing and encoding sound into a digital code, and a magnetic headpiece which transmits coded signals by a transcutaneous radiofrequency link to the internal part.

The internal part has a receiver stimulator which receives and decodes the data and conducts decoded signal to the electrode array. In the next step, there is a flexible silicone carrier, which has variable number of electrodes. The remaining cochlear nerve fibers are stimulated by the electrode array, which is surgically implanted in scala tympani of the cochlea.

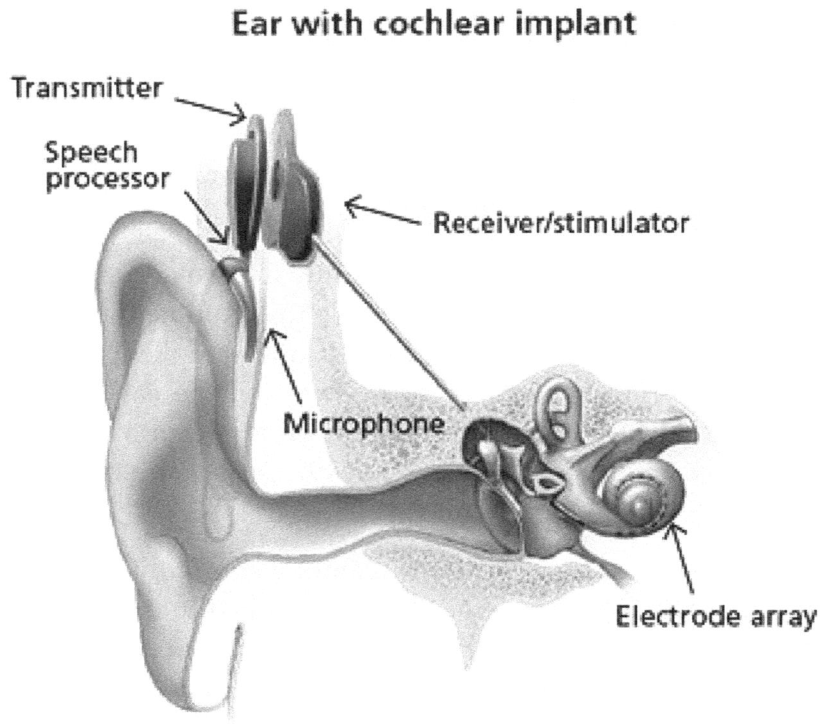

Figure 1. Different parts of cochlear implant (source: NIH/NIDCD https://www.nidcd.nih.gov/health/cochlear-implants).

3. Types of cochlear implants

3.1. Totally implantable cochlear implants

Currently available implants have an external part and need patients to wear it consisted of an external microphone, processor, and transmitting coil for empowering the electrode, which needs a dry and stable environment. Thus, development of totally implantable cochlear implants that make the whole system available underneath the skin is a new area of research. There are several challenges and requirements in the way of this progress including a tiny and sensitive microphone with ability to filter the endogenous noises, as well as a rechargeable battery with appropriate long life. There is a report of three patients with totally implantable cochlear implants [17].

3.2. Unilateral or bilateral cochlear implantation

Unilateral cochlear implantation was the only option offered at the beginning. Later, it was questioned if the patients would take more benefits from bilateral cochlear implants. Surprisingly, it was revealed that patients with bilateral cochlear implantation show better speech perception and improvement in "hearing in noise." Also, these patients showed a significantly better sound localization in comparison with their single-side implantation condition [18, 19].

Previous studies have concluded that there is no significant difference for audiologic outcomes between unilateral and bilateral cochlear implantation regarding surgical timing, as both ears can be implanted simultaneously or sequentially. Adult studies have shown that the second ear matches the first ear performance at 6 months [20]. The story has a difference when it comes to children, as it has been concluded that patients with simultaneous bilateral cochlear implantation have improved speech recognition and language when compared to children who were implanted sequentially [21].

The cost-effectiveness of bilateral cochlear implantation has remained controversial despite evident advantages of binaural stimulation. A Canadian study has reported that cochlear implantation is cost-effective in adults compared to no implantation; however, sequential bilateral cochlear implantation has a slight superiority in comparison with unilateral implantation [22]. Other studies have approved cost effectiveness of bilateral simultaneous pediatric implantation and unilateral adult cochlear implantation, although they have not approved cost-effectiveness of bilateral sequential pediatric implantation and bilateral (sequential or simultaneous) adult implantation [23].

4. Candidacy and patient selection

Selecting the right patient is the building block of a successful cochlear implantation. Therefore, a complete medical and audiologic workup is needed for evaluating candidacy of cochlear implantation and to make sure that the patient can tolerate anesthesia and surgical process. Patients are considered to take benefit from CI when they suffer from bilateral moderate to profound sensorineural hearing loss and when hearing aids cannot help them [24]. A combination of objective and subjective hearing tests is conducted to accurately identify the degree of hearing loss within audiometric frequencies. Currently available guidelines mention that children up to 2 years of age should have a bilateral profound sensorineural hearing loss, which is indicated by a pure tone audiometry (PTA) more than 90 dBHL for 500, 1000, and 2000 Hz frequencies, while patients older than 2 years of age should have bilateral sever to profound SNHL indicated by PTA more than 75 dBHL for 500, 1000, and 2000 Hz frequencies [25, 26]. Preoperative speech and language evaluation has the same importance for decision making regarding rehabilitation strategies and programs, as well as appropriateness of auditory performance, speech production, and mode of communication. Hearing loss is categorized to prelingual, postlingual, and perilingual types based on the time of onset. In prelingually deaf patients, hearing impairment occurs before gaining speaking skills, which is usually before 2 years of age, while it occurs after gaining complete speaking skills in postlingual patients which is usually after age of 5 years. In perilingual patients, hearing impairment occurs when some speaking skills are gained but are not completed usually between 2 and 5 years of age [16].

In addition, preoperative imaging and auditory testing are needed. Imaging modalities such as computed tomography (CT) scan, for assessing temporal bone, and magnetic resonance imaging (MRI), for evaluating brain anatomy and ruling out abnormalities of cochlear nerve, are conducted [15]. After scheduling patient for surgery, pneumococcal vaccines are administered according to FDA guidelines.

Current contraindications for cochlear implantation are two absolute and relative categories. Absence of cochlear development, deafness due to lesions of the central auditory pathway, and massive cochlear ossification that prevents electrode insertion are among absolute contraindications. Relative contraindications include aplasia of the acoustic nerve and medical conditions or developmental delays that would severely limit participation in aural rehabilitation.

5. Surgery

Cochlear implantation procedure is performed under general anesthesia associated with facial nerve monitoring. Surgeon needs to expose the mastoid, so a postauricular incision is made and soft tissue is dissected; latter, the surgeon makes a subperiosteal pocket for placement of implant magnet. A cortical mastoidectomy is performed associated with finding landmarks of temporal bone, such as incus, tegmen tympani, lateral semicircular canal, and sigmoid sinus. Then, the surgeon opens the facial recess, which is surrounded by chorda tympani, facial nerve, and incus buttress as its boundaries to identify the round window niche through the recess.

There are different methods for accessing scala tympani after finding the round window; in cochleostomy, the surgeon drills a separate hole and the anterior limit of the round window in extended cochleostomy. The implant is inserted into the cochlea, once the cochlea is opened. For making sure of the proper function of implant, an integrity test is performed by an audiologist at the end of the procedure. X-ray radiography is used to ensure proper location of cochlear implant by some surgeons. At the end, the patient is discharged the same day, and cochlear implant is usually activated 2–4 weeks postoperatively.

6. Complications

Cochlear implantation is generally a safe performed surgical procedure throughout the world with globally estimated complication rate of 16% [18]. Requiring additional surgery or cochlear explantation is categorized as major, and complications needing conservative medical management are classified as minor complications. Now, complication rates are decreasing due to improved experience, using smaller incisions and improvements in designing devices, and are generally calculated to be 11.8% for minor and 3.2% for major complications [27].

Infection is one of the most important major complications of cochlear implantation. Skin infection and acute otitis media are the most common type of implant-related infections ranging from 1 to 12% in the literature. Otitis media and soft tissue infection increase the risk of cochlear implant removal if leading to receiver stimulator infection. Also, it has been reported that cochlear implantation increases the risk of bacterial meningitis as 30-fold greater than general population; however, dawn of vaccination has made these cases sporadic [28]. Facial nerve palsy is another major complication of cochlear implantation, which is estimated to occur in 0.7% of cases due to heat induced by drill, cochleostomy, or reactivation of herpes virus as a result of surgery stress [29]. Finally, device failure is another major complication of cochlear implantation occurring in 2.5–6% of cases [18, 27]. Vestibular symptoms, such as vertigo and disequilibrium, are present in about one-third of patients postoperatively and are believed to last for more than 1 week after surgery. Most of these symptoms are resolved in weeks; however, patients over 70 years of age are more likely to have permanent vestibular weakness [30].

7. Hearing after cochlear implantation

Acoustic hearing remains preserved in more than half of the patients after cochlear implantation; however, previously, it was believed that insertion of electrode into the cochlea destroys the natural mechanism of hearing [31]. Preserving physiologic pathway of hearing has several advantages such as ability to localize the sound, recognize the speech, and hear in complex listening environments [32]. A variety of factors and approaches have been considered for improving hearing preservation after cochlear implantation. Previous studies have reported that full electrode insertion makes the hearing preservation possible; however, electrode insertion depth and length are determining factors for intracochlear trauma [24, 33].

Studies believe that the most hearing preservation achieves when the electrode is entirely located in scala tympani [34]. The most appropriate surgical approach has remained controversial; some previous studies have mentioned that there is no significant difference between round window and cochleostomy approaches regarding hearing outcomes [35, 36], while others reported that each method is superior for maximizing atraumatic scala tympani insertion. Eventually, preoperative prescription of steroids and steroid-eluting implants have been reported to improve hearing preservation up to 1 year from implantation [32].

In another retrospective analysis of cochlear implanted patients, researchers investigated the impact of related factors on hearing preservation. They reported an overall preservation likelihood of 39% for patients operated by refined soft surgery technique with a higher conservation rate at low frequencies when compared to high frequencies [37]. Age at the time of implantation, etiology of deafness, side of implant, electrode array model, and insertion technique, as well as type of cochleostomy, are investigated factors, which are considered to possibly affect hearing preservation; however, there are a variety of opinions on their effects, and further studies are required for conclusive results [36, 38–52].

8. Other applications of cochlear implant

8.1. Cochlear implantation for single-sided sensorineural hearing loss

Recently, a new topic has come up about cochlear implantation in setting of single-sided sensorineural hearing loss [53]. So far, options such as hearing aids, bone-anchored implants, and contralateral routing of signal (CROS) devices were applied for single-side deaf patients. While these options improve hearing by healthy ear, cochlear implantation restores hearing by deaf ear. Sound localization is a special challenge for patients with unilateral hearing loss.

A proper localization involves a good bilateral hearing and sound stimulation, as well as intraaural time differences, which allow complex processing of sounds. Recent studies have mentioned some advantages for cochlear implantation in unilateral hearing loss, and some has reported a better sound localization in comparison with bone-anchored implants [54]. Additionally, it has been shown that cochlear implants resolve tinnitus up to an acceptable extent in patients with single-sided deafness and may improve speech perception [34, 55].

8.2. Hybrid cochlear implants

A hybrid cochlear implant was developed by Gantz et al. with the aim of preserving residual hearing, which has only 10 mm of height [56]. This provides the possibility for stimulating the region responsible for high-frequency hearing in cochlea without stimulating regions responsible for low frequency hearing. Primary studies have revealed that hybrid implant application is associated with better hearing preservation and increased speech perception [35, 36, 57, 58]. In addition to the comparable performance of hybrid implants with conventional ones, patients with hybrid implants had improved music appreciation as a result of acoustic and electrical stimulation combination [56, 57]. Replacement of hybrid implant with full-length implant in a progressive hearing loss improves hearing and word recognition; however, it is associated with a notable additional cost [59, 60].

8.3. Cochlear implantation and Meniere's disease

Cochlear implantation has been utilized for Meniere's disease, a condition consisted of episodic attacks of tinnitus, hearing loss, and debilitating vertigo spells. Previous studies have shown resolution of related symptoms after cochlear implantation in Meniere's disease patients, although the hearing outcomes are not as acceptable as patients implanted for other reasons [61, 62].

9. Prospective of cochlear implantation

So far, some in vitro and animal studies have been conducted to resolve the hearing impairment problem using regenerative medicine; nevertheless, cochlear implantation remains as the most effective current treatment method. Further efforts are being put to cochlear implantation technology field in order to improve understanding speech in noise and music appreciations.

Abbreviations

CI	cochlear implant
CROS	contralateral routing of signal
dBHL	decibels hearing level

Hz	Hertz; unit of frequency
PTA	pure tone audiometry
SNHL	sensory-neural hearing loss

Author details

Mohammad Hossein Khosravi[1,2], Ali Kouhi[2,3], Sasan Dabiri[4], Pedram Borghei[5] and Masoumeh Saeedi[2,6]*

*Address all correspondence to: m.saeedi67@gmail.com

1 Student Research Committee (SRC), Baqiyatallah University of Medical Sciences, Tehran, Iran

2 International Otorhinolaryngology Research Association (IORA), Universal Scientific Education and Research Network (USERN), Tehran, Iran

3 Department of Otolaryngology—Head and Neck Surgery, Otorhinolaryngology Research Center, Tehran University of Medical Sciences, Tehran, Iran

4 Department of Otorhinolaryngology—Head and Neck Surgery, Amir Alam Hospital, Tehran University of Medical Sciences, Tehran, Iran

5 Otolaryngology Head and Neck Surgery, Tehran University of Medical Sciences, Tehran, Iran

6 Department of Otorhinolaryngology—Head and Neck Surgery, Faculty of Medicine, Baqiyatallah University of Medical Sciences, Tehran, Iran

References

[1] Roche JP, Hansen MR. On the horizon: Cochlear implant technology. Otolaryngologic Clinics of North America. 2015;**48**(6):1097

[2] https://www.nidcd.nih.gov/health/cochlear-implants

[3] Carlson ML, Driscoll CL, Gifford RH, McMenomey SO. Cochlear implantation: Current and future device options. Otolaryngologic Clinics of North America. 2012;**45**(1):221-248

[4] Ramsden RT. History of cochlear implantation. Cochlear Implants International. 2013; **14**(suppl. 4):3-5

[5] Volta A. XVII. On the electricity excited by the mere contact of conducting substances of different kinds. In a letter from Mr. Alexander Volta, FRS Professor of Natural Philosophy in the University of Pavia, to the Rt. Hon. Sir Joseph Banks, Bart. KBPRS. Philosophical Transactions of the Royal Society of London. 1800 Jan 1;**90**:403-431

[6] Eshraghi AA, Nazarian R, Telischi FF, Rajguru SM, Truy E, Gupta C. The cochlear implant: Historical aspects and future prospects. The Anatomical Record. 2012;**295**(11):1967-1980

[7] Wever EG, Bray CW. The nature of the acoustic response: The relation between stimulus intensity and the magnitude of cochlear responses in the cat. Journal of Experimental Psychology. 1938;**22**(1):1

[8] Djourno A, Eyries C, Vallancien B. Electric excitation of the cochlear nerve in man by induction at a distance with the aid of micro-coil included in the fixture. Comptes Rendus des Seances de la Societe de Biologie et de ses filiales. 1957;**151**(3):423

[9] Arts HA, Jones DA, Anderson DJ. Prosthetic stimulation of the auditory system with intraneural electrodes. Annals of Otology, Rhinology & Laryngology. 2003;**112**(9_suppl):20-25

[10] Eisen MD. Djourno, eyries, and the first implanted electrical neural stimulator to restore hearing. Otology & Neurotology. 2003;**24**(3):500-506

[11] Eshraghi AA, Gupta C, Ozdamar O, Balkany TJ, Truy E, Nazarian R. Biomedical engineering principles of modern cochlear implants and recent surgical innovations. The Anatomical Record. 2012;**295**(11):1957-1966

[12] Kiang NY, Moxon EC. Physiological considerations in artificial stimulation of the inner ear. Annals of Otology, Rhinology & Laryngology. 1972;**81**(5):714-730

[13] Bilger R, Black F. Auditory prostheses in perspective. Annals of Otology, Rhinology & Laryngology. 1977;**86**(3_suppl):3-10

[14] Clark GM, Tong YC, Martin LF. A multiple-channel cochlear implant: An evaluation using open-set cid sentences. The Laryngoscope. 1981;**91**(4):628-634

[15] Wilson BS, Finley CC, Lawson DT, Wolford RD, Eddington DK, Rabinowitz WM. Better speech recognition with cochlear implants. Nature. 1991;**352**(6332):236-238

[16] Vincenti V, Bacciu A, Guida M, Marra F, Bertoldi B, Bacciu S, et al. Pediatric cochlear implantation: An update. Italian Journal of Pediatrics. 2014;**40**(1):72

[17] Briggs RJ, Eder HC, Seligman PM, Cowan RS, Plant KL, Dalton J, et al. Initial clinical experience with a totally implantable cochlear implant research device. Otology & Neurotology. 2008;**29**(2):114-119

[18] Venail F, Sicard M, Piron JP, Levi A, Artieres F, Uziel A, et al. Reliability and complications of 500 consecutive cochlear implantations. Archives of Otolaryngology–Head & Neck Surgery. 2008;**134**(12):1276-1281

[19] Dunn CC, Tyler RS, Witt S, Ji H, Gantz BJ. Sequential bilateral cochlear implantation: Speech perception and localization pre-and post-second cochlear implantation. American Journal of Audiology. 2012;**21**(2):181-189

[20] Reeder RM, Firszt JB, Holden LK, Strube MJ. A longitudinal study in adults with sequential bilateral cochlear implants: Time course for individual ear and bilateral performance. Journal of Speech, Language, and Hearing Research. 2014;**57**(3):1108-1126

[21] Lammers MJ, Venekamp RP, Grolman W, Heijden GJ. Bilateral cochlear implantation in children and the impact of the inter-implant interval. The Laryngoscope. 2014; **124**(4):993-999

[22] Chen JM, Amoodi H, Mittmann N. Cost-utility analysis of bilateral cochlear implantation in adults: A health economic assessment from the perspective of a publicly funded program. The Laryngoscope. 2014;**124**(6):1452-1458

[23] McKinnon BJ. Cost effectiveness of cochlear implants. Current Opinion in Otolaryngology & Head and Neck Surgery. 2014;**22**(5):344-348

[24] Yawn R, Hunter JB, Sweeney AD, Bennett ML. Cochlear implantation: A biomechanical prosthesis for hearing loss. F1000prime Reports. 2015;**7**

[25] Heman-Ackah SE, Roland JT, Haynes DS, Waltzman SB. Pediatric cochlear implantation: Candidacy evaluation, medical and surgical considerations, and expanding criteria. Otolaryngologic Clinics of North America. 2012;**45**(1):41-67

[26] Forli F, Arslan E, Bellelli S, Burdo S, Mancini P, Martini A, et al. Systematic review of the literature on the clinical effectiveness of the cochlear implant procedure in paediatric patients. Acta Otorhinolaryngologica Italica. 2011;**31**(5):281

[27] Farinetti A, Gharbia DB, Mancini J, Roman S, Nicollas R, Triglia J-M. Cochlear implant complications in 403 patients: Comparative study of adults and children and review of the literature. European Annals of Otorhinolaryngology, Head and Neck Diseases. 2014;**131**(3):177-182

[28] Reefhuis J, Honein MA, Whitney CG, Chamany S, Mann EA, Biernath KR, et al. Risk of bacterial meningitis in children with cochlear implants. New England Journal of Medicine. 2003;**349**(5):435-445

[29] Fayad JN, Wanna GB, Micheletto JN, Parisier SC. Facial nerve paralysis following cochlear implant surgery. The Laryngoscope. 2003;**113**(8):1344-1346

[30] Enticott JC, Tari S, Koh SM, Dowell RC, O'leary SJ. Cochlear implant and vestibular function. Otology & Neurotology. 2006;**27**(6):824-830

[31] Carlson ML, Driscoll CL, Gifford RH, Service GJ, Tombers NM, Hughes-Borst BJ, et al. Implications of minimizing trauma during conventional cochlear implantation. Otology & Neurotology: Official Publication of the American Otological Society, American Neurotology Society [and] European Academy of Otology and Neurotology. 2011;**32**(6):962

[32] Gifford RH, Dorman MF, Skarzynski H, Lorens A, Polak M, Driscoll CL, et al. Cochlear implantation with hearing preservation yields significant benefit for speech recognition in complex listening environments. Ear and Hearing. 2013;**34**(4):413

[33] Bruce IA, Bates JEHM, Melling C, Mawman D, Green KMJ. Hearing preservation via a cochleostomy approach and deep insertion of a standard length cochlear implant electrode. Otology & Neurotology. 2011;**32**(9):1444-1447

[34] Vlastarakos PV, Nazos K, Tavoulari E-F, Nikolopoulos TP. Cochlear implantation for single-sided deafness: The outcomes. An evidence-based approach. European Archives of Oto-rhino-laryngology. 2014;**271**(8):2119-2126

[35] Adunka OF, Dillon MT, Adunka MC, King ER, Pillsbury HC, Buchman CA. Cochleostomy versus round window insertions: Influence on functional outcomes in electric-acoustic stimulation of the auditory system. Otology & Neurotology. 2014;**35**(4):613-618

[36] Havenith S, Lammers MJ, Tange RA, Trabalzini F, della Volpe A, van der Heijden GJ, et al. Hearing preservation surgery: Cochleostomy or round window approach? A systematic review. Otology & Neurotology. 2013;**34**(4):667-674

[37] Zanetti D, Nassif N, de Zinis LR. Factors affecting residual hearing preservation in cochlear implantation. Acta Otorhinolaryngologica Italica. 2015;**35**(6):433

[38] Skarzynski H, Lorens A, Piotrowska A, Anderson I. Partial deafness cochlear implantation in children. International Journal of Pediatric Otorhinolaryngology. 2007;**71**(9):1407-1413

[39] Causon A, Verschuur C, Newman TA. A retrospective analysis of the contribution of reported factors in cochlear implantation on hearing preservation outcomes. Otology & Neurotology. 2015;**36**(7):1137-1145

[40] Adunka OF, Buss E, Clark MS, Pillsbury HC, Buchman CA. Effect of preoperative residual hearing on speech perception after cochlear implantation. The Laryngoscope. 2008;**118**(11):2044-2049

[41] Skarzynski H, Lorens A, Piotrowska A, Anderson I. Preservation of low frequency hearing in partial deafness cochlear implantation (PDCI) using the round window surgical approach. Acta Oto-laryngologica. 2007;**127**(1):41-48

[42] Giordano P, Hatzopoulos S, Giarbini N, Prosser S, Petruccelli J, Simoni E, et al. A soft-surgery approach to minimize hearing damage caused by the insertion of a cochlear implant electrode: A guinea pig animal model. Otology & Neurotology. 2014;**35**(8):1440-1445

[43] Berrettini S, Forli F, Passetti S. Preservation of residual hearing following cochlear implantation: Comparison between three surgical techniques. The Journal of Laryngology & Otology. 2008;**122**(3):246-252

[44] Briggs RJ, Tykocinski M, Xu J, Risi F, Svehla M, Cowan R, et al. Comparison of round window and cochleostomy approaches with a prototype hearing preservation electrode. Audiology and Neurotology. 2006;**11**(Suppl. 1):42-48

[45] Sun CH, Hsu CJ, Chen PR, Wu HP. Residual hearing preservation after cochlear implantation via round window or cochleostomy approach. The Laryngoscope. 2015;**125**(7):1715-1719

[46] Lenarz T, James C, Cuda D, Fitzgerald O'Connor A, Frachet B, Frijns JH, et al. European multi-centre study of the nucleus hybrid L24 cochlear implant. International Journal of Audiology. 2013;**52**(12):838-848

[47] Gstoettner WK, Van de Heyning P, Fitzgerald O'Connor A, Morera C, Sainz M, Vermeire K, et al. Electric acoustic stimulation of the auditory system: Results of a multi-centre investigation. Acta Oto-laryngologica. 2008;**128**(9):968-975

[48] Souter MA, Briggs RJ, Wright CG, Roland PS. Round window insertion of precurved perimodiolar electrode arrays: How successful is it? Otology & Neurotology. 2011; **32**(1):58-63

[49] Di Nardo W, Cantore I, Cianfrone F, Melillo P, Rigante M, Paludetti G. Residual hearing thresholds in cochlear implantation and reimplantation. Audiology and Neurotology. 2007;**12**(3):165-169

[50] Rebscher SJ, Hetherington A, Bonham B, Wardrop P, Whinney D, Leake PA. Considerations for the design of future cochlear implant electrode arrays: Electrode array stiffness, size and depth of insertion. Journal of Rehabilitation Research and Development. 2008;**45**(5):731

[51] Di Nardo W, Cantore I, Melillo P, Cianfrone F, Scorpecci A, Paludetti G. Residual hearing in cochlear implant patients. European Archives of Oto-rhino-laryngology. 2007; **264**(8):855-860

[52] Jurawitz M-C, Büchner A, Harpel T, Schüssler M, Majdani O, Lesinski-Schiedat A, et al. Hearing preservation outcomes with different cochlear implant electrodes: Nucleus® hybrid™-L24 and nucleus freedom™ CI422. Audiology and Neurotology. 2014;**19**(5):293-309

[53] Kamal SM, Robinson AD, Diaz RC. Cochlear implantation in single-sided deafness for enhancement of sound localization and speech perception. Current Opinion in Otolaryngology & Head and Neck Surgery. 2012;**20**(5):393-397

[54] Nawaz S, McNeill C, Greenberg SL. Improving sound localization after cochlear implantation and auditory training for the management of single-sided deafness. Otology & Neurotology. 2014;**35**(2):271-276

[55] Kim D-K, Bae S-C, Park K-H, Jun B-C, Lee D-H, Yeo SW, et al. Tinnitus in patients with profound hearing loss and the effect of cochlear implantation. European Archives of Oto-Rhino-Laryngology. 2013;**270**(6):1803-1808

[56] Gantz BJ, Dunn CC, Walker EA, Kenworthy M, Van Voorst T, Tomblin B, et al. Bilateral cochlear implants in infants: a new approach—Nucleus Hybrid S12 project. Otology & Neurotology: Official Publication of the American Otological Society, American Neurotology Society [and] European Academy of Otology and Neurotology. 2010;**31**(8):1300

[57] Douchement D, Terranti A, Lamblin J, Salleron J, Siepmann F, Siepmann J, et al. Dexamethasone eluting electrodes for cochlear implantation: Effect on residual hearing. Cochlear Implants International. 2015;**16**(4):195-200

[58] Wanna GB, Noble JH, Carlson ML, Gifford RH, Dietrich MS, Haynes DS, et al. Impact of electrode design and surgical approach on scalar location and cochlear implant outcomes. The Laryngoscope. 2014;**124**:S1-S7

[59] Fitzgerald MB, Sagi E, Jackson M, Shapiro WH, Roland JT Jr, Waltzman SB, et al. Reimplantation of hybrid cochlear implant users with a full-length electrode after loss of residual hearing. Otology & Neurotology. 2008;**29**(2):168-173

[60] Carlson ML, Archibald DJ, Gifford RH, Driscoll CL, Beatty CW. Reimplantation with a conventional length electrode following residual hearing loss in four hybrid implant recipients. Cochlear Implants International. 2012;**13**(3):148-155

[61] Hansen MR, Gantz BJ, Dunn C. Outcomes following cochlear implantation for patients with single-sided deafness, including those with recalcitrant Ménière's disease. Otology & Neurotology: Official Publication of the American Otological Society, American Neurotology Society [and] European Academy of Otology and Neurotology. 2013;**34**(9):1681-1687

[62] McRackan TR, Gifford RH, Kahue CN, Dwyer R, Labadie RF, Wanna GB, et al. Cochlear implantation in Ménière's disease patients. Otology & Neurotology. 2014;**35**(3):421-425

13

Hearing Loss at High Frequencies and Oxidative Stress: A New Paradigm for Different Etiologies

Klinger Vagner Teixeira da Costa,
Kelly Cristina Lira de Andrade,
Maria Eduarda di Cavalcanti,
Ana Claudia Figueiredo Frizzo,
Aline Tenório Lins Carnaúba and
Pedro de Lemos Menezes

Abstract

The clinical assessment of hearing loss has been transformed and revised in terms of interpreting the characteristics of patterns found in relation to the relative frequency of certain diseases. However, increasing the threshold to 4 kHz as a starting point for hearing loss has shown to be common to different diseases such as noise-induced hearing loss. In noise-induced hearing loss, for example, six mechanisms can be considered: conversion of sound pressure level into hearing level, vascular failure in the cochlear region responsible for hearing at 4 kHz, sound wave propagation velocity is very high and causes the displacement amplitude in the cochlear duct, the structure anatomy of the cochlea causes a collision of fluids in the first curve of the cochlea, characteristics of auricular pavilion resonance and external auditory canal, and sound attenuation of the acoustic reflex. It is hoped that this new paradigm for the different hearing losses will result in a different approach to the physiological changes that affect the auditory system in the form of high-frequency hearing loss. As such, preventing, treating, and avoiding exacerbations are possibilities to be investigated in order to guarantee efficient communication and quality of life for individuals.

Keywords: hearing loss, noise-induced hearing loss, oxidative stress, presbycusis, chronic kidney disease

1. Introduction

Hearing is one of the primary means of human contact with the world, from the perception of acoustic signals that indicate danger through an alert system to the development of language and intellect. In the evolutionary process, the human auditory system underwent transformations that enabled it to capture, amplify (magnify), perceive, and discriminate sound, the last two achieved from the inner ear (cochlea) to the auditory cortex.

Human hearing perceives sounds ranging from 20 Hz to 16 kHz, and exhibits tonotopy from the cochlea to the auditory cortex, such that hearing frequencies are recognized in an organized manner along the auditory pathway. Under certain conditions that lead to hearing loss, initial and selective damage may occur at certain sound frequencies. This pattern of selective damage can be observed in a number of pathological conditions whose physiopathological foundation may be based on an oxidative stress model. Among these conditions are noise-induced hearing loss (NIHL), age-related hearing loss (presbycusis), ototoxic hearing loss, and hearing loss associated with chronic kidney disease (CKD).

2. Oxidative stress

Free radicals are species (molecules, ions) that contain free electrons (unpaired) in their structure and, as such, are usually highly reactive with other molecules [1]. Due to this reactivity, radicals can damage membranes and other cellular structures under oxidative stress conditions.

Oxidation reactions cause the formation of a variety of unstable reactive species that can trigger chain reactions in milliseconds, leading to disease and programmed cell death (apoptosis) [2]. Among the reactive species formed are reactive oxygen species (ROS), which participate in several physiological and pathological processes in the organism.

With the evolution of the cell and the use of molecular oxygen in energy metabolism, ROS began to play increasingly studied and significant roles in a number of diseases [3]. The main ROS are the superoxide anion radical (O_2^-), hydrogen peroxide (H_2O_2), and the hydroxyl radical (OH), the last being the most reactive and harmful [1].

Given that free radical production occurs naturally in the organism, an elaborate endogenous antioxidant system evolved to control the harmful effect of reactive species. This system includes antioxidant scavenger enzymes such as superoxide-dismutase (SOD) 1 and 2, catalase, glutathione (GSH), and related enzymes, including glutathione peroxidase (GPx), glutathione S-transferase (GST), and glutathione reductase (GSH-Red), which converts ROS into neutral, non-reactive molecules.

Thus, hearing losses with different etiologies have been studied at the cellular and molecular level, and there is a convergent tendency with respect to the association between them and oxidative stress.

3. Hearing losses

Over the centuries, man has advanced in a number of ways, but this progress has also introduced lifestyle habits that sometimes cause new risk factors for hearing loss.

Exposure to high levels of sound pressure (noise), both professionally and at leisure, can cause irreversible hearing loss, which is often progressive when an individual remains in contact with a daily sound source [4, 5].

Increased life expectancy means age-related hearing loss (presbycusis) has become more common and is one of the most prevalent chronic diseases worldwide.

The emergence of new drugs has led to the cure of numerous hitherto lethal diseases; however, the ototoxic effect of certain medications causes hearing loss and leaves sequelae in children and adults alike [6, 7].

Chronic kidney disease (CKD), which has multiple etiologies, can evolve with progressive hearing loss, representing yet another disability for kidney patients and compromising their quality of life. Moreover, the use of certain drugs for patients with CKD may worsen auditory function and be an aggravating factor for hearing loss [8].

These hearing disorders exhibit a sensorineural pattern due to the sites affected, which vary from the cochlea to the auditory cortical regions, with a preference for high sound frequencies. However, high-frequency damage is a starting point, and 4 kHz is seen as the border between frequencies that often remain preserved and those affected.

Assessment of the physiopathological model of these hearing losses shows that oxidative stress occurs under all the aforementioned conditions and emerges as a new paradigm that more deeply connects characteristic acoustic aspects common to all of them. The real reason for which hearing loss arises, preferentially and usually around 4 kHz, is not fully understood, but there may be a common point in molecular and physiopathological terms that leads to this spectral selectivity.

Starting with a model that considers oxidative stress, we will discuss each of the hearing loss conditions influenced by excess free radicals and expressed by an increase in high-frequency hearing thresholds.

3.1. Noise-induced hearing loss

Excessive exposure to noise induces sensorineural hearing loss resulting from damage to cochlear and neural structures in the inner ear, denominated NIHL. NIHL can be temporally classified into two types: hearing loss induced by chronic noise and acute acoustic trauma. Chronic NIHL is a hearing deficiency caused by continuous exposure to high levels of sound pressure that exert an average of 90 dBA, for eight hours a day, over several years or more [4], whereas acute acoustic trauma is hearing loss caused by short exposure to excessively loud sounds (100–150 dBA, decibel weighting curve A) [9].

Exposure to different sound levels leads to metabolic and mechanical damage. Metabolic damage could occur after exposure to noise between 85 and 115 dBA, whereas mechanical damage can emerge after exposure to sound levels above 115 dBA. Noise-induced hearing loss is due primarily to neural degeneration, which starts immediately after exposure to noise and progresses for several years after exposure [10].

Susceptibility to the harmful effects of noise differs significantly among individuals, that is, after identical exposure to noise, not all people suffer hearing loss, and when they do, the degree can vary. Thus, NIHL was classified as a disease resulting from external (environmental) causes, in addition to genetic predisposition [11].

Ciliated cells, particularly the more vulnerable external variety, are compromised in NIHL. There are around 12,000 external ciliated cells arranged in three rows in the basal region of the cochlea and in four or five rows in the apical region [12]. Thus, there are fewer ciliated cells at the cochlear base than the apex. With a sharp loss of ciliated cells, secondary neural degeneration is reflected in the auditory nerve and brainstem auditory nuclei [13].

The cochlea is a metabolically active organ and oxidative stress plays an important role in the pathogenic mechanisms of NIHL. The mitochondria generate energy to maintain cochlear metabolism; however, they are also the primary ROS generator. The fact that ciliated cells are highly energy-demanding during and after exposure to noise leads to a prolonged local release of free radicals, which may damage the cochlear epithelium, particularly if the antioxidant defense system is not efficient enough to neutralize them [11]. However, due to this exposure to ROS, as well as harmful environmental influences (noise), mitochondrial DNA (mtDNA) run the risk of maintaining mutations that may hinder the function of different organelles and lead to chronic diseases such as NIHL [14, 15].

Organ of Corti lesions occur primarily at the basal turn (Rosenthal's canal), in the area responsible for sounds between 3 and 6 kHz, regardless of the frequency range of aggressor noise, caused by six possible mechanisms [5]:

1. Conversion of dBA for sound intensity under the international guidelines to protect the auditory system into dBHL for hearing level;
2. Vascular failure in the cochlear region responsible for hearing at 4 kHz;
3. Sound wave propagation velocity is very high and causes the displacement amplitude in the cochlear duct to begin to grow in the 4 kHz region;
4. The structure anatomy of the cochlea causes a collision of fluids in the first curve of the cochlea;
5. Characteristics of auricular pavilion resonance and external auditory canal cause injury in the 4 kHz region.
6. Sound attenuation of the acoustic reflex occurs only for low frequencies.

The first mechanism raises the most speculation due to the dynamics of noise that exhibits the same intensity in dBA (decibel weighting curve A). This occurs because sound measures in dBA are the result of a weighted average of the amplitudes of each frequency that makes up the sound measured [16, 17]. **Table 1** illustrates an example of the necessary correction in dB in order to calculate sound intensity in dBA.

Table 1 shows that for a pure tone of 500 Hz to emit 100 dBA, it must exhibit 108.6 dB SPL. If the frequency were 4 kHz, sound should produce 101 dB SPL. As can be observed, for a complex sound to emit 100 dBA, different possible combinations of amplitudes by frequency exist.

The guidelines that protect workers in most of the countries that have such legislation include dB and weighting curve A as intensity measures. However, auditory assessments are conducted at dB hearing levels and depend on the specific earphones used in the assessment in order to match the dB hearing level and dB SPL. **Table 2** contains the reference values corresponding to 0 dBHL, by frequency, using Telephonics TDH-39 earphones, the most commonly found in audiometers.

Thus, for a person to have the sensation of hearing 0 dBHL, the sound must emit 7 dB SPL, if its frequency is 1 kHz. As such, for them to hear at 30 dBHL, at this frequency, the sound must produce 37 dB SPL [18].

Finally, **Figure 1** exhibits the correspondence curves, by frequency, for a sound in dBA, listened to through TDH-39 earphones and the matching result from one unit to another.

Figure 1 shows that the weighting differences and adjustments to dBHL result in greater weight for sound frequencies between 0.5 and 4 kHz. Thus, a sound that has different frequencies could exhibit higher physical intensities in the dB SPL band particularly, and more energy

Frequency (Hz)	dB SPL correction for dBA
250	−8.6
500	−3.2
1000	0
2000	1.2
4000	1
8000	−1.1

Table 1. dB correction to calculate intensity in dBA, by frequency.

Frequency (Hz)	Reference (dB SPL)
250	25.5
500	11.5
1000	7
2000	9
4000	9.5
8000	13

Table 2. Reference levels (dB SPL) for an intensity of 0 dBNA, by frequency.

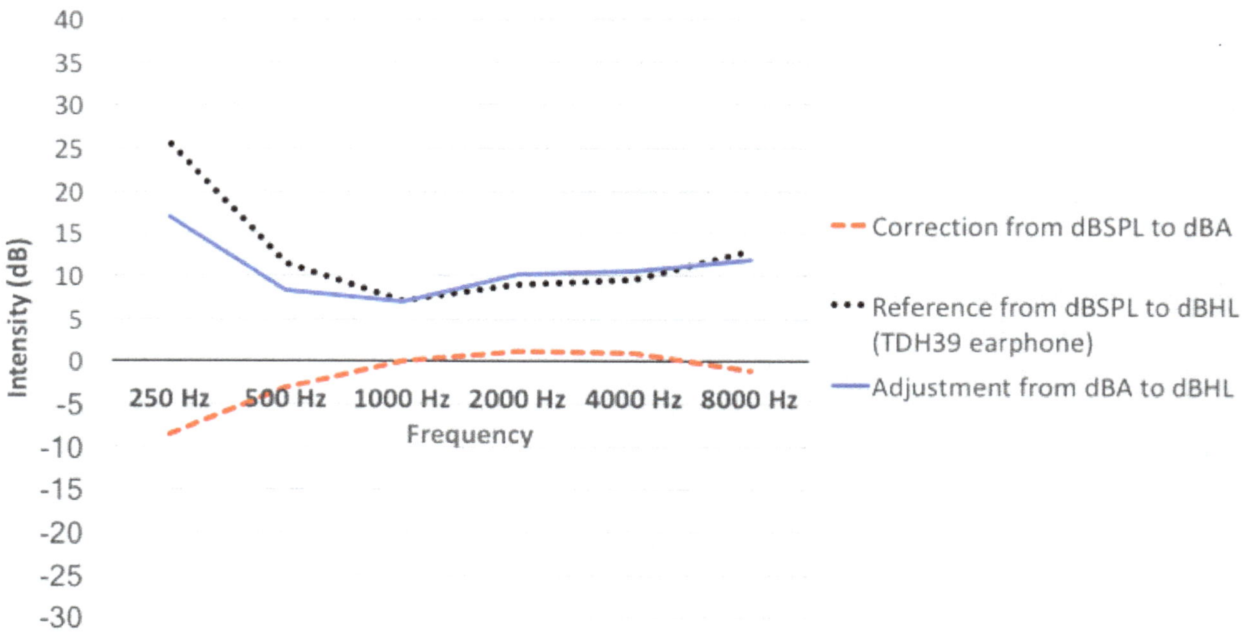

Figure 1. Adjustment from dBA to dBHL (TDH39 earphone).

could cause greater damage. However, it is necessary to know the other mechanisms in order to have a clearer understanding of the implications in the present topic.

The second, third, and fourth mechanisms described earlier explain why a frequency of 4 kHz is the first and most affected in terms of the degree of hearing loss [4, 5]. Furthermore, ciliated cells from the basal turn, the area responsible for high frequencies, are more susceptible to oxidative stress than those from the cochlear apex [19].

Even at a low oxidative stress levels, external ciliated cells from the basal turn are more vulnerable to damage, while internal and external ciliated cells from the middle and apical turns are more preserved [20]. The difference in antioxidant levels in basal turn to apical turn cells explains this greater susceptibility to lesions caused by ciliated cells from the base of the cochlea [19]. At the enzyme level, exposure to noise increases oxidase NADPHA (NOX) levels in the cochlea and a decline in SOD increases susceptibility to acoustic lesions. The accumulation of ROS subsequently triggers a complex cascade of biochemical processes including activation of c-Jun N-terminal kinase (JNK) and p38MAPK, the release of cytochrome and mitochondria and proca spase activation [3, 8, 9] (intrinsic apoptotic pathway) [21, 22].

Furthermore, the physiological mechanisms of resonance in the auditory system, primarily the concha and external auditory canal, are highly relevant in the audiometric configuration process of noise-induced hearing loss, especially at strong intensities [10]. The physiology of hearing studies the resonance in tubes in order to understand sound reception.

Resonance is closely related to the formation of stationary waves, which originate from a combination of two physical phenomena: reflection and interference [23] Resonance in the external auditory canal, calculated by the expression Vsound/4L (L = length of the canal), is around 3800 Hz, which can vary with temperature and be slightly higher or lower, due to the mobility of the tympanic membrane and the anatomic differences between subjects. As such, it can be concluded that, of the different sound frequencies that reach the ears, those around 3800 Hz are extraordinarily amplified. Since 3.8 kHz is not assessed in audiometry, these reflexes can be found at 4 and 3 kHz. **Figure 2** presents the results of pavilion (concha), external auditory canal (outer ear), and middle ear resonance studies, as well as attenuation caused by the stapedius reflex, which only has an effect at low frequencies [24–26]. **Figure 3** shows the gains resulting from the three physiological mechanisms.

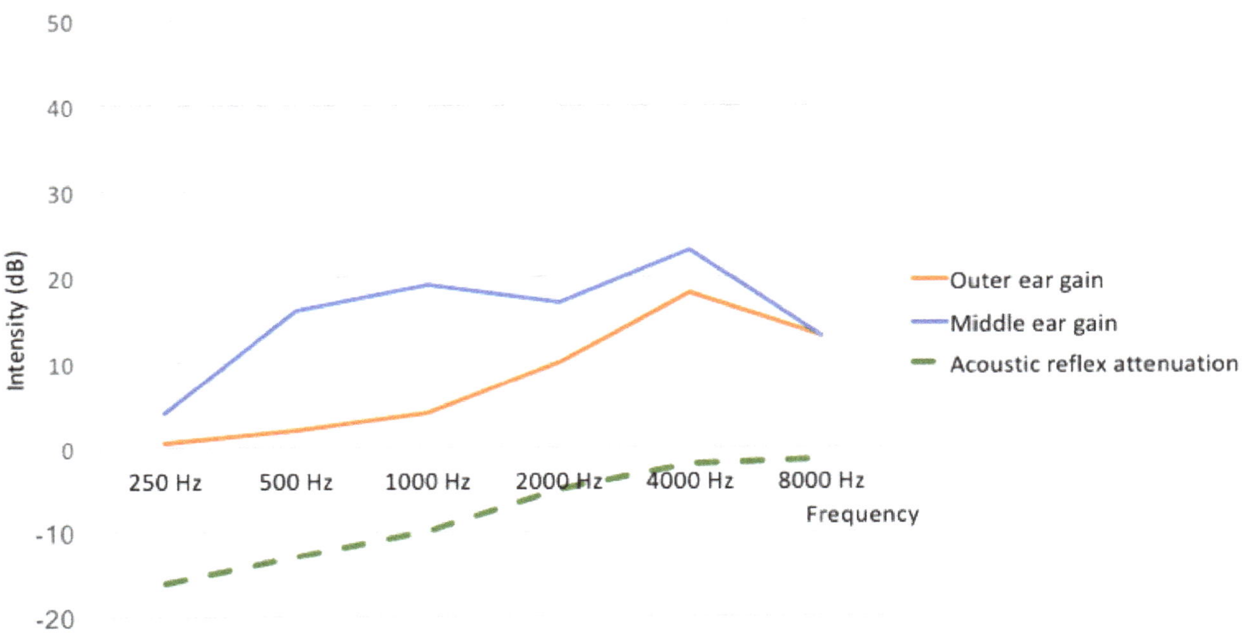

Figure 2. Outer/middle ear gain and acoustic reflex attenuation.

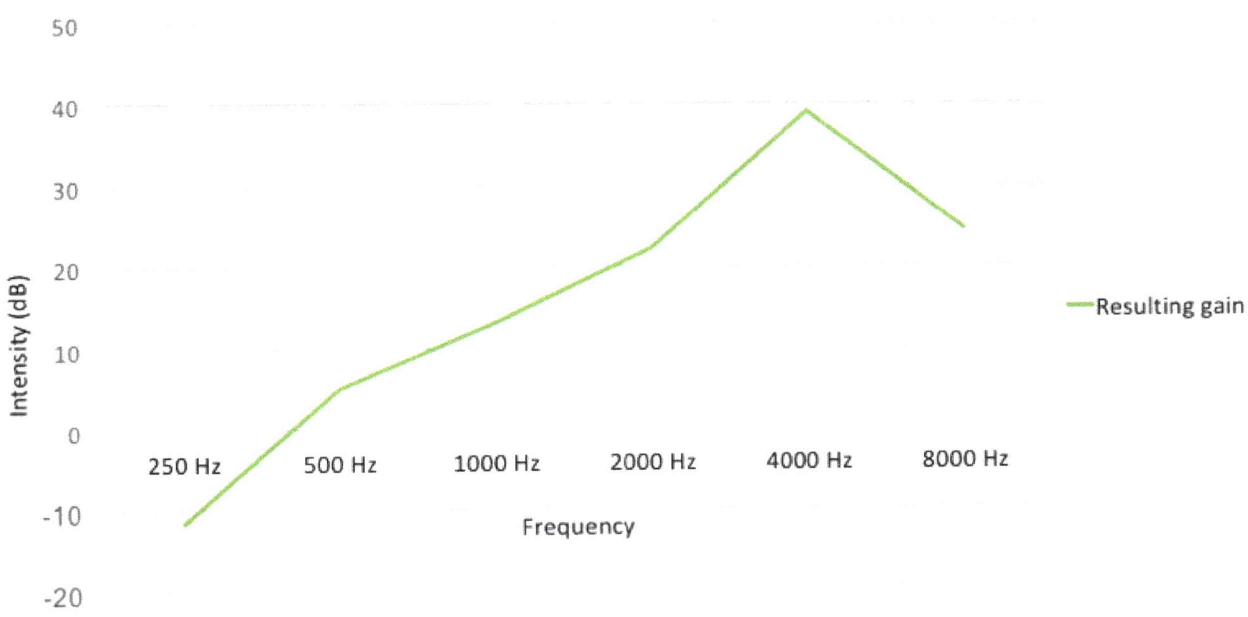

Figure 3. Resulting gain caused by the three physiological mechanisms.

Finally, relating the final physiological gain and the differences in adjustment between dBA and dBHL, despite knowing that there may be overlapping effects, and attempting to minimize errors and approach reality, **Figure 4**, which exhibits the result of the three physiological mechanisms, the dBA to dBHL adjustment, and the final result (orange line).

Finally, a sound input of 100 dBA illustrates how sound interacts with the auditory system and the spectrum resulting from this interaction (green line), as shown in **Figure 5**.

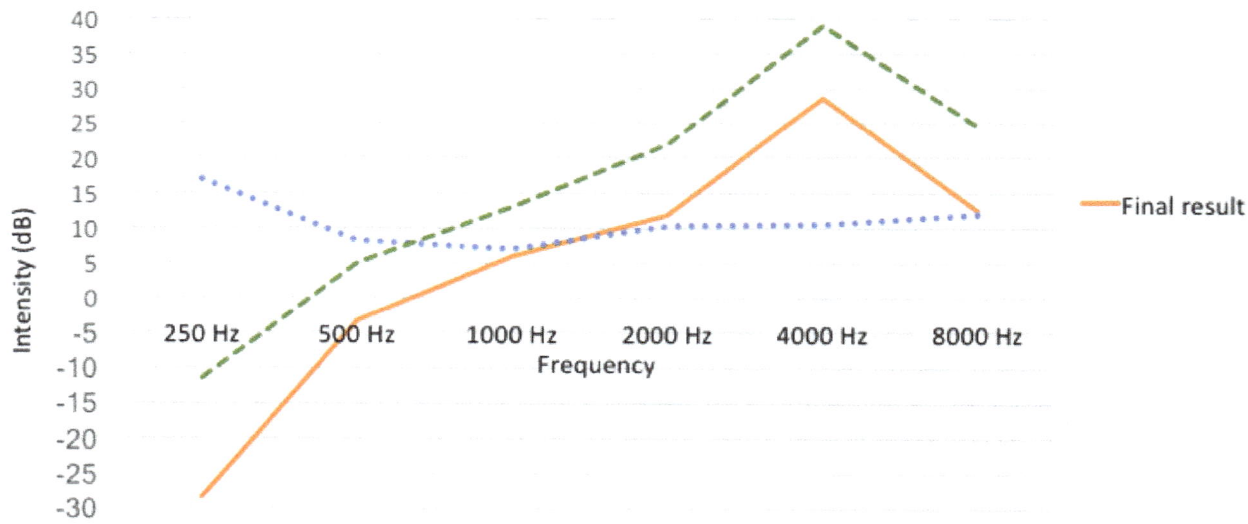

Figure 4. Final outcome, adjustment from dBA to dBHL, and physiological mechanisms.

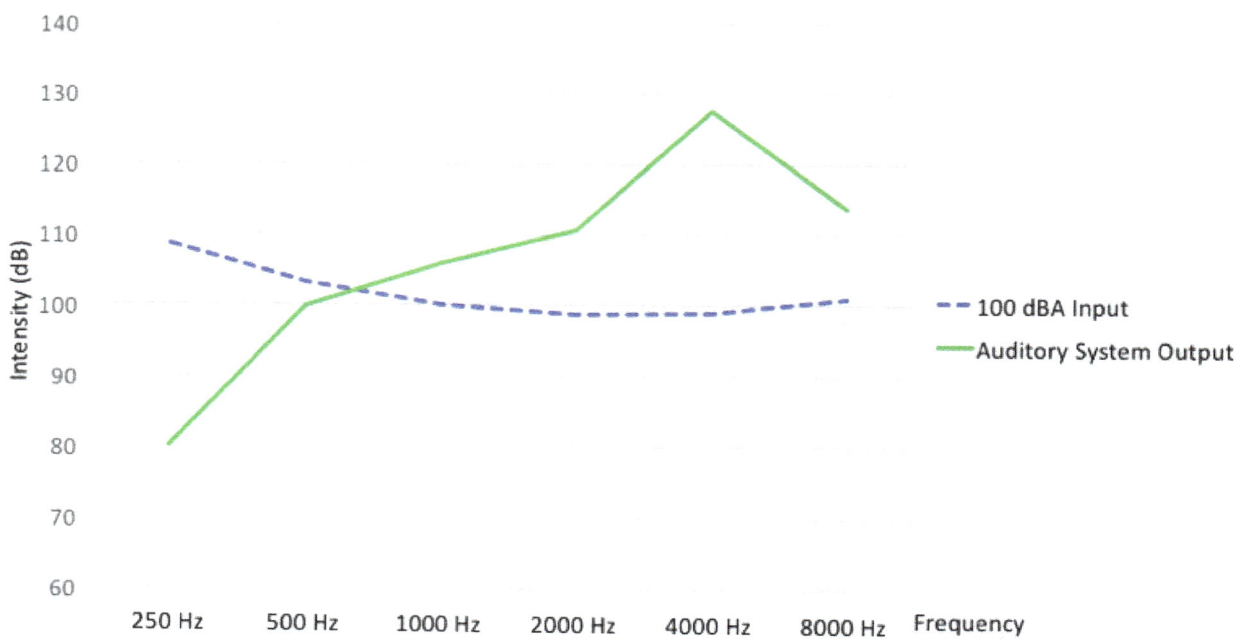

Figure 5. Final outcome: example of a 100 dBA input stimulus.

An input sound level of 100 dBA, resulting from weighting of 108.6, 103.2, 100, 98.8, 98, and 101.1 dB for 250, 500, 1, 2, 4, and 8 kHz, respectively, has an output of 80.2, 99.9, 106, 110.6, 127.5, and 113.7 dB, respectively. In other words, 4 kHz receives around 30 dB more than the original input, while at a frequency of 250 Hz, the intensity is approximately 28 dB lower.

Thus, considering the six aforementioned mechanisms, in addition to the lower number of external ciliated cells at the base of the cochlea and their increased susceptibility to oxidative stress, the audiometric profile of NIHL is defined as being at high frequencies, with the greatest effect at 4 kHz.

3.2. Presbycusis

Presbycusis is a highly complex multifactorial process involving hearing loss at high frequencies concomitantly with physical signs of aging [27].

It is the most common sensory disorder in the elderly, occurring in 25–40% of individuals aged 65 years or older and the prevalence tends to increase with age, ranging from 40 to 66% of people over 75 years old and more than 80% in those over the age of 85. The number of people with this disorder is expected to grow substantially due to the increase in life expectancy [28, 29].

Individuals with presbycusis exhibit reduced sensitivity and hearing comprehension in noisy environments, slow central processing of acoustic information and compromised sound source localization. As such, the limitations that emerge are proportional to the degree of auditory deficiency, affecting dialogue, musical appreciation, identification of warning signs, and, finally, participation in social activities [28] (**Table 3**).

The pathogenesis of presbycusis is not well understood. There is an association with extrinsic (noise, exposure to environmental ototoxic agents, traumatism, vascular injury, and diet), and intrinsic risk factors (metabolic changes, genetic factors, and physiological aging process) [31]. Furthermore, other changes have been proposed, such as altered vascular characteristics, a decrease in oxygen and nutrient supply and residue elimination, genetic mutations, and a significant increase in ROS production [28].

As stated earlier, mitochondria play a crucial role in maintaining cochlear energy homeostasis. Over the course of aging, a number of changes occur in the mitochondria and mitochondrial DNA (mtDNA), including (1) an increase in mitochondrial structural disorganization, (2)

Sensory	Atrophy occurs with loss of ciliated cells and supporting cells of the organ of Corti, starting in the basal turn of the cochlea and progressing slowly toward the apex
Neural	Neuronal atrophy occurs in the cochlea and central neural pathways. It is estimated that 2100 neurons are lost each decade
Metabolic/strial	Atrophy occurs in the stria vascularis, which normally maintains chemical, bioelectrical and metabolic equilibrium of the cochlea
Mechanical	Thickening of the basilar membrane occurs, more severely in the basal turn of the cochlea, where the basilar membrane is narrow

Table 3. Histologically, there are four types of presbycusis [23].

decline in their oxidative phosphorylation, (3) accumulation of mutations in the mtDNA, (4) rise in mitochondrial ROS production, and (5) increase in oxidative DNA, protein, and lipid damage [14].

Thus, the cellular environment in oxidative stress due to noise exposure is one of the main determinants of NIHL, since there may be multiple conditions causing this stress, all contributing to presbycusis in a same individual. The sensory and metabolic forms display a history of exposure to noise and the degree of impairment is greater at high frequencies [32]. In addition, the two forms exhibit an intrinsic cause and effect relationship with oxidative stress, while the mechanical and neural forms display different physiopathological mechanisms but are not exempt from the influence of excessive free radicals.

3.3. Ototoxic hearing loss

Ototoxic hearing loss is caused by the cochleotoxic effect of certain substances widely used in clinical practice. However, other substances present in professional activities also have harmful effects on the cochlea [33]. In addition to the cochleotoxic capacity of the drug, hearing loss is determined by other factors, including exposure to noise, genetic predisposition, malnutrition, advanced age, overall poor health, hypoacusis, and ringing in the ears [33, 34]. Genetic predisposition involves mitochondrial inheritance and oxidative stress [33] (**Table 4**).

The following drugs exhibit a cochleotoxic effect [33, 35–37].

Once inside the cell, aminoglycosides induce ROS production. They are considered "redox-inactive compounds" and, as such, need to be converted into the redox-active form to induce ROS formation. ROS generation involves the formation of an aminoglycoside-iron complex that catalyzes the oxidation of unsaturated fatty acids located in the internal layer of the plasma membrane [27].

The increase in ROS may be due to the depletion of thiol and antioxidant enzyme-reducing buffers and/or direct activation of ROS-producing systems. Cisplatin administration leads to reduced glutathione concentration in the cochlea and a significant decline in SOD activities, catalase, cochlear glutathione peroxidase, and glutathione reductase [27].

Aminoglycosides	Dihydrostreptomycin, neomycin, amikacin, and kanamycins A and B
Beta blocker	Propranolol
Diuretics	Etacrynic acid and furosemide cause reversible hearing loss and can exacerbate hearing loss caused by aminoglycosides
Non-steroidal anti-inflammatories	Salicylates and acetylsalicylic acid. Hearing loss is normally reversible
Cisplatin	Used in chemotherapy against cancer in both children and adults. In children, it can lead to delayed language development

Table 4. The following drugs exhibit a cochleotoxic effect [26, 28–30].

Under certain conditions, base disease in itself causes a condition of permanent oxidative stress in patients. Type 1 diabetes, pancreatitis, different metabolic syndromes, cardiovascular diseases, and chronic kidney failure are frequent examples of pathological conditions with permanent oxidative stress in which patients are more susceptible to hearing loss, and can be aggravated by the use of ototoxic drugs [38]. Hearing loss is normally bilateral, symmetrical, and greater at high frequencies.

3.4. Hearing loss associated with chronic kidney disease

Chronic kidney disease (CKD) is a metabolic syndrome caused by the progressive, irreversible and generally slow loss of renal excretory capacity [39]. In 2013, it was estimated that 2.5 million patients were in dialysis worldwide, a number that is expected to reach 6.5 million by 2030 [40].

The prevalence of hearing loss in patients with CKD, even children [41–45], is higher than in the general population [41]. The best-known association between CKD and hearing loss is Alport syndrome, which has a genetic origin [46]. However, in most cases, hearing loss in patients with CKD has no genetic origin but is due to anatomical, physiological, and pathological similarities between the nephron and stria vascularis of the cochlea [47]. Of CKD cases, 35% are caused by systemic hypertension (SHT) and 29% by diabetes mellitus (DM) [48].

Several factors lead to permanent oxidative stress in CKD, such as the base disease (hypertension, diabetes) that caused CKD, namely uremia. This state of oxidative stress can be aggravated in the inner ear when drugs with a potential ototoxic effect are used [38].

The primary lesion site of hearing loss in CKD is the cochlea [49]; however, some studies also report the involvement of retrocochlear pathways and the central nervous system [41, 50]. Hearing loss normally occurs symmetrically at high frequencies [8, 43, 51].

4. Oxidative stress as a new paradigm in hearing loss at high frequencies in different etiologies

The hearing losses under study are examples of pathological conditions in the inner ear that are clinically distinct, and often accumulate over a lifetime. Final expression is determined by molecular mechanisms based on oxidative stress. Assessing the different aspects such as etiology, clinical picture and treatment of these hearing disorders should not be restricted to pre-established immutable models that treat each of them separately without including the intrinsic and extrinsic factors that significantly influence auditory damage.

Prevention possibilities and rehabilitation perspectives for these hearing disorders have been discussed for decades. It is important to prevent NIHL by non-exposure to damaging sound levels, but this is not enough, since factors such as genetic predisposition to hearing loss and the use of ototoxic drugs may exacerbate the final audiological clinical condition. Presbycusis is the final product of different factors that are harmful to hearing during an individual's lifetime, such that its prevention is hindered by the limits in controlling these factors from childhood onward. Avoiding hearing loss caused by the use of ototoxic drugs is a challenge, since they cannot always be substituted by non-cochleotoxic medication due to the greater efficacy of the former in treating serious diseases, such as cancer. Maintaining good auditory acuity in chronic kidney patients is essential, since hearing loss becomes one more disorder for patients who depend on care and need good communication. Hearing loss related to CKD leads to restricted participation, as well as social and emotional impacts; however, the physio-pathology of CKD causes progressive and irreversible cochlear damage.

Some cell factors characterize the basal turn of the cochlea as a risk zone, justifying selective hearing loss at high frequencies in NIHL, presbycusis, ototoxic hearing loss, and CKD. The lower number of ciliated cells and their greater susceptibility in the basal turn make it a risk zone under aggressor conditions (noise, aging, ototoxic, CKD).

Furthermore, the acoustic reflex is efficient in protecting at frequencies below 2 kHz, leaving high frequencies under unfavorable conditions [52]. This reflex is defined as the contraction of middle ear muscles induced by intense acoustic stimulation. The tensor tympani muscle pulls the malleus (hammer) away from the eardrum and the stapedius muscle exerts force behind the stirrup, causing greater stiffness in the system and reducing sound transmission, primarily at low frequencies, that is, below 1 kHz. Thus, changes in middle-ear impedance, due to the aforementioned contractions, have little or no effect on frequencies above 2 kHz [53].

Studying hearing loss using a new model based on oxidative stress leads to new perspectives on how to prevent this disorder. Several factors display important limitations with respect to preventing auditory damage. However, when oxidative stress is present, understanding how it occurs and devising therapies to minimize it is a new prevention strategy that could be applied to workers exposed to intense noise, individuals with a family history of presbycusis, patients using ototoxic drugs and chronic kidney patients. Adjuvant antioxidant therapies represent a new method to help prevent hearing loss. This model serves as a potential alternative to treat the forms of hearing loss under study, and should be assessed more thoroughly for these and other hearing disorders.

5. Conclusions

NIHL, presbycusis, ototoxic hearing loss, and hearing loss associated with CKD may seem disconnected and quite different from one another, but oxidative stress emerges as a paradigm that helps reassess the reasoning behind these losses and better understand the environment of the cochlea when exposed to harmful intrinsic and extrinsic factors.

It is hoped that this new paradigm for the different hearing losses will result in a different approach to the physiological changes that affect the auditory system in the form of high-frequency hearing loss. As such, preventing, treating, and avoiding exacerbations are possibilities to be investigated in order to guarantee efficient communication and quality of life for individuals.

Conflict of interest

There is no conflict of interest.

List of the technical terms

CKD	chronic kidney disease
dBA	decibel weighting curve A
dBHL	decibel hearing level
DM	diabetes mellitus
GPx	glutathione peroxidase
GSH	glutathione
GSH-Red	glutathione reductase
GST	glutathione S-transferase
JNK	c-Jun N-terminal kinase
Hz	hertz
kHz	kilo hertz
L	length of the ear canal
NIHL	noise-induced hearing loss
NOX	noise increases oxidase
mtDNA	mitochondrial DNA
p38MAPK	the release of cytochrome and mitochondria and procaspase activation
ROS	reactive oxygen species
SHT	systemic hypertension

Author details

Klinger Vagner Teixeira da Costa[1,2], Kelly Cristina Lira de Andrade[1], Maria Eduarda di Cavalcanti[1,2], Ana Claudia Figueiredo Frizzo[3], Aline Tenório Lins Carnaúba[2] and Pedro de Lemos Menezes[1,2]*

*Address all correspondence to: pedrodelemosmenezes@gmail.com

1 CESMAC University Center, Brazil

2 Technology and Hearing Laboratory (LATEC), State University of Health Sciences of Alagoas State University, Maceió, Brazil

3 Júlio de Mesquita Filho Paulista State University (UNESP), Marília, Brazil

References

[1] Augusto O. In: Augusto O, editor. Radicais Livres—Bons, Maus E Naturais. São Paulo: Oficina de Textos; 2006

[2] Armstrong D. Introduction to free radical, inflammation, and recycling. In: Armstrong D, Stratton RD, editors. Oxidative Stress and Antioxidant Protection the Science of Free Radical Biology and Disease. New Jersey: Wiley Blackwell; 2016. p. 560

[3] Taysi S, Orkmez M, Saricicek E, et al. The effects of oral Ginkgo biloba supplementation on radiation-induced oxidative injury in the lens of rat. Pharmacognosy Magazine. 2011;**7**: 141-145. DOI: 10.4103/0973-1296.80673

[4] Araújo SA. Perda auditiva induzida pelo ruído em trabalhadores de metalúrgica. Revista Brasileira de Oto-Rino-Laringologia. 2002;**68**(1):47-52

[5] Nudelmann AA, Costa EA, Seligman J, Ibanez RN. PAIR Perda Auditiva Induzida Pelo Ruído. Porto Alegre: Bagagem Comunicação; 1997

[6] Villani V, Zucchella C, Cristalli G, et al. Vitamin E neuroprotection against cisplatin ototoxicity: Preliminary results from a randomized, placebo-controlled trial. Head Neck. 2016;**38** (S1):E2118-E2121. DOI: 10.1002/HED

[7] Freyer DR, Chen L, Krailo MD, et al. Effects of sodium thiosulfate versus observation on development of cisplatin-induced hearing loss in children with cancer (ACCL0431): A multicentre, randomised, controlled, open-label, phase 3 trial. The Lancet Oncology. 2016;**2045**(16):1-12. DOI: 10.1016/S1470-2045(16)30625-8

[8] da Costa KVT, Ferreira SMS, Menezes P de L. Hearing handicap in patients with chronic kidney disease: A study of the different classifications of the degree of hearing loss. Brazilian Journal of Otorhinolaryngology. 2016;**83**:580-589. DOI: 10.1016/j.bjorl.2016.08.008. [Epub ahead of print]

[9] Choi SH, Choi C. Noise-induced neural degeneration and therapeutic effect of antioxidant drugs. Journal of Audiology and Otology. 2015;**19**(3):111-119

[10] Kujawa S, Liberman MC. Acceleration of age-related hearing loss by early noise exposure: Evidence of a misspent youth. The Journal of Neuroscience. 2006;**26**(7):2115-2123

[11] Sliwinska-Kowalska M, Pawelczyk M. Contribution of genetic factors to noise-induced hearing loss: A human studies review. Mutation Research. 2013;**752**(1):61-65. DOI: 10.1016/j.mrrev.2012.11.001

[12] Kurk M, Amatuzzt MG. Anatomia e Fisiologia da Orelha Interna. In: Campos CAH de, Costa HO de O, editors. Tratado de Otorrinolaringologia. 1st ed. São Paulo: ROCA; 2003: 382-400

[13] Dobie RA. Perda auditiva Induzida pelo ruído. In: Bailey BJ, Johnson JT, Newlands SD, editors. Otorrinolaringologia—Cirurgia de Cabeça E Pescoço. 4th ed. Rio de Janeiro: Revinter; 2001. pp. 1097-1114

[14] Lee H, Wei Y. Mitochondria and aging. Advances in Experimental Medicine and Biology. 2012;**942**:311-327. DOI: 10.1007/978-94-007-2869-1

[15] Martin LJ. Biology of mitochondria in neurodegenerative diseases. Progress in Molecular Biology and Translational Science. 2012;**107**:355-415. DOI: 10.1016/B978-0-12-385883-2.00005-9

[16] IEC 61672-1:2013 Electroacoustics—Sound level meters—Part 1: Specifications. IEC. 2013

[17] Aarts RM. A comparison of some loudness measures for loudspeaker listening tests. Journal of the Audio Engineering Society. 1992;**40**(3):142-146

[18] Menezes PL, Caldas Neto S, Motta MA. Biofísica da audição. 1st ed. Lovise: São Paulo; 2005. 188 p

[19] Sha S, Taylor R, Forge A, Schacht J. Differential vulnerability of basal and apical hair cells is based on intrinsic susceptibility to free radicals. Hearing Research. 2001;**155**:1-8

[20] Baker K, Staecker H. Low dose oxidative stress induces mitochondrial damage in hair cells. The Anatomical Record. 2012;**295**:1868-1876. DOI: 10.1002/ar.22594

[21] Ohlemiller KK, McFadden SL, Ding D-L, et al. Targeted deletion of the cytosolic Cu/Zn-superoxide dismutase gene (Sod1) increases susceptibility to noise-induced hearing loss. Audiology & Neuro-Otology. 1999;**4**:237-246

[22] Ramkumar V, Whitworth CA, Pingle SC, Hughes LF, Rybak LP. Noise induces A 1 adenosine receptor expression in the chinchilla cochlea. Hearing Research. 2004;**188**:47-56. DOI: 10.1016/S0378-5955(03)00344-7

[23] Fuke LF, Shigekiyo CT, Yamamoto K. Os alicerces da física. 2nd ed. São Paulo: Saraiva; 1998. pp. 421-429

[24] Ballachanda BB. Theoretical and applied external ear acoustics. Journal of the American Academy of Audiology. 1997;**8**:411-420

[25] Nedzelnitsky V. Sound pressures in basal turns of cat cochlea. The Journal of the Acoustical Society of America. 1980;**68**:1676-1689

[26] Gridi-Papp M, Feng AS, Shen J, Yu Z, Rosowsk JJ, Narins PM. Active control of ultrasonic hearing in frogs. PNAS. 2008;**105**(31):11014-11019

[27] Poirrier AL, Pincemail J, Van Den Ackerveken P, Lefebvre PP, Malgrange B. Oxidative stress in the cochlea: An update. Current Medicinal Chemistry. 2010;**17**(30):3591-3604. DOI: 10.2174/092986710792927895

[28] Tavanai E, Mohammadkhani G. Role of antioxidants in prevention of age-related hearing loss: A review of literature. European Archives of Oto-Rhino-Laryngology. 2016;**274**:1821-1834. DOI: 10.1007/s00405-016-4378-6

[29] Arvin B, Prepageran N, Raman R. High frequency presbycusis–Is there an earlier onset? Indian Journal of Otolaryngology and Head & Neck Surgery. 2013;**65**(December):S480-S484. DOI: 10.1007/s12070-011-0356-x

[30] Schuknecht HF, Gacek MR. Cochlear pathology in presbycusis. The Annals of Otology, Rhinology, and Laryngology. 1993;**102**:1-16

[31] Yamasoba T, Lin FR, Someya S, Kashio A, Sakamoto T, Kondo K. Current concepts in age-related hearing loss: Epidemiology and mechanistic pathways. Hearing Research. 2013; **303**:30-38. DOI: 10.1016/j.heares.2013.01.021

[32] Schmiedt RA. The physiology of cochlear presbycusis. In: Gordon-Salant S, Frisina RD, Fay RR, Popper AN, editors. Springer Handbook Os Auditory Research. 34th ed. Baltimore: Springer; 2010. pp. 9-38. DOI: 10.1007/978-1-4419-0993-0

[33] de Oliveira JAA, Bernal TMO. Ototoxicidade de Aminoglicosídeos e Otoproteção. In: de Campos CAH, Costa HO de O, editors. Tratado de Otorrinolaringologia. 1st ed. São Paulo: ROCA; 2003

[34] Lautermann J, Mclaren J, Schacht J. Glutathione protection against gentamicin ototoxicity depends on nutritional status. Hear Research. 1995;**86**:15-24

[35] Packer RJ, Sutton LN, Elterman R, et al. Outcome for children with medulloblastoma treated with radiation and cisplatin, CCNU, and vincristine chemotherapy. Journal of Neurosurgery. 1994;**81**(5):690-698. DOI: 10.3171/jns.1994.81.5.0690

[36] Xie J, Talaska AE, Schacht J. New developments in aminoglycoside therapy and ototoxicity. Hearing Research. 2011;**281**:28-37. DOI: 10.1016/j.heares.2011.05.008.New

[37] Moore RD, Smith CR, Lietman PS. Risk factors for the development of auditory toxicity in patients receiving aminoglycosides. The Journal of Infectious Diseases. 1984;**149**(1):23-30 http://www.scopus.com/inward/record.url?eid=2-s2.0-0021365039&partnerID=tZOtx3y1

[38] Armstrong D, Stratton RD. Oxidative Stress and Antioxidant Protection—The Science of Free Radical Biology and Disease. New Jersey: John Wiley & Sons; 2016

[39] Draibe SA. Insuficiência renal crônica. In: Atualização Terapêutica de Prado, Ramos e Valle: Diagnóstico E Tratamento-2012/13. 2012. pp. 1092-1096 DOI: 10.1017/CBO9781107415324.004

[40] CARE FM. Fresenius Medical Care Annual Report 2013. Fresenius Med Care. 2014;**294**

[41] Thodi C, Thodis E, Danielides V, Pasadakis P, Vargemezis V. Hearing in renal failure. Nephrology, Dialysis, Transplantation. 2006;**21**(11):3023-3030. DOI: 10.1093/ndt/gfl472

[42] Mancini ML, Dello SL, Bianchi PM, Tieri L, Rizzoni G. Sensorineural hearing loss in patients reaching chronic renal failure in childhood. Pediatric Nephrology. 1996;**10**(1):38-40 http://www.ncbi.nlm.nih.gov/pubmed/8611353

[43] Nikolopoulos TP, Kandiloros DC, Segas JV, et al. Auditory function in young patients with chronic renal failure. Clinical Otolaryngology and Allied Sciences. 1997;**22**(3):222-225 http://www.ncbi.nlm.nih.gov/pubmed/9222626

[44] Samir M, Riad H, Mahgoub M, Awad Z, Kamal N. Transient otoacoustic emissions in children with chronic. Clinical Otolaryngology. 1998;**23**:87-90

[45] Stavroulaki P, Nikolopoulos TP, Psarommatis I, Apostolopoulos N. Hearing evaluation with distortion-product otoacoustic emissions in young patients undergoing haemodialysis. Clinical Otolaryngology and Allied Sciences. 2001;**26**(3):235-242. DOI: 10.1046/j.0307-7772.2001.00464.x

[46] Alport AC. Hereditary familial congenital haemorrhagic nephritis. British Medical Journal. 1927;**1**(16):504-506

[47] Pandey S, Gore G, Valame D, Mehta K. Audiometric profile in patients with chronic renal failure. Journal of Otolaryngology—Head & Neck Surgery. 2011;**40**(2):131-136. DOI: 10.2310/7070.2011.100109

[48] Sesso RC, Lopes AA, Thomé FS, Lugon JR, Martins CT. Brazilian chronic dialysis census 2014. Jornal Brasileiro de Nefrologia. 2016;**38**(1):54-61. DOI: 10.5935/0101-2800.20160009

[49] Ohashi T, Kenmochi M, Kinoshita H, Ochi K, Kikuchi H. Cochlear function of Guinea pigs with experimental chronic renal failure. The Annals of Otology, Rhinology, and Laryngology. 1999;**108**(10):955-962

[50] Antonelli AR, Bonfioli F, Garrubba V, et al. Audiological findings in elderly patients with chronic renal failure. Acta Oto-Laryngologica. Supplementum. 1991;**476**:54-68. DOI: 10.3109/00016489109127256

[51] Peyvandi A, Roozbahany NA. Hearing loss in chronic renal failure patient undergoing hemodialysis. Indian Journal of Otolaryngology and Head & Neck Surgery. 2013;**65**(Suppl 3):537-540. DOI: 10.1007/s12070-011-0454-9

[52] Cristina K, De AL, Dias E, et al. The importance of acoustic reflex for communication. Indian Journal of Otolaryngology and Head & Neck Surgery. 2011;**32**(3):221-227. DOI: 10.1016/j.amjoto.2010.02.002

[53] Zemlin WR. Princípios de Anatomia E Fisiologia Em Fonoaudiologia. Artmed: Porto Alegre; 2000

Permissions

All chapters in this book were first published in AEHL, by InTech Open; hereby published with permission under the Creative Commons Attribution License or equivalent. Every chapter published in this book has been scrutinized by our experts. Their significance has been extensively debated. The topics covered herein carry significant findings which will fuel the growth of the discipline. They may even be implemented as practical applications or may be referred to as a beginning point for another development.

The contributors of this book come from diverse backgrounds, making this book a truly international effort. This book will bring forth new frontiers with its revolutionizing research information and detailed analysis of the nascent developments around the world.

We would like to thank all the contributing authors for lending their expertise to make the book truly unique. They have played a crucial role in the development of this book. Without their invaluable contributions this book wouldn't have been possible. They have made vital efforts to compile up to date information on the varied aspects of this subject to make this book a valuable addition to the collection of many professionals and students.

This book was conceptualized with the vision of imparting up-to-date information and advanced data in this field. To ensure the same, a matchless editorial board was set up. Every individual on the board went through rigorous rounds of assessment to prove their worth. After which they invested a large part of their time researching and compiling the most relevant data for our readers.

The editorial board has been involved in producing this book since its inception. They have spent rigorous hours researching and exploring the diverse topics which have resulted in the successful publishing of this book. They have passed on their knowledge of decades through this book. To expedite this challenging task, the publisher supported the team at every step. A small team of assistant editors was also appointed to further simplify the editing procedure and attain best results for the readers.

Apart from the editorial board, the designing team has also invested a significant amount of their time in understanding the subject and creating the most relevant covers. They scrutinized every image to scout for the most suitable representation of the subject and create an appropriate cover for the book.

The publishing team has been an ardent support to the editorial, designing and production team. Their endless efforts to recruit the best for this project, has resulted in the accomplishment of this book. They are a veteran in the field of academics and their pool of knowledge is as vast as their experience in printing. Their expertise and guidance has proved useful at every step. Their uncompromising quality standards have made this book an exceptional effort. Their encouragement from time to time has been an inspiration for everyone.

The publisher and the editorial board hope that this book will prove to be a valuable piece of knowledge for researchers, students, practitioners and scholars across the globe.

List of Contributors

Maciej Ludwikowski
World Hearing Center, Institute of Physiology and Pathology of Hearing, Department of Teleaudiology, Kajetany/Warsaw, Poland

Piotr Henryk Skarżyński
World Hearing Center, Institute of Physiology and Pathology of Hearing, Department of Teleaudiology, Kajetany/Warsaw, Poland

Institute of Sensory Organs, Kajetany, Poland
Heart Failure and Cardiac Rehabilitation, Department of the Medical University of Warsaw, Poland
Center of Hearing and Speech, MEDINCUS, Kajetany, Poland

Fatih Oghan
Faculty of Medicine, Department of ORL&HNS, Dumlupinar University, Kutahya, Turkey

Ibrahim Erdim
Tokat Erbaa Hospital, Tokat, Turkey

Metin Çeliker
Recep Tayyip Erdogan University Research Hospital, Rize, Turkey

Muhammet Fatih Topuz, Ahmet Uluat, Onur Erdogan and Sinan Aksoy
SB DPU Evliya Celebi Research Hospital, Kutahya, Turkey

Agnieszka Pollak and Monika Ołdak
Department of Genetics, Institute of Physiology and Pathology of Hearing, Warsaw, Poland

Christiane Marques do Couto and Izabella dos Santos Brites
Department of Human Development and Rehabilitation, Faculty of Medical Sciences, University of Campinas - UNICAMP, Campinas, SP, Brazil

Harun Acıpayam
Department of Otolaryngology, Kanuni Sultan Süleyman Training and Research Hospital-Beylikdüzü Campus, İstanbul, Turkey

Hasan Emre Koçak and Mustafa Suphi Elbistanlı
Department of Otolaryngology, Bakırköy Sadi Konuk Training and Research Hospital, İstanbul, Turkey

Payton Lin
Centre for Biosystems, Neuroscience, and Nanotechnology (CBNN), City University of Hong Kong, Hong Kong SAR
Academia Sinica, Center for Information Technology Innovation, Taipei, Taiwan

Yu Tsao
Academia Sinica, Center for Information Technology Innovation, Taipei, Taiwan

Li-Wei Kuo
National Health Research Institute, Institute of Biomedical Engineering and Nanomedicine, Taiwan

Kenichi Takano
Department of Otolaryngology, Sapporo Medical University, School of Medicine, Sapporo, Hokkaido, Japan

Diego Zanetti and Federica Di Berardino
Audiology Unit, Department of Community Health and Clinical Sciences, Università degli Studi di Milano; Fondazione IRCCS Cà Granda, Ospedale Maggiore Policlinico Milano, Italy

Margherita Vezzani
Otorhinolaryngology Department, University of Milano-Bicocca, San Gerardo Hospital,Monza, Italy
Pediatric Otorhinolaryngology Department, Children's Hospital, Cincinnati, USA

Serena Gasperini and Rossella Parini
Rare Metabolic Diseases Unit, Department of Pediatrics, University of Milano-Bicocca, San Gerardo Hospital, Monza, Italy

Ryota Shimokura
Architecture and Production Design Engineering, Interdisciplinary Graduate School of Science and Engineering, Shimane University, Shimane, Japan

Pauliana Lamounier
Centro de Reabilitação e Readaptação Dr Henrique Santillo—CRER, Goiânia, GO, Brazil

Shumpei P. Yasuda and Yoshiaki Kikkawa
Mammalian Genetics Project, Tokyo Metropolitan Institute of Medical Science, Tokyo, Japan

Pedram Borghei
Otolaryngology Head and Neck Surgery, Tehran University of Medical Sciences, Tehran, Iran

Yuki Miyasaka
Mammalian Genetics Project, Tokyo Metropolitan Institute of Medical Science, Tokyo, Japan
Division of Experimental Animals, Center for Promotion of Medical Research and Education, Graduate School of Medicine, Nagoya University, Nagoya, Aichi, Japan

Mohammad Hossein Khosravi
Student Research Committee (SRC), Baqiyatallah University of Medical Sciences, Tehran, Iran
International Otorhinolaryngology Research Association (IORA), Universal Scientific Education and Research Network (USERN), Tehran, Iran

Ali Kouhi
International Otorhinolaryngology Research Association (IORA), Universal Scientific Education and Research Network (USERN), Tehran, Iran
Department of Otolaryngology—Head and Neck Surgery, Otorhinolaryngology Research Center, Tehran University of Medical Sciences, Tehran, Iran

Sasan Dabiri
Department of Otorhinolaryngology—Head and Neck Surgery, Amir Alam Hospital, Tehran University of Medical Sciences, Tehran, Iran

Masoumeh Saeedi
International Otorhinolaryngology Research Association (IORA), Universal Scientific Education and Research Network (USERN), Tehran, Iran
Department of Otorhinolaryngology—Head and Neck Surgery, Faculty of Medicine, Baqiyatallah University of Medical Sciences, Tehran, Iran

Kelly Cristina Lira de Andrade
CESMAC University Center, Brazil

Aline Tenório Lins Carnaúba
Technology and Hearing Laboratory (LATEC), State University of Health Sciences of Alagoas State University, Maceió, Brazil

Klinger Vagner Teixeira da Costa, Maria Eduarda di Cavalcanti and Pedro de Lemos Menezes
CESMAC University Center, Brazil
Technology and Hearing Laboratory (LATEC), State University of Health Sciences of Alagoas State University, Maceió, Brazil

Ana Claudia Figueiredo Frizzo
Júlio de Mesquita Filho Paulista State University (UNESP), Marília, Brazil

Index

P

R

S

T

V